CARDIOPULMONARY PHYSIOLOGY IN ANESTHESIOLOGY

NOTICE

Medicine is an ever-changing science. As new research and clinical experience broaden our knowledge, changes in treatment and drug therapy are required. The authors and the publisher of this work have checked with sources believed to be reliable in their efforts to provide information that is complete and generally in accord with the standards accepted at the time of publication. However, in view of the possibility of human error or changes in medical sciences, neither the authors nor the publisher nor any other party who has been involved in the preparation or publication of this work warrants that the information contained herein is in every respect accurate or complete, and they are not responsible for any errors or omissions or for the results obtained from use of such information. Readers are encouraged to confirm the information contained herein with other sources. For example and in particular, readers are advised to check the product information sheet included in the package of each drug they plan to administer to be certain that the information contained in this book is accurate and that changes have not been made in the recommended dose or in the contraindications for administration. This recommendation is of particular importance in connection with new or infrequently used drugs.

CARDIOPULMONARY PHYSIOLOGY IN ANESTHESIOLOGY

Michael G. Levitzky, Ph.D.

Professor of Physiology and Anesthesiology
Louisiana State University Medical Center

Stanley M. Hall, M.D., Ph.D.

Clinical-Professor of Anesthesiology
Louisiana State University Medical Center
Co-Director Anesthesiology Department
Children's Hospital of New Orleans

Kathleen H. McDonough, Ph.D.

Professor of Physiology
Louisiana State University Medical Center

McGRAW-HILL
Health Professions Division

New York   St. Louis   San Francisco
Auckland   Bogotá   Caracas   Lisbon   London
Madrid   Mexico City   Milan   Montreal   New Delhi
San Juan   Singapore   Sydney   Tokyo   Toronto

McGraw-Hill

A Division of The McGraw·Hill Companies

CARDIOPULMONARY PHYSIOLOGY IN ANESTHESIOLOGY

Copyright © 1997 by *The* **McGraw-Hill** *Companies, Inc.* All rights reserved. Printed in the United States of America. Except as permitted under the United States Copyright Act of 1976, no part of this publication may be reproduced or distributed in any form or by any means, or stored in a data base or retrieval system, without the prior written permission of the publisher.

1 2 3 4 5 6 7 8 9 0   DOC DOC   9 8 7 6

This book was set in Times Roman by Progressive Information Technologies.
The editors were Martin J. Wonsiewicz and Pamela Touboul;
the production supervisor was Richard Ruzycka;
the cover designer was Edward Schultheis;
R. R. Donnelley & Sons was printer and binder.

ISBN 0-07-037534-8

Library of Congress Cataloging-in-Publication Data

Levitzky, Michael G.
    Cardiopulmonary physiology in anesthesiology / Michael G. Levitzky, Stanley M. Hall, Kathleen H. McDonough.
        p.   cm.
    Includes bibliographical references and index.
    ISBN 0-07-037534-8
    1. Cardiopulmonary system—Physiology.   2. Anesthetics—Physiological effect.   I. Hall, Stanley M.   II. McDonough, Kathleen H.   III. Title.
    [DNLM: 1. Cardiovascular System—physiology.   2. Respiration—physiology.   3. Anesthesia.   WG   102   L666c   1997]
    RD82.L48   1997
    617.9'6—DC20
    DNLM/DLC
    for Library of Congress

This book is dedicated

to the memory of

Stephen S. Hall

CONTENTS

PREFACE

The boredom to sheer terror ratio for clinical anesthesiology is commonly given as 99:1, although it sometimes seems reversed for new residents and freshman student nurse anesthetists. However, this proportion can be favorably increased (say to the range of 99.9:0.1) by a better understanding of the physiology and pathophysiology that produce undesirable perioperative events. By anticipating (or at least being able to explain) problems, more appropriate and timely interventions can be provided.

The goals of anesthesiology include providing patient safety, patient comfort, and a stable operative field. Also, surgeons need anesthesiology to blame for surgical misadventures. Indeed, we know a spine surgeon who frequently asks intraoperatively, "anesthesia, what are you doing to make 'em bleed?"

While anesthesia is intended to block or diminish the physiologic responses to painful stimuli, as well as the perception of pain, the neurologic effects are not the only important consideration. Circulatory and respiratory effects of anesthesia and perioperative events are also vital concerns. Additionally, interactions with the patient's pathophysiology can crucially affect the anesthetic course.

This book is primarily intended for anesthesia care providers in training and those preparing for certification. Anesthesiology departments with large research components frequently employ clinical physiologists for their expertise in experimental designs and techniques; the clinical practice of anesthesiology is possibly the area of patient care that has the profoundest and most rapidly changing effects on human physiology.

The authors would like to thank Beverly Smith and Betsy Giaimo for their valuable assistance in preparing this manuscript and our families for their patience and understanding.

Part 1
CARDIOVASCULAR PHYSIOLOGY

1

FUNCTION AND STRUCTURE OF THE CARDIOVASCULAR SYSTEM

PHYSIOLOGY OF THE CARDIOVASCULAR SYSTEM

The main function of the cardiovascular system is to transport materials such as hormones and nutrients to the cells of the body and to remove secretions and waste products. The energy of the heart's contractions propels the blood through the blood vessels to all of the tissues of the body. The arteries carry blood away from the heart and branch into progressively smaller vessels. The smallest vessels are the capillaries, with walls consisting of only one cell layer of simple squamous endothelium. The systemic capillaries are the site of exchange of materials between the blood and body tissues. The pulmonary capillaries are the site of exchange between the blood and the alveolar gas. The capillaries are so numerous and well distributed that almost no cell in the body is greater than 70μ from a capillary.

Certain substances (such as oxygen, nutrients, and hormones) contained in the blood pass either through the capillary endothelium or through the spaces where endothelial cells meet. These substances diffuse through the interstitial fluid (outside the capillary) that bathes the cells of the tissues (Claude Bernard's *Internal Milieu*). Once in the interstitial fluid, these materials interact with receptors on the cell membrane or pass through the cell membrane into the cell. Carbon dioxide; metabolic waste products; and secretory products such as hormones, autacoids (biologically active substances such as prostaglandins), and stored nutrients released for use elsewhere in the body follow the same route but in the opposite direction. Concentration gradients determine the direction of movement.

The systemic arterial blood vessels play an important role in maintaining the blood pressure and in distributing the blood flow to the different vascular beds by changing the tone of the smooth muscle in their walls. Elasticity of the vessel walls also helps to change the pulsatile input from the heart into a steady flow through the capillaries. The smooth muscle of the vessel walls also acts to stop

3

hemorrhage by vasoconstriction at times when the vessels are injured (the vascular endothelium and the blood also play major roles in hemostasis).

The hemoglobin in the red blood cells is important because it greatly increases the ability of the blood to carry oxygen to the tissues. Other important functions of the blood include protection of the body against foreign material and organisms and maintenance of the body's homeostasis.

ANATOMY OF THE CARDIOVASCULAR SYSTEM

Although the heart is a single organ anatomically, physiologically it acts as two pairs of pumps arranged in series. The right side of the heart consists of a thin-walled, weakly pumping right atrium and a thicker-walled, stronger right ventricle. The right atrium receives venous blood from the tissues of the body via the superior and inferior vena cava, as well as via the coronary sinus, which drains some of the blood from the coronary arteries. Venous return and the weak right atrial contraction push blood through the right atrioventricular (AV) valve (the tricuspid valve) into the right ventricle. The right ventricle pumps the blood through the pulmonic valve and into the pulmonary arteries. The relatively short pulmonary arteries branch many times until the blood finally reaches the pulmonary capillaries, which lie between the alveoli of the lung. There are about 1000 pulmonary capillaries in the wall of each alveolus, thus making for a large surface area for gas exchange between the body and the alveolar air. The pulmonary capillaries drain into the pulmonary venules, which merge to form lobar veins. These, in turn, combine to form the four main pulmonary veins. These veins carry the blood to the left side of the heart. The left atrium pumps the blood returning via the pulmonary veins through the left AV valve (the mitral or bicuspid valve) into the left ventricle. The left ventricle ejects the blood through the aortic valve into the thick-walled elastic aorta, which then branches to form the major arteries. They supply every organ of the body (including the lungs, which also get the output of the right ventricle). The smaller muscular arteries (such as the radial or renal artery) then divide into smaller arterioles from which the capillaries originate. Draining the capillaries, the venules form larger veins, which ultimately combine to form the superior and inferior vena cava.

The components of the cardiovascular system are the heart, the vessels, and the blood. The heart is the muscular pump that forces the blood through the pulmonary and systemic circulations. The blood is the medium for transportation of nutrients, gases, waste products of metabolism, and cellular secretions. Blood also constantly replenishes the interstitial fluid with a filtrate of plasma that leaks through and around the endothelial cells of the capillaries. Interstitial fluid is also produced by the metabolism of the cells of the tissues. The excess interstitial fluid is drained via the lymphatic vessels back into the venous circulation, mostly via the thoracic duct.

The Heart

The heart is contained within a nondistensible sac (the pericardium), the inner surfaces of which are lined with simple squamous epithelium (mesothelium). The pericardial sac usually contains only a few milliliters of fluid, which act as a lubricant. The visceral pericardium, which lines the surface of the heart, slides against the parietal pericardium, which lines the inner surface of the pericardial sac. The pericardium helps to prevent overdistention of the ventricles should venous return acutely increase. Excess fluid in the pericardial sac or constriction by the pericardial sac can interfere with cardiac filling (cardiac tamponade). This is a life-threatening emergency that can be greatly complicated by anesthesia. Proper management is discussed in Chapter 22.

The heart is composed mostly of cardiac muscle cells with little connective tissue. The outer surface of the heart is called the *epicardium*. The muscular wall is called the *myocardium*. The innermost portion of the heart which faces the blood is called the *endocardium*. The coronary vessels run from the epicardium to the endocardium, and so the endocardium is at greatest risk of ischemia (actually, the subendocardium because the very innermost layers of cells can receive their nutrients from the blood within the chambers).

The major structures of the heart are shown in Fig. 1-1. The atria are separated from the muscular ventricles by a fibrous ring that contains the four cardiac valves. (This fibrous ring also acts as an electrical-mechanical barrier separating each atrial depolarization and contraction from the ventricular depolarization and contraction.) The one-way cardiac valves consist of cusps of nondistensible collagen covered by a layer of endothelium. Atrioventricular valves separate the atria from the ventricles. The right AV valve is tricuspid, while the left AV valve (mitral) is bicuspid. The cusps of the AV valves are attached to the fibrous rings that separate the atria from the ventricles. The free margins of the cusps are attached to the papillary muscles (projections of the ventricular myocardium) by threadlike strands of collagen (chordae tendineae). The chordae keep the valves from prolapsing (opening backwards into the atria) and causing regurgitation of the blood back into the atria during systole. If the chordae are too long, the valve leaflets may sometimes bulge into the atrium during systole, contacting the atrial wall, and produce arrhythmias, chest pain, and endocarditis. The valve leaflets are very thin and delicate and appear translucent or nearly transparent in healthy individuals.

The thin-walled right atrium receives blood from the superior and inferior vena cava. The inferior vena cava is partially separated from the right atrium by an incomplete (eustachian) valve. This valve acts to partially separate the blood returning to the heart so that truly mixed venous blood (which is needed for measurements when performing the shunt equation and other calculations) can be obtained only from the pulmonary artery. The right atrium also receives blood from the coronary sinus, which opens into the right atrium between the orifice of the inferior vena cava and the tricuspid valve. Withdrawal of a Swan-Ganz catheter can injure the tricuspid valve, if the catheter becomes entangled in the

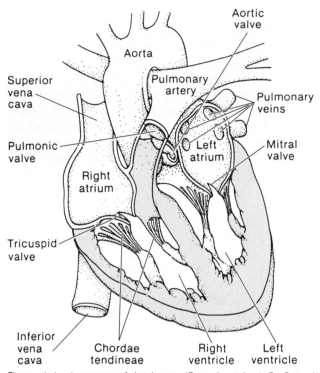

Figure 1-1   Anatomy of the heart. (From Levitzky MG, Cairo JM, Hall Sr: *Introduction to Respiratory Care* Philadelphia, Saunders, 1990, with permission.)

chordae tendineae (especially if the catheter balloon is inflated during withdrawal).

The atria possess appendages (auricles) that can be used to provide surgical access to the inside of the heart without causing significant impairment of cardiac function. Entry through the auricle of the right atrium is performed to divert the venous return to the heart for cardiopulmonary bypass. Entry through the right auricle can also be used to provide surgical access to the tricuspid valve. The inner surface of the atria is irregular and unsmooth due to the presence of musculi pectinati (blood clots frequently adhere to these structures during atrial fibrillation). The right atrium contracts during the end of ventricular diastole to provide the "atrial kick" that adds about 25 percent of the right ventricular end-diastolic volume.

Although the right ventricle is much thicker walled than the right atrium, the right ventricular wall is only one-third as thick as the wall of the left ventricle in the normal adult. This is due to differences in afterload that the two chambers must attain. In neonates, the walls of the two ventricles are approximately the same thickness because the afterload of the two ventricles is similar before birth. The two ventricles share a common wall, the ventricular septum, and the portion of the septum near the apex is thicker and more muscular while the portion near the valvular ring is thinner, membranous, and more likely to be the site of ventricular septal defects (VSD).

During right ventricular contraction, when the ventricular chamber pressure exceeds right atrial pressure, the AV valve bulges backwards into the atrium and closes. Isometric contraction of the right ventricle continues to raise the pressure until the pulmonary valve opens and ejection occurs. After traversing the pulmonary circulation, the blood returns to the left atrium via the four pulmonary veins. There are no valves between the pulmonary artery and the thin-walled left atrium. The two atria share a common wall (the atrial septum).

During embryologic development (Fig. 1-2), the two atria are connected by an opening in the atrial septum (foramen ovale), which allows blood to enter the left side of the heart, bypassing the high resistance of the pulmonary circulation in the uninflated fetal lung. At birth, decreased pulmonary vascular resistance and pressures allow closure of this foramen ovale. Unexpected neurologic injuries following anesthesia have been explained as resulting from "paradoxical embolism" (emboli gaining access to the left side of heart through a patent foramen ovale and then entering the cerebral circulation). Better monitoring of tissue oxygenation seem to have greatly decreased the incidence of these devastating events (or have at least provided alternate explanations).

In a manner similar to the right side, the pulmonary venous return and left atrial contraction fill the left ventricle during diastole. Ventricular contraction closes the mitral valve, then opens the aortic valve as ventricular pressure increases.

The Vessels

Blood vessels are more than mere conduits that carry blood from the heart to the other tissues and back. Vessels play an important role in maintenance of blood pressure, distribution of blood flow, and hemostasis. The systemic circulation receives blood from the left ventricle and drains into the right atrium while the pulmonary circulation (which has lower blood pressures) receives about the same amount of blood per time from the right ventricle and delivers it to the left atrium. The lymphatic vessels transport excess interstitial fluid back to the veins, mainly via the thoracic duct.

Systemic Circulation   The thick-walled elastic aorta ascends as it leaves the left ventricle, then arches toward the left side of the body, and finally descends toward the lower extremities. The two coronary arteries leave the aorta immediately distal to the aortic valve. The blood supply to the head and upper extremities leaves the aorta at its arch via the brachiocephalic (innominate) artery, which gives rise to the right subclavian artery and the right common carotid artery, and via the left subclavian artery and the left common carotid artery, which also branch off the aorta. Blood supply to the chest wall and intercostal muscles leaves

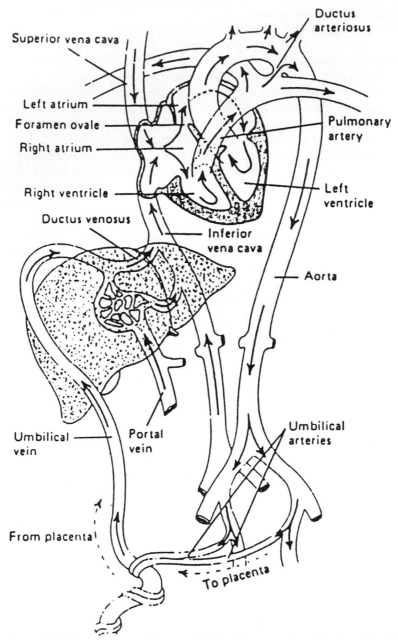

Figure 1-2 Fetal circulation: Oxygenated blood returning from the placenta via the umbilical vein can either enter the portal circulation or continue directly to the inferior vena cava (via the ductus venosus). Most of the oxygenated blood entering the heart from the inferior vena cava is deflected by the eustachian valve through the foramen ovale (in the intraatrial septum) and then ejected by the left ventricle to the head and upper extremities. Deoxygenated blood returning via the superior vena cava passes through the tricuspid valve, right ventricle, pulmonary artery, ductus arteriosus, and then into the aorta distal to the take off of the vessels to the head and upper extremities. (Reprinted with permission from Ganong, WF. *Review of Medical Physiology*, 13th. ed. Norwalk, CT; Appleton & Lange, 1987.)

the proximal part of the descending aorta via the intercostal arteries. The larger airways of the lung receive their nutrient blood flow via the bronchial arteries which also exit the aorta above the diaphragm.

The thoracic and cervical portions of the spinal cord receive their perfusion via the vertebral arteries, which are branches of the subclavian. Below the diaphragm, the anterior portion of the spinal cord receives its blood supply via a branch of the aorta called the *radicular artery of* Adamkiewicz. Prolonged cross-clamping of the aorta in the chest can result in thrombosis of this anterior spinal artery and loss of lower extremity motor function, resulting in paraplegia. Other branches of the aorta and their corresponding vertebral level of branching from the aorta are depicted in Fig. 1-3. The largest systemic arteries, such as the aorta and its major branches, have much more elastic tissue and collagen in their walls and fewer smooth muscle cells than smaller arteries and arterioles. This elastic tissue allows them to stretch when the heart ejects the stroke volume. Stretching the vessel walls tends to keep systemic arterial systolic blood pressure lower than it would be if these vessels were less distensible. Additionally, the recoil of these vessels' walls (*windkessel* vessels) maintains diastolic pressure and blood flow through the arteries and capillaries.

The arterial tree terminates in the small muscular arterioles The tone of the arterioles in different vascular beds helps determine the distribution of blood flow to the tissues. The arterioles are the site of greatest resistance to blood flow in the systemic circulation. Thus, the decrease in pressure that occurs as blood flows from the systemic arteries to the veins is greatest in the arteriolar segments of the systemic circulation. As the arterial tree divides, the total cross-sectional area of the various branches increases dramatically and reaches its peak in the capillaries. Net cross-sectional area decreases as veins merge to form larger vessels. Because the amount of blood flow through the various segments is the same, when net cross-sectional area increases, the linear velocity of blood flow decreases. Thus, the capillary segment has the slowest blood flow. The largest fraction of blood volume is normally found in the veins because they are the most compliant segment of the systemic circulation.

The microcirculation consists of vessels less than 100μ in diameter, including the terminal arterioles, metarterioles, capillaries, and postcapillary venules. The metarterioles, which contain smooth muscle, either give rise to the capillaries or can act as a direct connection between an arteriole and a venule. A small band of smooth muscle (precapillary sphincter) found at the origin of many capillaries can act to open or close off sections of capillary beds. They are under "local" control (they dilate or constrict in response to alterations in levels of oxygen, carbon dioxide, pH, metabolites, ions, and the temperature of the immediate environment). The larger vessels are under neural control. Certain organs, such as the skin or portions of the gastrointestinal tract, have arteriovenous shunt vessels directly connecting an artery and vein, allowing diversion of blood flow away from larger sections of the capillary bed.

The organization and structure of the capillary beds vary considerably in different organs. Some organs, such as the liver, have leaky capillaries with many pores called *fenestrations*. Others have capillaries with few fenestrations. The capillaries of the cerebral circulation have virtually no fenestrations, thereby forming the blood-brain barrier.

The pores allow large molecules and substances that cannot pass through the capillary endothelial cells to be exchanged between the interstitial fluid and the blood. Certain large insoluble particles are transported through the capillary wall by a process called *endocytosis,* in which the endothelial cell membrane surrounds the particles to form vesicles that are then used to transport them

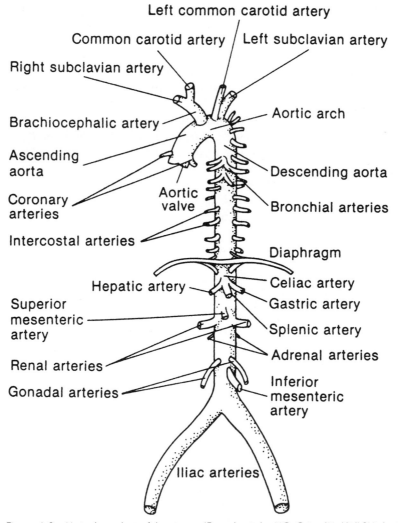

Figure 1-3 Major branches of the aorta. (From Levitzky MG, Cairo JM, Hall SM: *Introduction to Respiratory Care*, Philadelphia, Saunders, 1990, with permission.)

through the cell. The material leaves the cell and enters the interstitial space by a process called *exocytosis*.

The capillaries, metarterioles, and shunt vessels all drain into the venules, which are slightly larger in diameter than their corresponding arterioles but have much thinner walls. Exchange between the blood and the interstitial space can probably continue through the thin walls of the venules. The venules, as well as the larger veins that they form, have smooth muscle that is under neural (and possibly humoral) control.

There are usually at least two veins for every corresponding artery. Each vein usually has a greater internal diameter and is much easier to distend (at least at lower volumes) than their companion arteries. Thus the total cross-sectional area for the veins is greater than that of the companion arteries, and the flow is therefore much slower through the veins. The veins are often referred to as capacitance vessels because of their capacity to store blood. The volume of blood in the veins is therefore normally much greater than that in the arteries. Similarly the arterioles, with their large component of smooth muscle are frequently referred to as resistance vessels. Stimulation of the sympathetic innervation of the veins reduces their intravascular volume.

The veins of the extremities have delicate crescent-shaped valves which allow one-way flow of blood to the heart. Although there is not sufficient blood pressure in the veins to push the blood "uphill" to the heart, compression of the veins by contraction of the skeletal muscle squeezes the blood toward the great veins and right atrium. The veins of the thorax, abdomen, and brain have no valves.

Pulmonary Circulation When compared to the vessels of the systemic circulation, pulmonary vessels are generally short and thinned-walled and have large lumens. In addition, the pulmonary circulation has relatively little smooth muscle. As a consequence, pulmonary circulation normally offers much less resistance to blood flow than does the systemic circulation. This results in a much lower pulmonary artery blood pressure than that of the systemic arteries, even though the right and left ventricular output is nearly identical. The smooth muscle that is present in the pulmonary circulation is innervated by the sympathetic nervous system and is also affected by local factors, as discussed in Part 2.

The short arteries of the pulmonary circulation branch rapidly, ultimately forming as many as 280 billion pulmonary capillaries surrounding the alveoli. Except for the pulmonary valve, there are no other valves in the pulmonary circulation. The surface area of the pulmonary capillary-alveolar interface is about 60 to 80 m^2 in a normal adult. This large area for gas exchange helps explain why patients with lung disease do not become symptomatic until the problem is fairly severe.

The Lymphatic System The lymphatic system serves important transport and defense functions. It helps drain the interstitial space by returning fluids and other materials into the systemic venous system, mainly via the thoracic duct. The rate of lymph flow through the thoracic duct of the adult is about 100 ml of lymph per hour. About 20 ml of lymph enter the venous circulation at other points for a total of 120 ml of lymph flow per hour. This relatively low lymph flow shows that although large amounts of fluid leak out at the high pressure arterial end of the capillaries most of the fluid reenters the lower pressure venous end, with only a small portion drained via the lymphatics.

The interstitial space receives fluid from two sources: water and other by-products of cellular metabolism leave the cells of the tissue; and fluid leaks from the capillaries through the endothelial cells or through the pores between the endothelial cells. About one-tenth of the plasma that enters the capillaries leaks through the cells or pores into the interstitial space. Most of this fluid is taken back up at the venous ends of the capillary (as discussed later in Chap. 7). The plasma filtrate that is not reabsorbed by the capillaries is drained from the interstitial space, along with the excess water produced by the cells, via the lymphatics.

The lymphatic vessels start with blind-ending vessels that are similar in structure to the systemic capillaries. Fluid and particles enter these vessels, which drain into larger lymph vessels comparable to the systemic veins. The lymphatic vessels have many valves, which can even be found at the very tips of the terminal lymphatic capillaries. The movement of lymph toward the venous circulation is aided by contraction of small amounts of smooth muscle around the larger lymphatic segments, which squeezes the lymph through the valve and into the next lymphatic segment. The contraction of skeletal muscle, movement of the body limbs, arterial pulsations, and compression of the tissues by objects outside the body all act to help propel the lymph forward into the next segments and toward the venous system. The thoracic duct drains into the systemic venous circulation at a point near where the left subclavian vein joins the left jugular vein.

The Blood

Blood is a suspension of different kinds of cells (and cell fragments such as platelets) in an aqueous medium called *plasma*. The cells (formed elements) can be easily separated from the plasma by centrifugation because they have a greater density than plasma. The ratio of the volume of the blood cells to the total volume of blood (expressed as a percentage) is called the *hematocrit*. The hemoglobin level in grams per deciliter can be fairly accurately estimated by dividing the hematocrit by 3. The normal hematocrit for an adult male is about 45 percent (hemoglobin = 15 g/dl), and for an adult female about 39 percent (with a hemoglobin of 13 g/dl). One percent of the blood consists of white blood cells and platelets. This layer (buffy coat) appears between the plasma and the more dense red blood cells following centrifugation.

Plasma   Plasma is a clear, straw-colored solution that is about 90 percent water. Plasma is the liquid portion of blood that has not undergone coagulation;

serum refers to the liquid portion of blood obtained after coagulation has occurred and many of the clotting factors have been consumed. Plasma contains many kinds of proteins that have several functions. Albumin is an important transport protein which combines with materials (such as certain hormones or drugs) in the plasma, reducing their uptake by the other tissues of the body. Additionally, albumin plays a major role in the oncotic Starling forces acting to retain fluid within the capillaries. Albumin molecules are slightly too large to leak through the endothelial pores, so they help keep fluid from moving into the interstitium. Certain plasma proteins also can serve enzymatic functions such as pseudochol-inesterase and other nonspecific esterases (such as those responsible for break-down of ester local anesthetics and labetalol). The protein fraction also contains several proteins important in the body's clotting system: both procoagulants and anticoagulants. The other major group of proteins in the plasma consist of the immunoglobins, which are produced by cells in the lymphoid tissues. These im-munoglobins such as IgG are also called antibodies. Another group of proteins (the complement group) also participates in immunologic reactions by stimulating and attracting white blood cells (chemotaxis). The concentration of electrolytes in the plasma is essentially the same as that of the interstitial fluid. Other dissolved substances in the plasma such as carbon dioxide and oxygen, as well as nutrients and waste products, are in approximately the same concentration as in the inter-stitial fluid.

The Blood Cells   The most common cell in the blood is the red blood cell with about 5 million cells per cubic millimeter. There are normally approximately 5,000 to 10,000 white blood cells per cubic millimeter of blood, while the normal platelet count is 150,000 to 450,000 per cubic millimeter.

Erythrocytes   The erythrocytes are biconcave disks that average about 7μ in diameter and about 2μ at their thickest part. They therefore have a high surface area to volume ratio, which aids in the diffusion of oxygen and carbon dioxide into and out of the cells. Erythrocytes are deformable, which allows them to change shape as they pass through small vessels. The average life span of eryth-rocytes in the body is 120 days, while banked blood can be kept for 30 to 45 days depending on the preservative. Hemoglobin (a conjugated protein with a molecular weight of about 64,500 daltons) is the major component of the eryth-rocyte. In addition to transporting oxygen, hemoglobin plays an important role in carbon dioxide transport and hydrogen-ion buffering. Although the red blood cells lack a nucleus and many organelles, they are able to metabolize nutrients such as glucose.

Leukocytes   There are several types of white blood cells (Table 1-1) with the most common type being the neutrophil, also called polymorphonucleocyte (PMN). Neutrophils and the other white blood cells (eosinophils and basophils), which come from the bone marrow (*myelogenous*), are called *granulocytes,* which refers to the granules contained in the vesicles of their cytoplasm. The agranu-

Table 1-1   Normal Percentages of the Different Types of White Blood Cells

Neutrophils	62.0
Eosinophils	2.3
Basophils	0.4
Monocytes	5.3
Lymphocytes	30.0

locytes (lymphocytes and monocytes) are formed in the lymph nodes. The granulocytes and monocytes protect the body against invading organisms by ingesting them by the process of phagocytosis. The phagocytic cells destroy the ingested bacteria with lytic enzymes found in intracellular organelles known as lysosomes. Leukocytes also participate in inflammatory reactions. They are attracted to sites of tissue injury by chemotatic factors. The number of neutrophils greatly increases during an acute infection and immature neutrophils ("bands" and "stabs") increase in the circulation. Increased numbers of eosinophils are associated with allergic reactions and parasitic infections. Basophils can leave the vessels and enlarge about five times in size to become tissue mast cells (which contain large amounts of heparin and histamine and play a role in anaphylactic reactions).

The lymphocytes are specialized white blood cells that provide immune function. They are subdivided into "T" cells (originating in the thymus) and "B" cells (originating in the bursa which is an organ found in birds but not mammals). When B-lymphocytes were first identified, they were discovered in birds and found to arise from the bursa. Their origin in mammals is more diffuse and so they are said to arise from the "bursal" equivalent. These cells are responsible for the "humoral" immunity: that is, the secretion of antibodies such as immunoglobins. The T-cells are subdivided into "helper" T-cells and "killer" T-cells. The helper T-cells regulate the populations of other immune cell types by secreting chemical signals. The killer T-cells recognize, phagocytize, and eliminate material to which they are sensitized. Monocytes are the largest white blood cells and also assist the immune system by processing antigens so that the B-lymphocytes can produce specific antibodies to them.

Thrombocytes   Platelets (thrombocytes) are about 2μ in diameter and come from the megakaryocytes (large multinucleated cells) in the bone marrow. When the platelets contact collagen, they swell and become irregular and adhesive. They secrete adenosine diphosphate (ADP) and enzymes causing the formation of thromboxane A, which activates other platelets. Thromboxane A is formed from arachidonic acid using the cyclooxygenase enzyme pathway. The platelets have a life span of about 10 days, which explains why aspirin ingestion, which irreversibly blocks the formation of thromboxane A, is contraindicated for 2 weeks preceding surgery. When a blood vessel is injured, the blood comes in contact with the collagen in the connective tissue surrounding the blood vessels and activates the clotting cascade that ends in the formation of fibrin which, with platelets, form the clot.

REFERENCES

Agur AMR: *Grants Atlas of Anatomy.* 9th ed. Baltimore, Williams & Wilkins.

Berne RM, Levy MN: *Physiology.* 2nd ed. St. Louis, CV Mosby, 1988.

Cote CJ, Ryan JF, Todres ID, Goudsouzian NG: *A Practice of Anesthesia for Infants and Children.* Philadelphia, Saunders, 1990.

Ganong WF, *Review of Medical Physiology.* 13th ed. Norwalk, Appleton & Lange, 1987.

Levitzky MG, Cairo JM, Hall SM: *Introduction to Respiratory Care.* Philadelphia, Saunders, 1990.

Moore KL: *Before We Are Born: Basic Embryology and Birth Defects* (Rev Reprint). Saunders, Philadelphia, 1977.

Netter FH: *The CIBA Collection of Medical Illustrations, Heart,* vol 5, Summit, NJ, CIBA, 1979.

Sadler TW: *Langman's Medical Embryology,* 7th ed. Williams & Wilkins, Baltimore, 1995.

2

ELECTROCARDIOGRAPHY

A standard for basic anesthetic monitoring notes, "Every patient receiving anesthesia shall have the electrocardiogram continuously displayed from the beginning of anesthesia until preparing to leave the anesthetizing location." * The continual evaluation of the patient's circulation (also an anesthetic monitoring standard) requires an understanding of the physiologic events represented by the electrocardiogram (ECG). Note that *continual* is defined as "repeated regularly and frequently in steady rapid succession" whereas *continuous* means "prolonged without any interruption at any time."

ELECTROPHYSIOLOGY OF MYOCARDIAL CELLS

The ECG is a graphic representation of the net electrical activity of the heart associated with the action potentials of the myocardial cells. An understanding of action potentials of individual myocardial cells is necessary to interpret the electrical events depicted in the ECG. The excitable cells of the body, such as muscle and nerve, characteristically exhibit action potentials — changes in the cell membrane's electrical charge from the preexisting resting membrane potential. All living cells in the body have a resting membrane potential due to the presence of relatively more negatively charged ions (anions) inside the cell than outside. This imbalance of charges is caused by three factors:

1   The resting cell membrane is 50 to 100 times more permeable to potassium than to sodium.
2   The sodium/potassium adenosine triphosphotase (Na/K ATPase) pump, which creates a gradient for diffusion of these ions across the cell membrane by actively transporting potassium into the cell and sodium out of the cell.

* American Society of Anesthesiologists

3   The presence of many intracellular anions (such as proteins, phosphates, and sulfates) that cannot diffuse through the cell membrane or diffuse poorly.

Potassium passively leaks from the cell much more rapidly than sodium diffuses into the cell. As the positively charged potassium ions leave the cell, the poorly diffusible anions are left intracellularly, resulting in a negative resting membrane potential (approximately -85 to -100 mV). At the same time, sodium is continuously actively transported out of the cell while potassium is transported into the cell. These factors are combined in order to calculate the approximate resting membrane potential using the *Nernst Equation:*

$$EMF = -61 \log \frac{\text{ion concentration inside} \times P}{\text{ion concentration outside} \times P}$$

where P = permeability of the membrane and EMF = electromotive force.
   The Nernst Equation depends on the following:

1   The polarity of the electrical charge of each ion (cation or anion)
2   The permeability of the membrane to each ion
3   The concentrations of the respective ions on the two sides of the membrane

Resting membrane potentials calculated using the Nernst equation are very close to those actually measured in laboratory studies.
   Certain membrane events (such as electrical stimulation, application of chemicals, mechanical stimulation, heat, or cold) can alter the permeability of the myocardial cell membrane to sodium. The diffusion of sodium into the cell suddenly increases by the opening of the *fast sodium channels* producing the depolarization phase of an action potential. The increase in permeability to sodium is called *activation* of the membrane. The fast sodium channels are open for only a few 10,000ths of a second, causing the abrupt onset of the action potential observed in ventricular muscle. Sodium leaks inward through multiple membrane channels, producing an action potential once threshold voltage is reached. Enough sodium rushes into the cell to make the inside of the cell positive with respect to the outside (reversal potential). This is followed by a prolonged influx of calcium and sodium ions via *slow calcium channels,* which is associated with a simultaneous decrease in potassium efflux. This maintains the positive intracellular charge (for 150 to 300 ms). The decreased permeability to potassium prevents rapid repolarization of the membrane. When the slow calcium channels close, the permeability to potassium increases, causing repolarization as the cell returns to the resting potential and ending the action potential. A representative diagram of a ventricular myocardial cell action potential is shown in Fig. 2-1. The action potential is subdivided into phases 0 to 4, representing the permeability changes

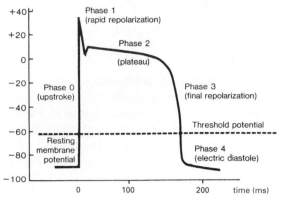

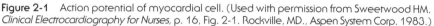

Figure 2-1   Action potential of myocardial cell. (Used with permission from Sweetwood HM. *Clinical Electrocardiography for Nurses*, p. 16, Fig. 2-1. Rockville, MD., Aspen System Corp. 1983.)

in the cell membrane. Phase 0 represents depolarization (caused by the rapid influx of sodium). Phase 1 is the brief interval when sodium influx slows, while chloride enters and potassium leaves the cell. Phase 2 is the plateau (lasting up to 150 ms) caused by the closure of sodium channels and entry of calcium via its slow channels. Permeability to potassium rapidly increases during phase 3, restoring the transmembrane potential to -70 to -90 mV. Following repolarization, phase 4 starts once the negative transmembrane potential is restored and lasts until the next action potential begins.

In contrast to the aforementioned ventricular cell action potential, the membrane potential of a sinus nodal cell normally possesses much greater automaticity. Between discharges (during phase 4), the sinus nodal cell membrane potential is only -55 to -60 mV as opposed to -85 to -90 mV for a ventricular cell. Additionally, the sinus nodal cell's membrane is inherently leakier than ventricular cell membranes and this leakiness increases over time until threshold voltage is achieved. Normally, ventricular muscle cell membrane permeability to sodium does not increase nearly as rapidly. Because sinus nodal cells start at a higher resting potential and that potential increases much more rapidly than those of ventricular muscle cells (due to nodal cell's increasing permeability to sodium), sinoatrial (SA) nodal cells arrive at threshold voltage earlier.

The heart rate is increased by increasing the frequency of depolarization of pacemaker cells. This can occur by increasing the slope of phase 4, by reduction of threshold potential (making it more negative), or by elevating the resting membrane potential (making it less negative). Norepinephrine increases heart rate by increasing the slope of phase 4; lidocaine reduces the slope of phase 4, especially in ventricular muscle cells (reducing the incidence of premature ventricular contractions). Vagal stimulation reduces heart rate by hyperpolarizing pacemaker cells (making their transmembrane potential more negative) and by reducing the slope of phase 4.

REFRACTORY PERIOD

Following depolarization, the sodium channels close, becoming one of two non-conducting states known either as *resting* or *inactivated*. Resting sodium channels may activate to become open channels, while inactivated channels must first undergo transition to the resting state. Due to the presence of a large number of inactivated sodium channels during much of the action potential, the membrane is completely refractory to further stimulation (*the absolute refractory period*). The absolute refractory period occurs during phases 1, 2, and part of 3. During the latter portion of phase 3 of an action potential, a stronger than normal stimulus could evoke a second action potential (*the relative refractory period*). This reflects the need to activate a critical number of sodium channels to trigger an action potential.

T TUBULES AND CALCIUM

As is true in other excitable cells, the action potential spreads over the entire cardiac muscle fiber cell membrane, including the *T tubules*. The T tubules are indentations of the cell membrane penetrating deeply into the cardiac muscle cell. The T tubules of cardiac muscle cells are about five times larger in diameter but fewer in number than the T tubules of skeletal muscle cells. Adjacent to the T tubules are the *cisternae*, which are modified portions of the sarcoplasmic reticulum. The cisternae contain highly concentrated calcium, which they release when an action potential spreads over the cell membrane. The calcium binds to troponin, which abolishes the inhibitory effect of troponin on the interaction between actin and myosin. In the presence of ATP, the actin and myosin filaments bind and slide along each other, causing muscular contraction. Additionally, the calcium that enters the myocardial cells via slow calcium channels is essential in determining the strength of the contraction. Thus, extracellular calcium concentration directly affects cardiac muscle contraction while having little effect on the contraction of skeletal muscle (which relies almost entirely on the calcium ions released from the cisternae). When the slow calcium channels close, calcium pumps return the calcium to the inside of the sarcoplasmic reticulum or else pump it out of the cell to terminate contraction. The duration of contraction is mainly a function of the duration of the action potential—approximately 0.15 s in atrial muscle and 0.3 s in ventricular muscle. Note that changes in heart rate can affect the duration of contraction. Tachycardia decreases the duration of each individual systole, but the heart spends more total time in the contracted state. At a heart rate of 72, the heart spends about 40 percent of the time in systole, while at a heart rate of 210, 62 percent of the time is spent in systole. As diastolic time decreases, ventricular filling can be reduced, resulting in a decreased cardiac output; the time available for coronary blood flow to the ventricle is also reduced.

MYOCARDIAL SYNCYTIUMS

The muscle cells of the atria are very similar in structure to those of the ventricles. These cells contain large amounts of organized actin and myosin filaments that give a striated appearance. The excitatory and conductive cells are modified myocardial cells but contain few contractile filaments. Although the heart's conducting system is affected by autonomic nerves and may seem to conduct impulses in a manner similar to nerve cells, the conducting system is not composed of neurons. Instead impulses are conducted directly from one myocardial cell to an adjacent cell because they are essentially fused together, separated by only a thin portion of modified cell membrane called the *intercalated disc*. Action potentials travel directly from one cardiac muscle cell to another (without using neurotransmitters) through intercalated discs, which have only about 1/400th the resistance of the regular cell membrane. Myocardial cells are arranged in a lattice with intercalated discs the sites where one cell meets another. Thus, the heart chambers are electrically a *syncytium* of many individual heart muscle cells that are so interconnected that when one of these cells becomes excited, the action potential spreads throughout the entire lattice. The walls of the heart chambers are composed almost entirely of cardiac muscle cells but contain some connective tissue and blood vessels.

The two atria are electrically isolated from the two ventricles by fibrous tissue (at the level of the endocardial cushion) surrounding the valvular openings between the atria and ventricles. The two atria act as a syncytium during depolarization and during contraction. The ventricles are also joined syncytially but function separately from the atria. The only communications between the atria and ventricles are via the three internodal pathways. The velocity of conduction of cardiac muscle in the heart chamber walls is 0.3 to 0.5 m/s, while in the specialized conducting system the speed of conduction ranges from as slow as 0.02 (at the atrioventricular (AV) node) to as much as 4 m/s.

SELF-EXCITATION OF THE SINOATRIAL NODE

The contractile cells of the atrial syncytium and the ventricular syncytium have a relatively stable resting membrane potential. For the self-excitatory cells of the nodes and conducting system, the cell membrane potential is not as flat (and so not really "resting") during the intervals between action potentials. In the nodal and conducting cells, the cell membrane potential increases and triggers the action potentials.

As previously mentioned, the cell membrane's inward leakiness to sodium is one of the factors responsible for establishment of the resting membrane potential. However, in the SA node cells, the inward permeability spontaneously changes, producing the self-excitation. The increasing inward leak of sodium ions causes a rising membrane potential of sinus nodal cells. When it reaches the *threshold potential* of about -40 mV, the slow calcium-sodium channels become activated, allowing the very rapid entry of both calcium and sodium, which causes the depolarization phase of the action potential.

Normally, the slope of phase 4 is steepest in the cells of the SA node, so this site acts as the origin of myocardial action potentials. Conditions such as hypoxia or electrolyte imbalances can cause the slope of phase 4 to become steeper in other areas of the heart, resulting in an ectopic origin of the heart's depolarization (such as a nodal contraction or a premature ventricular contraction).

CONDUCTING SYSTEM

The SA node is where the normal rhythmic self-excitatory impulse is generated (Fig. 2-2). This crescent-shaped group of modified myocardial cells makes up part of the lattice of the superior lateral wall of the right atrium immediately below and lateral to the opening of the superior vena cava. Its blood supply is via the SA nodal artery, which usually is a branch of the right coronary artery. The sinus node normally depolarizes first (as discussed earlier) and from here the impulses spread throughout the rest of the atrial lattice and also through the *internodal pathways*.

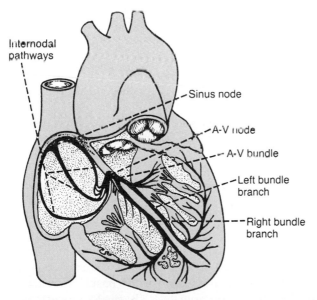

Figure 2-2   The sinus node and the Purkinje system of the heart showing also the A-V node, the atrial internodal pathways, and the ventricular bundle branches.

The internodal pathways consist of three small bundles of specialized conducting fibers called the anterior, middle, and posterior internodal pathways. These pathways conduct the impulse from the sinus node to the AV node. The anterior internodal pathway divides into two branches: *Bachmann's bundle* travels to the left atrium to deliver the impulse there; and the descending branch connects the SA and the AV node. The middle internodal tract *(Wenckebach's bundle)* runs posteriorly within the interatrial septum. The posterior internodal track is called *Thorel's pathway* and runs posterolaterally. Anomalous accessory pathways can connect the atria directly to the ventricle or interconnect other areas of the conducting system and produce preexcitation syndrome. *Kent's bundle* directly connects the left atrium and left ventricle.

The AV node (Fig. 2-2) is contained in the posterior septal wall of the right atrium directly behind the tricuspid valve, adjacent to the opening to the coronary sinus. Blood supply to the AV node is from a branch of the right coronary artery called the AV nodal artery. Before the impulse enters the AV node, there is a slight delay that helps allow the atria to pump their contents forward into the ventricles before ventricular systole begins. This delay is due to the transitional fibers that connect the internodal pathways to the AV node. Conduction velocity is also quite low in the AV node, as well as in the fibers that connect the AV node to the AV bundle (the bundle of His, which distributes the impulse to the ventricles). The total delay between the start of the atrial impulse and the start of the ventricular impulse is about 0.16 s, with about 0.13 s of this delay occurring in conducting fibers in and immediately surrounding the AV node. This delay in conduction is due to the small diameter of the fibers and few intercalated discs connecting successive fibers in this part of the pathway. Additionally, the resting membrane potentials of these cells are much less negative than the normal resting membrane potentials of other cardiac muscle cells. The low voltage of these conducting cells results in resistance to the development of action potentials due to the low ion gradients.

After the delay at the transitional fibers, AV node, and penetrating portion of the AV bundle, conduction proceeds rapidly through the very large diameter Purkinje fibers of the distal portion of the AV bundle and bundle branches. These structures then distribute the impulse throughout both ventricles. The Purkinje fibers are on the endocardial surfaces of both ventricles, and so the action potential as well as contraction begins endocardially and then spreads outward through the wall of the heart.

The conducting system of the heart (Table 2-1) acts to prevent dysrhythmias. In addition, it spreads depolarization rapidly so ventricular muscle cells contract simultaneously to produce a forceful contraction. This simultaneous contraction of ventricular muscle cells does not occur with much slower cell to cell conduction, resulting in less forceful contractions. The rapid transmission of cardiac impulses means that the fibers stimulated first are still refractory at the time the last fibers are stimulated. A delay in transmission of cardiac impulses throughout the ventricle makes it possible for impulses from the last excited ventricular muscle fiber to reenter the first muscle fiber and produce ventricular fibrillation.

Table 2-1   The Excitatory and Conductive System of the Heart

Sinoatrial node
Internodal Pathways
  Anterior
  Middle
  Posterior
Transitional fibers
Atrioventricular node
Penetrating portion of the atrioventricular bundle
Atrioventricular bundle (bundle of His)
Right and left bundle branches of Purkinje fibers

The endocardial location of the Purkinje fibers produces a depolarization of the myocardium that spreads from the inside of the heart to the outside. Normally action potentials of the interior cells are of longer duration than those of the epicardial cells. Thus depolarization spreads from inside to outside, whereas repolarization travels from outside to inside.

The ion flux for depolarization of a single cell (Na^+ travels into the cell) is in the opposite direction of that during repolarization (K^+ travels out of the cell). This can be represented on a graph of an action potential as forces moving in opposite directions (upstroke and downstroke).

The ECG is a graphic representation of the net electrical activity caused by the action potentials of the myocardial cells. When the active (sensing) electrode detects depolarization moving in its direction, it is represented graphically on the ECG as an upstroke. The electrical events of ventricular depolarization are represented on the ECG by the QRS complex while ventricular repolarization is displayed by the T wave. If the myocardium depolarized from inside to outside and was represented as an upstroke on the ECG, then repolarization would be a downstroke if it also occurred from inside to outside. However, because repolarization occurs from outside to inside, its graphic representation is usually in the same direction as that for depolarization. During certain heart diseases such as myocardial ischemia, the endocardial cells are unable to sustain their depolarization and so repolarization occurs from inside to outside producing inverted T waves or S-T elevation (Fig. 2-3A). Atrial depolarization is depicted by the P wave on the ECG, but atrial repolarization is concealed because it normally occurs concurrently with the QRS caused by ventricular depolarization. The names of the different ECG waves are given in Fig. 2-3B.

When cardiac depolarization begins in the SA node and is delivered normally by the conducting system at a heart rate appropriate for the patient's age, the heart is said to be in normal sinus rhythm (Fig. 2-4). Normal heart rate tends to decrease with age until adulthood. The range for sinus rhythm is 85 to 250 from birth to 3 months, 100 to 190 from 3 months to 2 years, 60 to 140 from 2 years to 10 years, and 60 to 100 for ages greater than 10 years.

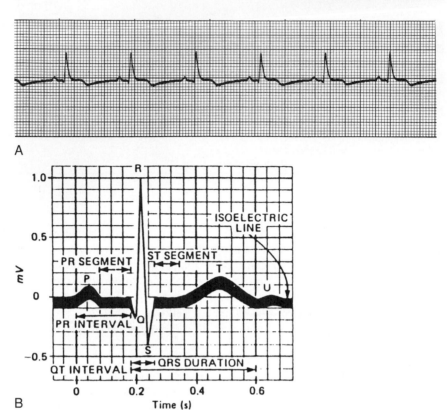

B

Figure 2-3 A. S-T elevation. B. Normal waves and intervals on the electrocardiogram. (Used with permission from Stoelting RK. *Pharmacology and Physiology in Anesthetic Practice,* 2d ed. Philadelphia, Lippincott, 1991 p. 708, Fig. 48-1.)

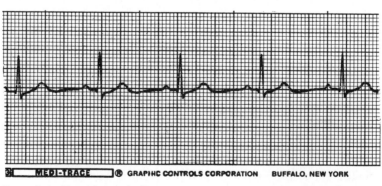

Figure 2-4 Normal sinus rhythm.

Table 2-2   Electrocardiogram Changes Associated
with Electrolyte Abnormalities

Electrolyte Abnormality	ECG Effect
Hypokalemia (Alkalosis produces the same ECG effects)	ST depression T-wave flattening Q-T prolongation Pronounced U wave
Hyperkalemia (Acidosis produces the same ECG effects)	Peaked T wave P-R prolongation ST depression QRS widening Ventricular fibrillation or standstill
Hypocalcemia	Prolonged Q-T interval Flat prolonged ST PR and QRS shortening
Hypercalcemia	Short Q-T interval ST segment may disappear Widened T wave AV conduction disturbances
Hypomagnesemia	Prominent U waves Diminished P and QRS Dysrhythmias especially with hypokalemia or digitalis
Hypermagnesemia	P-R prolongation QRS widening T-wave elevation

EFFECTS OF ELECTROLYTES ON THE ELECTROCARDIOGRAM

Electrolyte abnormalities usually produce ECG changes (Table 2-2). The ECG is profoundly affected by the relative amounts of intra- and extracellular potassium. Moderate hypokalemia (3 to 3.5 mEq/liter) produces flattening (and occasional inversion) of T waves and tall U waves (U waves are deflections that follow T waves). With severe hypokalemia, ST depression is also observed. Hyperkalemia produces narrow, peaked T waves with a shortened Q-T interval. Increasing potassium levels produce widening of the QRS complex and simulate left bundle branch block (described later in this chapter). Further potassium increases will lengthen the P-R interval until eventually the wave is lost. Ventricular asystole or fibrillation occurs when potassium levels are greater than 10 to 12 mEq/liter.

Hypocalcemia sometimes produces a prolonged Q-T interval by elongating the ST segment. The absence of the U wave differentiates hypocalcemia from hypokalemia. With hypercalcemia, the P-R interval is prolonged, the QRS complex is wide, the Q-T interval is shortened with an abrupt takeoff of the widened T-wave. The ECG changes associated with hypocalcemia are exaggerated by hypomagnesemia and corrected by hypermagnesemia. Decreased magnesium levels are characterized by tall, peaked T waves and a normal Q-T interval. Other characteristics mimic hypokalemia and may include prominent U waves and diminished voltage of P waves and QRS complexes. Hypermagnesemia produces prolonged P-R interval increased width of the QRS complex and elevation of the 'T' wave and possibly sinus or AV blocks. Alkalosis produces the same ECG findings as hypokalemia, whereas acidosis produces findings similar to hyperkalemia.

ELECTROCARDIOGRAM MONITORING IN THE OPERATING ROOM

Lead II is used most commonly for routine surgery because normally the P wave is easily seen, facilitating detection of junctional or ventricular dysrhythmias (Fig. 2.5).

For operating room ECG monitors with only three electrodes, rearranging the location of the electrodes will produce a lead called MCL_1 (modified chest lead one), which is very useful for detecting intraoperative dysrhythmias. This is done by placing the left arm electrode over the left upper chest. The left leg electrode is placed in the V_1 position (fourth intercostal space to the right of the sternum). The right arm electrode remains in the usual location. The MCL_1 lead is viewed by selecting lead III on the ECG monitor.

Intraoperative ECG monitors with five electrodes are used routinely during heart surgery or during surgery when there is an increased risk of myocardial ischemia. The four standard electrodes are located on the shoulders and hips while the V_5 electrode is in the left fifth intercostal space in the anterior axillary line. Leads II and V_5 are usually displayed simultaneously but any of leads I, II, III, aV_R, aV_L, aV_F, or V_5 can be selected.

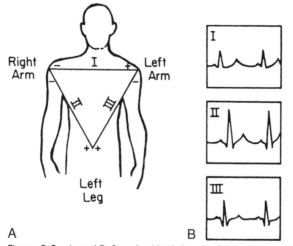

Figure 2-5 A and B. Standard limb leads of the electrocardiogram and typical recordings. (Stoelting RK. *Pharmacology and Physiology in Anesthesiology Practice*, 2d ed. Philadelphia, Lippincott, 1991, p. 708, Fig. 48-2.)

MONITORING FOR MYOCARDIAL ISCHEMIA

ST-segment trend analysis, usually of two or three leads (especially II and V_5), is frequently used for detecting intraoperative left ventricular ischemia. Analysis of lead V_{5R} (the chest electrode is located in the right fifth intercostal space in the anterior axillary line) is useful to monitor the occasional patient whose disease renders them more likely to develop right ventricular ischemia.

Changes in pulmonary capillary wedge pressure or the appearance of V waves on the Swan-Ganz catheter tracing provide some information concerning myocardial ischemia. However, these methods have largely been supplanted by the use of intraoperative transesophageal echocardiography. Assessment of new regional wall motion abnormalities by transesophageal echocardiography is much more sensitive than ECG or pulmonary arterial pressure monitoring for the detection of acute ischemia.

DYSRHYTHMIAS

Dysrhythmias occurring during surgery or in the postoperative period can seriously compromise perfusion or can progress to complete cardiac arrest. First the dysrhythmia must be correctly identified. Precipitating causes should be removed (e.g., endobronchial intubation or traction on the extraocular muscles, carotid sinus, brain stem, bowel, or heart). Only then should treatment be considered.

Treatment under anesthesia is usually unnecessary unless one of the following occurs:

1 The dysrhythmia cannot be controlled by treating underlying causes.
2 Hemodynamic function is compromised.
3 The dysrhythmia predisposes to more serious cardiac dysrhythmias.

Chronic dysrhythmias are commonly disease related and relatively stable. Their presence should be noted during the preoperative ECG. Preoperative cardiology consultation will reveal if the dysrhythmia is adequately controlled and antidysrhythmic medications are at optimal levels. Chronic dysrhythmias are usually associated with heart disease such as myocardial ischemia, heart failure, Wolff-Parkinson-White (WPW) syndrome, long QT syndromes, and mitral valve prolapse. Dysrhythmias can also be related to other systemic diseases (thyrotoxicosis, tetanus, stroke, or chronic lung disease).

Dysrhythmias of acute onset are more likely to be reversible. Dysrhythmias developing intraoperatively can be due to hypoxemia, acidosis, alkalosis, hypokalemia, hyperkalemia, hypocarbia, hypercarbia, hypothermia, hyperthermia, endotracheal intubation, or myocardial irritation by intracardiac catheters. Intraoperative onset of dysrhythmias can also be related to myocardial infarction, cardiac contusion secondary to chest trauma, or thoracic, cardiac, adrenal, or neurosur-

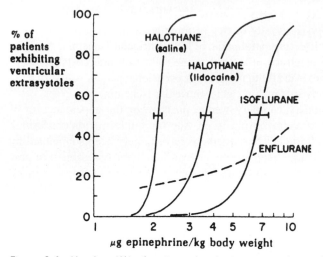

Figure 2-6   Number (%) of patients developing ventricular cardiac dysrhythmias with increasing doses of submucosal epinephrine injected during administration of 1.25 MAC concentrations of the volatile anesthetic. (Reprinted with permission from Johnston RR, Eger EI, Wilson A. An isoflurane and halothane in man. *Anesth Analg* 1976;55:709–12.)

gical procedures. The patient's preoperative anxiety can also induce dysrhythmias.

Drug-induced dysrhythmias can be exacerbated by anesthetic agents and succinylcholine chloride. Perioperative dysrhythmias can result from digitalis intoxication, tricyclic antidepressants, theophylline, catecholamines (including those that are topical and over the counter), anorexiants, and cocaine (Fig. 2-6).

Inhalational anesthesia, especially with ether agents, can cause suppression of the SA node activity and emergence of latent pacemakers within or below the AV node. Halothane sensitizes the myocardium to catecholamines, increasing the likelihood of PVCs (Figure 2-7).

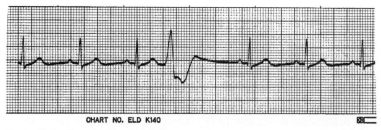

CHART NO. ELD K140

Figure 2-7   Sinus rhythm with PVC.

PRINCIPLES OF ANTIDYSRHYTHMIC DRUG THERAPY

1   Do not discontinue antidysrhythmic drugs preoperatively.
2   Identify dysrhythmias and correct any precipitating factors.
3   Use antidysrhythmic drugs with a clear understanding of their indications, toxicity, and clinical pharmacology.

Dysrhythmia detection and identification is the principal goal of intraoperative ECG monitoring. Although several studies have shown that the majority of patients develop some type of rhythm disturbance during surgery, the majority of intraoperative dysrhythmias are not treated with the administration of antidysrhythmic drugs but are only noted and sometimes treated by changing anesthetic agents or depth of anesthesia.

Supraventricular Dysrhythmias

Sinus Dysrhythmia   Sinus dysrhythmia usually refers to variations in heart rate associated with the changing phases of ventilation (the rate increases during inspiration) but rarely can occur without relationship to ventilation (Fig. 2-8). Treatment is not necessary.

Premature Atrial Contractions   Premature atrial contractions (PACs) arise from an atrial site other than the SA node and depolarize the atria before the next normal SA nodal impulse. They appear as a premature, abnormally shaped P wave and usually a normal QRS complex, although aberrant conduction can make the QRS complex appear widened (like a PVC) but with the same axis as the normal QRS complex (Fig. 2-9). Occasionally the P-wave is so early that the ventricle is refractory. Consequently, conduction does not occur and there is no QRS complex. Frequent PACs can lead to other supraventricular tachydysrhythmias. Intraoperative treatment with a beta blocker or calcium channel blocker may be necessary if the dysrhythmia is causing poor hemodynamic function.

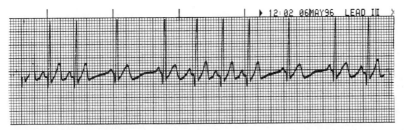

Figure 2-8   Sinus Dysrhythmia.

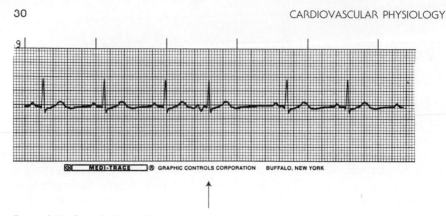

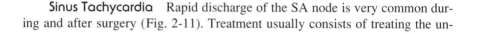

Figure 2-9   Sinus rhythm with premature atrial contraction (PAC) indicated by arrow.

Sinus Bradycardia   The SA node depolarizes at a slower than normal rate (Fig. 2-10). Occasionally ventricular ectopic pacemaker sites take over, causing "premature" contractions (PVCs) that usually disappear when the sinus rate is accelerated. Sinus bradycardia can result from athletic conditioning so treatment is unnecessary in this situation. For the patient with ischemic heart disease, a slow heart rate is the goal of beta blocker therapy. However, bradycardia can be the result of narcotics, anticholinesterases, or overly deep inhalational anesthesia and can lead to profound hypotension and cardiac arrest. It is important to remember that bradycardia in adults is indicated by a heart rate less than 60, whereas bradycardia in patients younger than 2 years old is indicated when the heart rate falls below 100 beats per minute. Bradycardia, especially when the heart rate is below 40 beats per minute and is producing hypotension, PVCs, or decreased systemic perfusion usually requires treatment. Atropine for adults and epinephrine for pediatric patients are the first line drugs for treatment. Rarely infusion of a beta$_1$ agonist drug or placement of a pacemaker is required.

Sinus Tachycardia   Rapid discharge of the SA node is very common during and after surgery (Fig. 2-11). Treatment usually consists of treating the un-

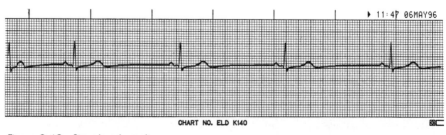

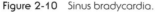

Figure 2-10   Sinus bradycardia.

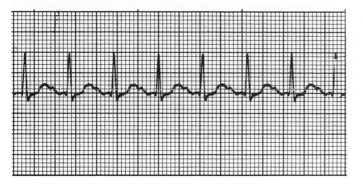

Figure 2-11   Sinus tachycardia.

derlying cause but frequently the cause is difficult to pinpoint. Etiologies include pain (light anesthesia), hypovolemia, anxiety, fever (including malignant hyper-thermia), hyperthyroidism, and heart failure. After the anesthesiologist determines the cause, a beta blocker can be used in patients with ischemic heart disease to help prevent further myocardial ischemia. Heart rates of approximately 150 beats per minute can be caused by sinus tachycardia, paroxysmal supraventricular tachycardia (PSVT), and atrial flutter with a 2:1 block. Diagnostic maneuvers to determine which of the three dysrhythmias is present include carotid massage, administration of edrophonium chloride, and atrial or esophageal ECG leads to better identify the P waves. Edrophonium or carotid massage produces a slight-to-no effect on sinus tachycardia, whereas a PSVT will usually convert to sinus rhythm (but may be unaffected). These manuevers in the presence of atrial flutter with 2:1 block can increase the heart block and make the flutter waves more apparent.

Paroxysmal Supraventricular Tachycardia   A PSVT refers to a rapid se-quence of supraventricular premature beats originating from a site other than the SA node. This was formerly known as paroxysmal atrial tachycardia (PAT; Fig. 2-12). The rate can be very rapid and lead to severe myocardial ischemia.

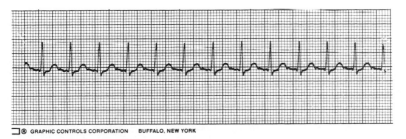

® GRAPHIC CONTROLS CORPORATION   BUFFALO, NEW YORK

Figure 2-12   Paroxysmal supraventricular tachycardia.

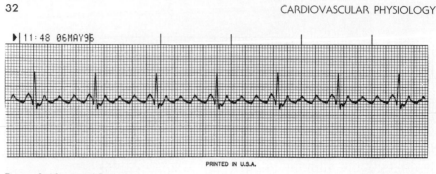

Figure 2-13   Atrial flutter.

This dysrhythmia can be associated with the WPW syndrome, in which an abnormal internodal conduction pathway (the bundle of Kent) is present. Adenosine administration by rapid peripheral intravenous (IV) bolus (for adults, 6 mg initially, then 12 mg if the PSVT is not eliminated within 1 to 2 min; in children, 0.05 to 0.25 mg/kg is the dosage used) is the treatment of choice. Other treatments include carotid massage, edrophonium, phenylephrine, propanolol, lidocaine, quinidine, procainamide, rapid overdrive pacing (then progressively slowing the rate once the ectopic focus is "captured"), and cardioversion. Surgical ablation of accessory conduction pathways is sometimes necessary.

Atrial Flutter   An irritable focus in the atria usually with a more rapid depolarization rate (250 to 350 beats per minute) than for PSVT produces atrial flutter (with a "sawtoothed" pattern called "F" waves instead of P waves), which is typically associated with AV block (Fig. 2-13). The atrial rhythm is regular, but the ventricular rhythm may be regular with a fixed block or irregular with a variable block. Commonly 2 : 1 block exists with a atrial rate of 300 and a ventricular rate of 150, but the block can vary between 2 : 1 and 8 : 1. A rapid ventricular response with a low cardiac output and poor coronary perfusion can be slowed by pharmacological means using digitalis or a beta blocker, but acute decompensation usually can be effectively treated using cardioversion (25 Joules).

Atrial fibrillation   Atrial fibrillation is an extremely rapid and irregular atrial focus, which produces no P waves on the ECG but instead a fine fibrillatory pattern called "f" waves (Fig. 2-14). The ventricular rhythm is usually irregularly irregular and is frequently associated with a pulse deficit. Conditions that cause atrial dilatation (e.g., mitral stenosis or regurgitation) are frequently associated with atrial flutter or fibrillation. Treatments include digitalis, beta blockers, and cardioversion. (Note: Anticoagulation is necessary before cardioverting patients with long-standing fibrillation).

Nodal Rhythm   The nodal rhythm impulse originates at the AV node or His Bundle and travels down into the ventricles normally and also travels retro-

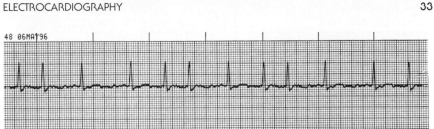

Figure 2-14   Atrial fibrillation.

gradely into the atrium (Fig. 2-15). Depending on the location of impulse formation, the P wave can occur simultaneously with the QRS (and will be obscured
by the QRS), immediately before the QRS (P-R interval less than 0.1 s), or it can
follow the QRS complex. Nodal rhythms are common during anesthesia using
inhaled agents. They decrease blood pressure and cardiac output by about 15
percent in normal patients but by a higher percentage in patients with heart disease. If hypotension or hypoperfusion occurs, atropine, ephedrine, or other beta$_1$
agonists can increase the activity of the SA node. Nodal rhythm is also called
junctional rhythm. Wandering atrial pacemaker is a type of nodal rhythm where
multiple irritable sites in the atria or AV node act as the pacemaker.

Ventricular Dysrhythmias

   Premature Ventricular Contractions   Premature ectopic beats arising
from a focus below the AV junction are common during anesthesia and in patients
with cardiac disease. A wide QRS complex with an ST segment that slopes in
the opposite direction of the QRS and a compensatory pause is associated with
these premature beats (Fig. 2-16A). The rhythm is irregular, and no P wave is
seen for this beat. This dysrhythmia is potentially dangerous because it can pro-
ceed to ventricular tachycardia and/or fibrillation. Multifocal PVCs (from many
irritable sites), coupled PVCs (bigeminy as seen in Fig. 2-16B; PVC's from two
identifiable pacemakers), short runs of PVCs (a run of more than 3 is sometimes
considered to be ventricular tachycardia), or R-wave-on-T-wave phenomenon is
especially dangerous. Initial treatment consists of correcting underlying abnor-

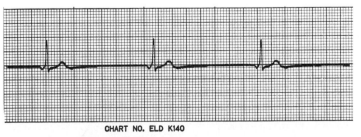

CHART NO. ELD K140

Figure 2-15   Nodal rhythm.

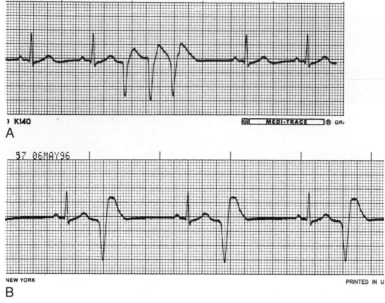

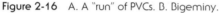

Figure 2-16   A. A "run" of PVCs. B. Bigeminy.

malities such as electrolyte imbalances, light anesthesia, or hypoxemia. Lidocaine is the drug of choice with an initial dose of 1.5 mg/kg IV bolus. Lidocaine infusion (1 to 4 mg/min), procainamide, bretylium, or beta blockers are sometimes necessary for recurrent PVCs.

Ventricular Tachycardia   An acute run of more than three ectopic beats (Fig. 2-17) can be life-threatening, although chronic ventricular tachycardia is tolerated by some patients. The danger of ventricular tachycardia is due to its tendency to progress into ventricular fibrillation. Ventricular tachycardias with rates up to 250 beats per minute decrease cardiac output and coronary perfusion. Treatments include lidocaine bolus and cardioversion (50 J). *Torsades de pointes* (twisting of the points) is a ventricular tachycardia with the ventricular complexes appearing to twist or spiral around the isoelectric line. It can be associated with drug interactions such as that between certain H_1 blockers and antibiotic or an-

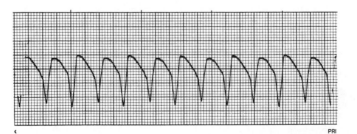

Figure 2-17   Ventricular tachycardia.

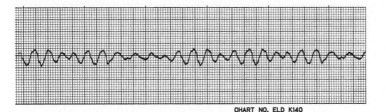

CHART NO. ELD K140

Figure 2-18   Ventricular fibrillation.

tifungal agents and can even result from certain antidysrhythmics such as amio-
darone, quinidine, or procainamide.

Ventricular Fibrillation   Chaotic asynchronous depolarization of the ventricles produces no effective cardiac output. No recognizable QRS complexes are
seen on the ECG (Fig. 2-18). This dysrhythmia can be caused by myocardial
ischemia, electrolyte imbalance, hypoxemia, and hypothermia. During cardiac
surgery, fibrillation is induced intentionally to produce better operating conditions. Treatment includes immediate cardiopulmonary resuscitation with defibrillation (200 to 400 J externally or 10 to 60 J internally) as the definitive treatment. Occasionally propranolol, bertylium, or lidocaine is useful.

Ventricular Asystole   The complete absence of ventricular activity produces a straight line on the ECG (although P waves can still be present). Discon-
necting the ECG from the patient must be ruled out. Ventricular asystole can be
caused by vagal stimulation, extremely deep inhalational anesthesia (especially
with halothane), or drugs such as succinylcholine. Hyperkalemic cardioplegic
solutions are infused into the coronary circulation to produce asystole during
cardiac surgery in order to reduce myocardial oxygen requirements.

Treatment consists of cardiopulmonary resuscitation while trying to convert
asystole to ventricular fibrillation (which is more responsive to treatment). Persistent asystole is poorly responsive to treatment although transvenous pacemaker
insertion is sometimes helpful.

Heart Blocks

Cardiac impulses can be delayed or blocked anywhere in the conducting system
due to ischemia or necrosis of conducting fibers, the effects of drugs, or other
pathological conditions such as myocardial infarction. Heart blocks can be subdivided into either AV heart blocks or intraventricular conduction disturbances,
even though many blocks identified as AV blocks are due to blockage in the
intraventricular conduction system. The AV blocks are classified as first, second,
or third degree. The bundle branch blocks, hemiblocks, and multifascicular blocks
make up the intraventricular conduction delays.

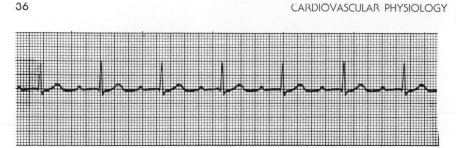

Figure 2-19   First degree heart block.

First Degree Heart Block   A prolonged delay in passage of the impulse through the AV node produces a P-R interval greater than 0.2 s (one large square on the ECG). There are no dropped QRS complexes, and treatment is unnecessary (Fig. 2-19).

Second Degree Heart Block   There are two types of second degree heart block: Mobitz type I involves AV nodal disturbance (Fig. 2-20A), and Mobitz type II involves disturbance of the bundle of His and Purkinje conducting tissues (Fig. 2-20B). For both of these blocks not all P-waves are followed by QRS complexes. During Mobitz type I heart block, P-R intervals change and, sometimes, conduction to the ventricle does not occur resulting in no QRS complex. Wenckebach is a type I second degree heart block where the P-R interval progressively increases until the QRS is dropped. During a Mobitz type II heart block, the P-R intervals do not change but there are dropped QRS complexes. This type has a more serious prognosis because it frequently progresses to third degree heart block.

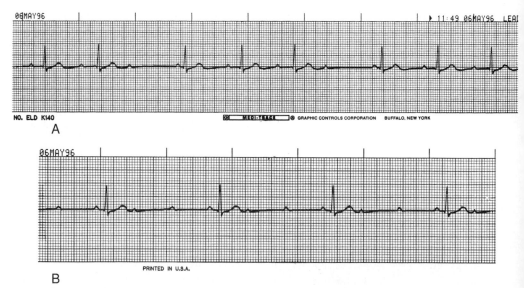

Figure 2-20   A. Second degree Heart block, type I. B. Second degree heart block, type II.

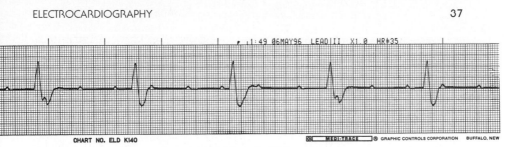

CHART NO. ELD K140

Figure 2-21   Third degree heart block with wide QRS complexes.

Third Degree Heart Block   In third degree heart block, there is no relationship between the P waves and the QRS complexes, hence the names complete
heart block or AV dissociation (Fig. 2-21). The ventricular rate (30 to 40 beats
per minute) is too slow to maintain adequate perfusion. Syncope (Stokes-Adams
Syndrome) and heart failure frequently occur, requiring pacemaker insertion, although atropine or $beta_1$ agonists can temporarily increase the heart rate.

Right Bundle Branch Block   Right bundle branch block can be clinically
insignificant. Depolarization of the left ventricle is normal, but late slow propagation of impulses from the left ventricle toward the right ventricle produces a
tall, wide R′ (double-peaked) wave in V_1 and late, wide S waves in V_5 and V_6.

Left Bundle Branch Block   Left bundle branch block occurs when the impulse reaches the ventricles exclusively through the right bundle branch, making
the QRS complex widen to more than 0.21 s (Fig. 2-22). Although right ventricular propagation is normal, its depolarization normally produces a small amount
of current. The impulse then spreads from right to left, causing deep, wide S
waves in V_1 and wide, tall R waves in the left ventricular leads. Incomplete left
bundle branch block produces a QRS that is slightly less widened. The LBBB is
always associated with heart disease.

Hemiblocks   If only one of the branches of the left bundle branch is impaired, the resulting conduction disturbance is called a hemiblock. A left anterior
hemiblock (LAH) results from pathology of the anterior (superior) division of the
left bundle branch. When the conduction disturbance is in the posterior (inferior)
division of the left bundle branch, it is termed a *left posterior hemiblock* (LPH).

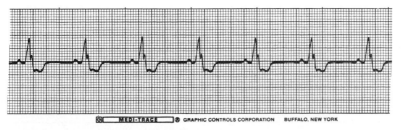

MEDI-TRACE ® GRAPHIC CONTROLS CORPORATION   BUFFALO, NEW YORK

Figure 2-22   Left bundle branch block.

Bifascicular and Trifascicular Block   When a right bundle branch block exists in combination with LAH or LPH, it is termed a *bifascicular block*. When a bifascicular block is combined (or present) with a first degree or second degree AV block, a trifascicular block is said to be present. These blocks tend to progress into complete heart block.

Antidysrhythmic Drugs

Although there are many drugs classified as antidysrhythmics, only a handful are used perioperatively. Prompt speed of onset, titratability, and intravenous administration are some of the characteristics desirable in antidysrhythmics given by anesthesiologists. Traditionally, antidysrhythmic drugs are classified according to the drug's effect on the action potentials of a single myocardial cell (Table 2-3).

Anesthesia and conditions associated with surgery (e.g., anxiety, pain, and vagal stimulation) can cause suppression of the SA node and emergence of latent pacemakers within the AV node or lower in the conducting system. Additionally, development of reentry circuits can occur.

As already noted, dysrhythmias must first be identified and then precipitating causes are treated or removed (e.g., traction on extraocular muscles or endobronchial intubation). Treatment, if necessary, can comprise changing anesthetic depth or agent, physical techniques such as pacemaker insertion, defibrillation or cardioversion, or drug administration, including chronotropes or traditional antidysrhythmics.

Table 2-3   Classes of Antidysrhythmic Drugs

Classes	Mechanism	Examples
I	Membrane stabilizers (sodium channel blockers)	
IA	Slow conduction—Moderate	Quinidine
		Procainamide
		Disopyramide
IB	Slow conduction—Mild	Lidocaine
		Tocainide
		Mexiletine
		Phenytoin
IC	Slow conduction—Marked	Flecainide
		Encainide
		Lorcainide
II	Beta-adrenergic antagonists	Propranolol
III	Prolonged repolarization	Bretylium
		Amiodarone
IV	Calcium entry blockers	Verapamil
		Diltiazem
V	Cardiac glycosides-parasympathomimetic, increased automaticity, increased slope of phase 4	Digoxin

Certain antidysrhythmics can produce other dysrhythmias as a side effect. Use of beta blockers to treat sinus tachycardia can result in sinus bradycardia. Phenytoin is rarely administered perioperatively for its antidysrhythmic action but is occasionally given as seizure prophylaxis, especially with neurosurgical procedures. Rapid administration of phenytoin can produce heart block, brady-cardia, and asystole, making slow infusion mandatory.

Atropine   Atropine is useful in the treatment of asystole, bradycardia, or heart block in adult patients but may cause tachydysrhythmias or myocardial ischemia. When used in pediatric patients, a minimum dose of 0.1 mg IV or ET should be given because atropine's weak peripheral cholinergic receptor agonist effect in smaller doses causes additional slowing of the heart rate.

Beta₁ Agonists   Epinephrine and isoproterenol are useful for treating at-ropine-refractory bradycardia or heart block. Epinephrine is recommended as first choice over atropine for pediatric patients, especially neonates. Isoproterenol should not be used during cardiopulmonary resuscitation because it reduces per-fusion pressure. Tachydysrhythmias or myocardial ischemia can result from the use of these drugs especially in patients with coronary narrowing.

Lidocaine   A dose of 1.0 mg/kg IV can be used to treat ventricular ectopy or stable ventricular tachycardia. The same dose can be used to prevent recurrence of ventricular fibrillation following defibrillation during cardiopulmonary resus-citation (see American Heart Association's treatment algorithm). It is the drug of choice for acute suppression of most ventricular dysrhythmias but also possesses negative inotropic effects. Side effects (grand mal seizures and asystole) are the same as seen with accidental intravenous administration of local anesthetics dur-ing regional techniques. The dose should be reduced in patients with congestive heart failure or hepatic disease as well as in geriatric or pediatric patients.

Procainamide   The drug of choice for acute treatment of lidocaine-resist-ant ventricular dysrhythmias, procainamide can produce hypotension, AV block, and QRS widening. The dose should be reduced in patients with congestive heart failure or renal failure.

Bretylium   Bretylium is more effective for the treatment of ventricular tachycardia or fibrillation than it is for suppression of ventricular ectopy. It is commonly used after lidocaine and procainamide have failed to control the dys-rhythmia. The dose is 5 mg/kg IV or ET with an additional 10 mg/kg every 15 min for a total dose of 30 mg/kg if needed. Side effects include postural hypo-tension, nausea, and vomiting. Bretylium causes an initial period of hypertension and worsening dysrhythmias due to norepinephrine (NE) release, which is then followed by hypotension due to subsequent inhibition of NE release. It should be used with caution in patients with digitalis toxicity and avoided in patients with pulmonary hypertension and pheochromocytoma.

Adenosine   Adenosine can restore normal sinus rhythm in patients with PSVT including those associated with reentry due to accessory bypass tracks (WPW syndrome). It does not convert atrial flutter, atrial fibrillation, or ventricular tachycardia to normal sinus rhythm. It must be injected rapidly because it is metabolized in less than 1 min. The usual dose is 6 mg IV with 12 mg given every 2 min twice thereafter (for children, 50 to 200 μg/kg) for a total of 3 doses. Transient heart block or brief asystole frequently follows its administration.

Verapamil   Verapamil is useful for treating PSVT by delaying conduction through the AV node and prolonging AV nodal refractoriness. Atrial fibrillation or flutter also responds to its administration. The dose is 5 to 10 mg IV over 3 to 5 min and can be repeated after 15 min if necessary. Ventricular dysrhythmias are not affected by verapamil. It also is a coronary and peripheral arterial vasodilator so it is useful for treatment of angina pectoris. It must be used with caution in patients with congestive heart failure or hypotension and in the presence of beta blockade. Verapamil should be avoided in patients with sick sinus, preexisting AV heart block, or WPW with preexcitation.

Propranolol   Propanolol is a nonselective, competitive beta antagonist useful for treatment of PSVT, atrial fibrillation, flutter, sinus tachycardia, and catecholamine-mediated dysrhythmias such as ventricular ectopy. It is also used to prevent reflex tachycardia caused by vasodilators such as nitroprusside (and allows use of lower nitroprusside infusion rates which reduces the risk of cyanide toxicity). It blocks renin release and decreases cardiac output. Titrate cautiously in patients with heart failure, bronchoconstriction, or insulin-dependant patients with diabetes. (It can mask the sympathetic-mediated signs of hypoglycemia.) It is not recommended for use in WPW with preexcitation. Dosage is 0.1 to 1.0 mg IV titrated to a total dose of 0.1 mg/kg.

Esmolol   This beta$_1$ selective blocker has the same indications and cautions as for propranolol but is much shorter acting. Its elimination half-time is 4 min because it is rapidly hydrolyzed in the plasma by red cell esterases. Dosage is 0.1 to 0.5 mg/kg IV bolus and infusion of 25 to 200 μg/kg/min titrated to effect.

REFERENCES

American Society of Anesthesiologists, *Standards for basic anesthetic monitoring,* Approved by House of Delegates on October 21, 1986, and last amended on October 13, 1993. 1996 ASA Directory of Members, Section 4: *Basic Standards.* Park Ridge, IL. ASA 1966.

Guyton A: *Textbook of Medical Physiology,* 8th ed, Philadelphia, Saunders, 1991.

Hurst JW, Logue RB, Rackley CE, et al: *The Heart.* New York, McGraw-Hill, 1982.

Katz AM: Cardiac action potential, in Katz AM: *Physiology of the Heart.* New York, Raven Press, 1977.

Marriot HJL: Electrical axis, in Marriot HJL (ed): *Practical Electrocardiography*. Baltimore, Williams & Wilkins, 1983.

Sumikawa K, Ishizaka N, Suzaki M: Arrhythmogenic plasma levels of epinephrine during halothane, enflurane, and pentobarbital anesthesia in the dog. *Anesthesiology,* 58: 322–325, 1983.

Thys DM, Hillel Z, Goldman ME, et al: A comparison of hemodynamic indices derived by invasive monitoring and two dimensional echocardiography. *Anesthesiology,* 1987.

Atlee JL, Bosnjakzj. Mechanism for Cardiac Dysrythmias. *Anesthesiology,* 72:347–74, 1990.

3

CARDIAC OUTPUT AND CARDIAC CYCLE

CARDIAC OUTPUT

Cardiac output (CO) is the volume of blood pumped by the left ventricle (or right ventricle) per minute. The volume of blood pumped per beat is called the stroke volume (SV).

$$CO = SV \times HR$$

where HR = heart rate.

The output of the two ventricles is essentially equal over a period of time (minutes), whereas the SV for any one beat can be different for the two ventricles. Cardiac output, during resting conditions, can be estimated as 80 ml per kilogram of body weight or 8 percent of the body weight in kilograms. For a man weighing 70 kg, the CO is approximately 5600 ml/min or 5.6 liters/min under resting conditions. Cardiac output can increase four- or fivefold depending on the metabolic requirements of the body. As O_2 consumption by the body increases, as with exercise, CO increases proportionally in order to deliver more O_2 to the active tissues (Fig. 3-1). As O_2 consumption by the body decreases, as with sleep, CO also decreases.

In order to normalize the CO in patients of different body sizes, CO is divided by the body surface area. This value is called the cardiac index (CI), and its units are liters per minute per square meter of body surface area. Body surface area can be estimated from the height (cm) and weight (kg) of an individual. The CI for the man weighing 70 kg with a body surface area of 1.7 m² equals 3.3 liters/min/m².

Measurement of Cardiac-Output

Flow Probes Cardiac output can be measured either invasively or noninvasively. One common method in animal research is to place a flow probe

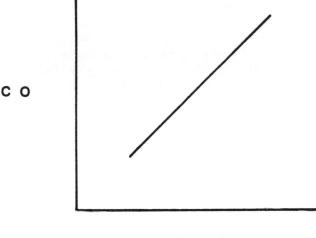

CO

WORK / O$_2$ CONSUMPTION

Figure 3-1   The relation between cardiac output (CO) and whole body oxygen consumption or work performed by the body. In a normal individual with a normal heart, CO is determined by the amount of work that all of the systemic tissues are performing or the total amount of oxygen that is required by the tissues to perform that work.

around the ascending aorta (or the main pulmonary artery). Ultrasonic and electromagnetic flow probes generally measure the velocity of flow (centimeters per second). Volume flow is calculated by multiplying the measured velocity (centimeters per second) by the blood vessel cross-sectional area (square centimeters):

$$\text{cm/s} \times \text{cm}^2 = \text{cm}^3/\text{s} = \text{ml/s}$$
$$\text{ml/s} \times 60 \text{ s/min} = \text{ml/min}$$

Fick Principle   Less invasive methods of measuring CO generally require catheterization of at least one blood vessel. The Fick principle (Adolph Fick, 1870) states that the uptake of a substance (X) by an organ is equal to the blood flow to that organ multiplied by the difference between the arterial and venous concentration of that substance [X].

$$\text{Uptake of X} = \text{BF} \times [\text{Art}_{[X]} - \text{Ven}_{[X]}]$$

This principle also applies to the whole body. The uptake or use of a substance (X) by the whole body is equal to the blood flow to the body multiplied by the arteriovenous difference in [X]. If blood flow to the body is the CO, then

$$CO = \text{uptake (X)} / (\text{Art}_{[X]} - \text{Ven}_{[X]})$$

Measurement of body uptake (or consumption) of O_2 is easily performed with a spirometer. Therefore, O_2 uptake or consumption and the arteriovenous difference in O_2 are used for calculating CO. The arterial concentration of O_2 can be measured in blood from any artery if the blood sample is taken anaerobically. Estimates of venous blood $[O_2]$ must be made on a sample of mixed venous blood since the different organs of the body extract different amounts of O_2 and, thus, venous blood $[O_2]$ varies in different organs. For example, the heart extracts 75 percent of the O_2 from the arterial blood, whereas the resting skeletal muscle may extract only 20 to 25 percent of the O_2. Venous blood mixes in the right atrium and ventricle; therefore the best site for sampling mixed venous blood is the pulmonary artery. This sample must also be taken anaerobically. Normally, O_2 consumption is measured over a 5-min period, and the arterial and venous blood samples are taken simultaneously at 2½ min. For example, whole body O_2 consumption is measured as 275 ml of O_2 per minute.

$$\text{Arterial } O_2 = 20 \text{ vol \% or 20 ml } O_2/100 \text{ ml blood}$$

$$\text{Pulmonary Artery } O_2 = 15 \text{ vol \% or 15 ml } O_2/100 \text{ ml blood}$$

$$CO = O_2 \text{ consumption} / (\text{Art } [O_2] - \text{Ven } [O_2])$$

$$CO = 275 \text{ ml } O_2/\text{min} / (20 \text{ ml } O_2/100 \text{ ml blood}$$
$$- 15 \text{ ml } O_2/100 \text{ ml blood})$$

$$CO = 5500 \text{ ml/min}$$

An important assumption made in using the Fick principle to estimate CO is that the individual is in a steady state. Instantaneous changes in CO cannot be measured.

Indicator Dilution   *Dye Dilution, Cardiogreen*   Dye dilution (Stewart-Hamilton, 1897) is based on the principle that the dilution of a bolus of dye by the CO can be measured in a peripheral artery, and that one can then calculate the CO if the following applies:

1   The amount of dye that is injected is known.
2   The average concentration of the dye during one pass through the circulation is determined.
3   The time for one pass of the dye through the circulation is determined.

Two catheters are needed. One is introduced into the right atrium via a peripheral vein and is used for injection of dye. The other catheter is introduced into an artery, and the tip of the catheter is positioned in the ascending aorta to sample the blood for dye concentration. For example, 5 mg of cardiogreen is injected into the right atrium. The arterial concentration of dye is monitored over time and the average dye concentration, as illustrated in Fig. 3-2, is 0.25 mg per 100 ml of blood. The time for one pass of dye through the circulation is determined to be 12 s.

$$CO = 5 \text{ mg}/[(0.25 \text{ mg}/100\text{ml blood}) \times 12 \text{ s}]$$
$$= 167 \text{ ml/s}$$

$$167 \text{ ml/s} \times 60 \text{ s/min} = 10,000 \text{ ml/min}$$

The use of this method assumes that the individual is in a steady state, that the dye is not removed too rapidly from the circulation, and that the dye does not itself alter the CO or the cardiovascular system. Determination of CO by dye dilution takes less time than does measurement of cardiac output by the Fick method.

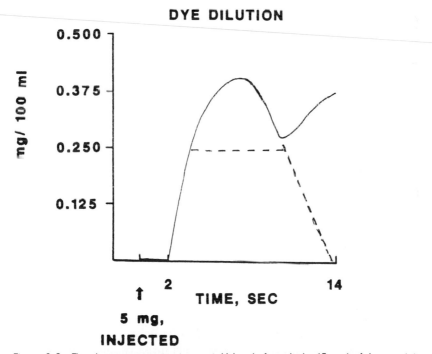

Figure 3-2   The dye concentration in arterial blood after a bolus (5 mg) of dye was injected into the right atrium. The second increase in dye concentration occurs when dye returns to the heart from short circulation pathways and is then recirculated. Thus to measure the average dye concentration in one pass of dye through the circulation, the descending curve is extrapolated to the abscissa and the the average dye concentration is calculated. As shown by the dashed horizontal line, the average concentration was 0.25 mg/100 ml blood and it took 12 s for the first pass of dye through the circulation.

Thermodilution   Thermodilution is a special type of indicator dilution in which the indicator is temperature. A known amount of solution at a known temperature is injected as a bolus into the right atrium. The temperature of the blood is monitored by a thermistor probe located, usually, in the pulmonary artery. As the cold solution is diluted by the CO, the thermistor probe measures changes in blood temperature. A CO computer uses the thermodilution curve, the volume of cold solution injected, the time for generation of the dilution curve, and temperature exchange factors to calculate the CO.

With the advent of the Swan-Ganz catheter, CO measurement can be readily performed with the use of only one catheter. This catheter can be introduced via the jugular vein into the right heart and pulmonary artery. Within the Swan-Ganz catheter there are several lumens, a thermistor probe, and a balloon near the tip. One lumen opens into the right atrium when the tip of the catheter is positioned in the pulmonary artery. Proper positioning can be assessed because another lumen of the catheter opens at the tip of the catheter. With this lumen attached to a pressure transducer, the position of the tip of the catheter as it is introduced into the right atrium, right ventricle, and, then, the pulmonary artery can be followed by the pressure changes as shown in Fig. 3-3. The balloon near the end of the catheter can be inflated with gas and assists in directing the catheter in the direction of the blood flow. With the tip of the Swan-Ganz catheter located in the pulmonary artery, a known volume of solution with a known temperature is injected into the right atrium. The thermistor probe, also located in the pulmonary artery, measures blood temperature. These data are used by the computer to calculate CO.

This technique is used clinically because it has several advantages over dye dilution:

1   One venous catheter is used.
2   Multiple determinations can be made in short periods of time because the cold solution is diluted into the total blood volume and total body heat.

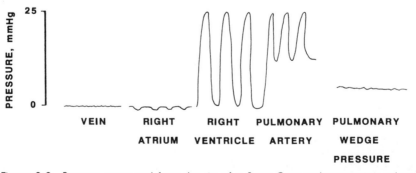

Figure 3-3 Pressure measured from the tip of a Swan-Ganz catheter as it is advanced through the venous circulation, right atrium, right ventricle, into the pulmonary artery, and finally the pulmonary capillary wedge pressure.

3   Use of a dye requires removal of this foreign substance from the body; thermodilution adds only water and glucose (or isotonic saline) to the body.

Noninvasive Techniques   Echocardiography, radionuclide imaging, and radiographic techniques currently are used clinically to estimate ventricular volume during contraction (systole) and relaxation (diastole). The difference between these two volumes gives SV and can thus be used to estimate CO.

CARDIAC CYCLE

The cardiac cycle is divided into two major stages: contraction or systole and relaxation or diastole. Each of these stages is further subdivided to describe or coincide with changes in muscle mechanics or blood flow velocity.

Ventricular Pressure

The initial stage of ventricular contraction occurs after the ventricle has been filled with blood and the spread of the action potential through the Purkinje fibers has resulted in ventricular depolarization and calcium influx. Contraction begins, and, when ventricular pressure exceeds atrial pressure, the atrioventricular (AV) valves close (Fig. 3-4, point A). Since the semilunar valves are also closed (ventricular pressure is lower than aortic or pulmonary artery pressure), the initial phase of contraction (points A to B) is called isovolumic or isovolumetric. The volume of blood in the ventricle does not change, although the ventricular muscle cells are developing tension and ventricular pressure is rapidly increasing. When ventricular pressure exceeds the pressure in its respective outflow tract (point B), the semilunar valve opens. For the left ventricle this occurs at approximately 80 mmHg or torr. For the right ventricle this occurs at approximately 8 torr. With the opening of the semilunar valves, blood is ejected from the ventricles. The first third of the ejection occurs at a high velocity, with subsequent ejection being less rapid. When the ventricular cells undergo repolarization, the muscle cells decrease tension and ventricular pressure falls rapidly. When ventricular pressure is lower than aortic (or pulmonary artery) pressure, the semilunar valves close and systole ends (point C). Since semilunar valves and AV valves are closed, this relaxation stage is isovolumic. Tension and pressure fall, but ventricular volume remains constant. When ventricular pressure is less than atrial pressure, the AV valves open and the ventricles begin to fill with blood. The initial stage of filling is very rapid. As diastole progresses, the filling rate slows until the last third of diastole when the atria contract and push more blood into the ventricles. Atrial contraction is probably important in increasing ventricular diastolic volume in older individuals and also in cases in which the ventricle is stiff, as with scar tissue deposition after myocardial infarction.

PRESSURE TRACING

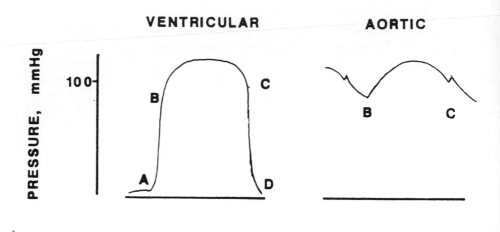

TIME

Figure 3-4 Left ventricular pressure and aortic pressure during one cardiac cycle. Point A represents closure of the mitral valve; Point B indicates opening of the aortic valve; Point C indicates closure of the aortic valve, and Point D represents opening of the mitral valve.

Ventricular Volume and Pressure

Under resting conditions, at the end of diastole (Fig. 3-5, point A), ventricular volume is great (~120 ml), and pressure is low (0 to 5 mmHg). Since the AV valves are open, atrial pressure is similar to ventricular end-diastolic pressure. Right atrial pressure equals right ventricular end-diastolic pressure, which is approximately 0 mmHg. Left atrial pressure equals left ventricular end-diastolic pressure, which is approximately 2 to 5 mmHg. When the ventricles begin developing tension and the mitral and tricuspid valves have closed, ventricular volume remains constant (points A to B). Pressure increases rapidly (to ~80 torr in the left ventricle and ~8 torr in the right ventricle), opens the aortic or pulmonic valve, and ejection begins. Probably 70 percent of the SV (approximately 80 ml) is ejected from the left ventricle during the rapid ejection phase (first one-half of ejection); the other 30 percent is ejected more slowly over the rest of systole. In our example, the SV (points B to C) equals 80 ml. The SV as a percent of the end-diastolic volume is called the ejection fraction (EF). End-diastolic volume was 120 ml; EF = 80 ml/120 ml = .67 or 67 percent. The volume of blood remaining in the ventricle when ejection ends is called the end systolic volume. The pressure in the ventricle just prior to relaxation is called end-systolic pressure. End-systolic volume is 40 ml in Fig. 3-5. Note that during ejection, ventricular and aortic pressures increase. Aortic pressure increases because blood is being pumped into it. Ventricular pressure increases to match the aortic pressure so that ejection can continue. As blood flows down the aorta, aortic pressure begins to fall and ventricular pressure again falls to match aortic pressure. The ventricle develops only the pressure that is necessary to just exceed aortic pressure so that blood is pumped from the ventricle into the aorta (or pulmonary artery).

With the initiation of relaxation (due to repolarization of the ventricular muscle cells), ventricular pressure declines very rapidly. With closure of the semilunar valves at the very beginning of relaxation, the rapid decline in pressure occurs with no change in ventricular volume (points C to D). Volume remains at ~40 ml, and pressure drops in the left ventricle from ~90 mmHg to ~0 mmHg in ~50 ms. When the AV valves open, ventricular filling occurs, rapidly at first and more slowly during the middle third of diastole. Approximately 70 percent of the filling will occur in the first third of diastole. In a steady state, the SV (80 ml) will be replaced during diastole. During the final third of diastole, atrial contraction will complete the filling of the ventricle.

End-diastolic volume of the ventricle is not always set at 120 ml but rather can vary with such factors as venous return or blood flow back to the heart; how forcefully the ventricle contracts and therefore how much blood is pumped out per beat; and, to some extent, on heart rate. As heart rate increases, the time in diastole decreases. At high heart rates (~180 beats per minute), there may be too little time for the ventricle to fill normally such that end-diastolic volume decreases.

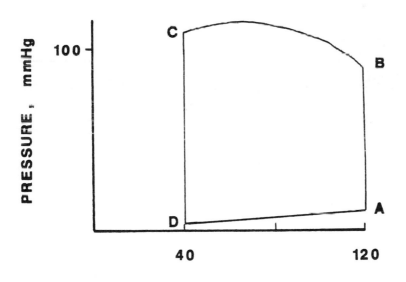

VOLUME, ml

Figure 3-5   The pressure and volume changes occurring in the left ventricle during a cardiac cycle. As in Fig. 3-4, Point A represents closure of the mitral valve, Point B opening of the aortic valve; Point C closure of the aortic valve, and Point D opening of the mitral valve. Segment D to A represents the venous return to the ventricle during that cardiac cycle and segment B to C represents stroke volume ejected during that cardiac cycle. In a steady state these two volumes are the same.

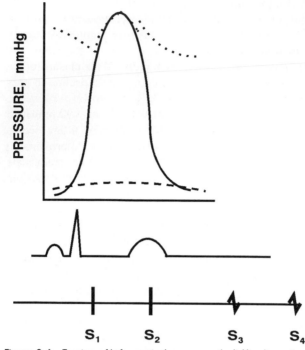

S_1 S_2 S_3 S_4

Figure 3-6 Tracing of left ventricular pressure (solid line), aortic pressure (small dashed line), atrial pressure (long dashed line), electrocardiogram and heart sounds (S_1 through S_4) during one cardiac cycle. Time is represented on the x-axis.

Changes in end-diastolic volume elicit changes in cardiac muscle force of contraction, which will be discussed in Chapter 4.

Electrocardiogram

Figure 3-6 shows electrical activity monitored on the surface of the body in conjunction with the pressure and volume changes during the cardiac cycle. The P wave represents atrial depolarization and initiates atrial contraction. The QRS complex represents ventricular depolarization and marks the initiation of ventricular contraction. It occurs prior to, and possibly extends through, isovolumic contraction. Ventricular depolarization leads to isovolumic relaxation.

Heart Sounds

Theoretically four heart sounds can be detected with a phonocardiogram (a graphic record of the vibrations or sounds made when a microphone is placed over the chest wall). At least two of these (and many times three) can be heard with auscultation. The first audible sound, S_1, occurs at the time when the AV valves close. It can be split into a mitral component (M_1) and a tricuspid component (T_1), since normally the mitral valve closes slightly before the tricuspid valve. Anything that delays right ventricular contraction, such as right bundle branch block, can exaggerate the split between M_1 and T_1 and make the split audible. The actual sound of S_1 probably occurs as a result of several factors:

1   Turbulence: As pressure in the ventricle increases and closes the AV valve, the blood is forced against the valve and turbulent flow is initiated.
2   Vibration: Blood pushed back against the AV valves sets up vibration in the valve leaflets.
3   Ventricular muscle contraction: It may generate its own sound.

The second heart sounds occurs at the time that the semilunar valves close and the AV valves open. This sound also consists of two components, one in conjunction with closure of the aortic valve (A_2) and the other in conjunction with the closure of the pulmonic valve (P_2). Again, any condition that delays or prolongs right ventricular ejection will cause a splitting of these two components of S_2. Normal physiologic splitting of S_2 can occur with inspiration when the venous return to the right side of the heart is increased and, therefore, right ventricular ejection is slightly prolonged. With expiration, S_2 may seem to be only one sound.

The third audible heart sound, S_3, occurs in the middle of diastole. It probably results from filling of the ventricle when it is slightly less compliant. In early diastole, during rapid filling, the ventricle is very compliant such that large changes in ventricular volume are accompanied by minimal changes in ventricular pressure. As ventricular volume increases, ventricular compliance tends to decrease so that blood entering the ventricle during the middle third of diastole can cause turbulence. This sound is not heard routinely but can be heard more clearly in children (with a thinner chest wall) and in individuals with stiffer or less compliant ventricles.

The fourth heart sound, S_4, occurs in conjunction with atrial contraction. This sound is rarely heard in younger individuals but can be heard in older individuals in whom atrial contraction plays a more important role in filling the ventricle. Accentuation of S_3 or S_4 leads to the so-called gallop rhythm and may be indicative of myocardial contractile and structural changes subsequent to myocardial ischemia and infarction.

The heart sounds, especially when there are abnormalities of the valves, can be best distinguished at certain anatomical sites, as illustrated in Fig. 3-7. The mitral component of S_1 is best heard over the apex of the left ventricle. The tricuspid component of S_1 is best heard on the left side of the sternum. Both sounds are most readily heard over the ventricle with which the turbulence is associated. The aortic and pulmonic components of S_2 are best heard along the great vessel with which they are associated. Thus, P_2 is best heard at the upper left border of the sternum and A_2 is best heard at the upper right border of the sternum.

Murmurs

Abnormal hearts sounds can occur when the AV or semilunar valves undergo pathologic changes. Two such changes are stenosis or failure of the valves to open completely and insufficiency or failure of the valves to close completely. With stenosis of a valve, a greater pressure is required to pump a normal SV across a restricted valve opening. With greater pressures across a stenotic valve, turbulence occurs and thus abnormal sounds are produced. With failure of a valve to close completely, flow occurs across the incompetent valve and again turbulence occurs and abnormal sounds are produced. The most common murmurs occur either during systole or during diastole. The period during the cardiac cycle in which the murmur occurs can help establish the site of the abnormality. For example, during systole murmurs can occur if the aortic or pulmonic valve is stenotic. Thus greater than normal ventricular pressures are required to eject a normal SV across a smaller orifice. With stenosis of either of the semilunar valves, the intensity of the abnormal sound is greatest during the most rapid phase of ejection. Systolic murmurs can also occur if one of the AV valves does not close completely. During ventricular contraction, blood is not only ejected into the aorta or pulmonary artery but is also forced across the patent AV valve into the atrium. Again, abnormal sounds will occur during systole. Diastolic murmurs will occur when a semilunar valve does not close properly. During ventricular relaxation, blood normally is entering the ventricle only from its respective atrium. However, if, for example, the aortic semilunar valve is patent during diastole, since aortic pressure is greater than ventricular pressure, blood will flow from the aorta back into the ventricle (as well as in the normal direction into the periphery). Turbu-

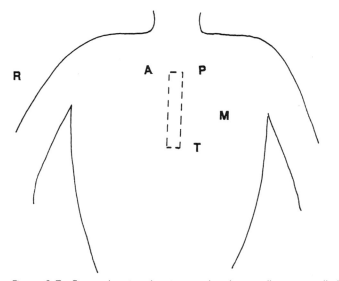

Figure 3-7 Figure showing the sites on the chest wall to optimally hear heart sounds, especially abnormal heart sounds or murmurs. A = aortic valve, P = pulmonic valve, T = tricuspid valve, M = mitral valve. R indicates the right side of the body.

lence will occur, and sound will be produced. Another diastolic murmur that can occur is that which is produced by a stenosis of the AV valve. This sound will be most prominent during the rapid filling phase of diastole or during atrial contraction with its associated rapid pumping of blood into the ventricle. The source of the murmur can be partially localized by the time during the cardiac cycle in which it occurs and also by the site on the chest wall where the murmur can be best heard, as shown in Fig. 3-7.

BIBLIOGRAPHY

Berne RM, Levy MN: *Physiology* 3rd ed., St. Louis, Mosby Year Book, 1993, pp 410–415.

Guyton AC, Hall JE: *Textbook of Medical Physiology* 9th ed. Philadelphia, W.B. Saunders Company, pp 110–113; 239; 250–251.

Rhoades RA, Tanner GA: *Physiology,* Boston, Little, Brown and Company, 1995, pp 260–263; 269–272.

4

THE HEART PUMP

As already presented in Chapter 1, the function of the heart is to pump blood from the venous system into the arterial system from which it can be distributed to the capillaries of the tissues. The heart is made up of cardiac muscle which is striated due to the orderly arrangement of actin and myosin within the cell. Muscle contraction occurs when the actin and myosin head interact as a result of removal of hindrance imposed by troponin-tropomyosin. Calcium binding to troponin results in the change in configuration of the contractile proteins thus allowing binding of actin to the appropriate binding site on the myosin head and sliding of actin across the myosin filaments.

The contractile properties of cardiac muscle are important to discuss in order to understand how the heart functions effectively as a pump. The two primary contractile properties of muscle to be discussed are the length-tension relationship and the force-velocity relationship.

LENGTH-TENSION

If a strip of cardiac muscle is studied in an isometric configuration (i.e., in such a manner that the muscle is stretched prior to stimulation, is not allowed to shorten during contraction, but its tension development can be measured), the results shown in Fig. 4-1 can be derived. Resting tension (Points A to B) is the tension present during the unstimulated state and is due to components of the cell that are noncontractile. Upon stimulation, tension is developed (Points B to C) because of the actin-myosin cross-bridge interaction, but the muscle is not allowed to shorten. The muscle then relaxes to its original state and resting tension (Points C to D). As the resting muscle is stretched, i.e., as the sarcomeres are lengthened, the passive (resting or nonstimulated) tension progressively increases (Fig. 4-2). If the muscle is stimulated to contract, it develops tension. From a greater resting length, greater tension can be developed. This relationship between muscle length and active tension also occurs in skeletal muscle and in smooth muscle to some

54

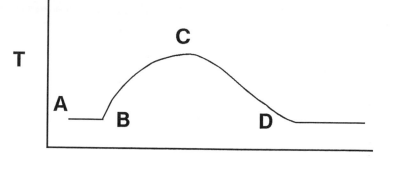

TIME

Figure 4-1   Tension as a function of time in a papillary muscle stimulated to contract under conditions in which there is tension development but no muscle shortening (isometric contraction).

extent The probable mechanisms by which increasing muscle length allows for increasing tension development is that the number of cross bridges that can be formed is determined by the length of the muscle just prior to stimulation. There is some optimum length (some estimate that optimum sarcomere length is 2.2 μ) at which the maximum number of cross bridges that can be formed will be formed. At lengths below this optimum, fewer cross bridges can interact and, therefore, less tension can be developed. Above the optimum length, again, fewer cross bridges can form and less tension can be developed. At lower lengths, overlap

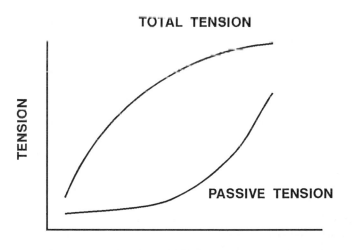

TOTAL TENSION

TENSION

PASSIVE TENSION

LENGTH

Figure 4-2   Muscle tension as a function of resting muscle length. As resting muscle length increases, both passive (resting tension) and total muscle tension increase. The difference between total tension and passive tension is the active tension that is generated by actin and myosin cross-bridge interaction.

occurs between actin filaments; at greater than optimum lengths, the actin-myosin overlap regions have been pulled apart. Under both circumstances fewer cross bridges can interact.

The correlate of the length-tension relationship in the intact heart, studied as a pump, is that on stretching the heart, i.e., filling the ventricle to greater volumes at the end of diastole, the subsequent contraction will be more forceful. In the intact organism, an increase in cardiac muscle length resulting from increased ventricular filling would result in a more forceful contraction and an increase in stroke volume (SV). This relationship between ventricular end-diastolic volume and force of contraction was first characterized in amphibian hearts by Otto Frank in the late 1890s and in mammalian hearts by Ernest Starling and coworkers in the early 1900s. The length-tension relationship in cardiac muscle has thus been termed the *Frank-Starling relationship*. The parameter that mainly determines end-diastolic length in the whole heart is end-diastolic volume. Ventricular end-diastolic pressure and atrial pressure estimate end-diastolic volume and therefore estimate end-diastolic sarcomere length. End-diastolic pressure gives an approximation of end-diastolic volume because the ventricle is compliant during diastole and there is a somewhat linear relationship between end-diastolic volume and end-diastolic pressure especially at physiologic end-diastolic volume (Fig. 4-3). If the compliance of the ventricle were to change, such as with scar tissue formation resulting from a myocardial infarction, end-diastolic pressure would be a less accurate estimate of myocardial end-diastolic fiber length since high end-diastolic pressure might be associated with low end-diastolic volume and thus short sarcomere lengths.

Left (or right) atrial pressure is indicative of left (or right) ventricular end-diastolic pressure since at the end of diastole, the atrioventricular (AV) valves are

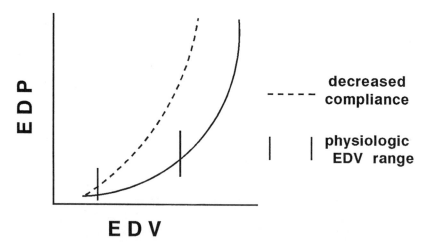

Figure 4-3 Ventricular end-diastolic pressure (EDP) as a function of ventricular end-diastolic volume (EDV). The normal heart is very compliant and functions at relatively low end-diastolic volumes and end-diastolic pressures. A decrease in compliance, as might occur with a myocardial infarction, shifts the curve to the left such that end-diastolic pressure may be elevated.

open and there is a minimal pressure difference between the atrial and ventricular chambers. As with the inexactness of end-diastolic pressure in estimating end-diastolic volume, atrial pressures also suffer the same inaccuracy. However, atrial pressures are useful estimates of end-diastolic volume, especially at high atrial pressures which would generally indicate an elevated filling of the ventricle. This increased ventricular filling might occur with infusion of large volumes of fluid into an organism or with an inability of the ventricle to pump efficiently thus leaving higher than normal volumes in the ventricle after ejection.

Under normal conditions, cardiac muscle, at the end of diastole, is at lower than the optimum length. Therefore, under normal conditions there is cardiac reserve in that greater filling of the ventricle can result in greater output by the ventricle. There are estimates that a left ventricular end-diastolic pressure of 10 mmHg in a normal heart represents the optimum length for tension development. Of course this presumes a normal compliance of the ventricle. In a ventricle stiffened by scar tissue, a higher end-diastolic pressure might be required for the optimum Frank-Starling effect.

The length of the cardiac fibers at the end of diastole represents the preload of the heart. In isolated cardiac muscle preparations, one can measure the length of the muscle prior to the onset of contraction. In the intact heart, length or preload is determined by how full the ventricle is just prior to contraction, i.e., preload in the intact heart is the volume in the ventricle at the end of diastole. A greater end-diastolic volume represents a greater stretch of cardiac fibers and therefore a greater preload. A smaller end-diastolic volume represents a lesser preload. Again, end-diastolic pressure and left atrial pressure or right atrial pressure estimate end-diastolic volume and end-diastolic fiber length or preload.

FORCE-VELOCITY

In order to understand the force-velocity relationship in cardiac muscle, isotonic contractions are studied, i.e., the muscle shortens and the rate of shortening is measured (velocity of shortening). In this preparation the initial length of muscle (preload) is held constant but the muscle can shorten on contraction. The effect of putting greater load on the muscle can be assessed by measuring the shortening and velocity of shortening. The load that the muscle must "lift" in order to shorten is the afterload. This load is not "sensed" by the muscle until *after* it is stimulated to contract. The muscle generates enough tension to equal the load it must lift (Fig. 4-4, stage A). This stage of the contraction is thus an isometric contraction, i.e., there is no change in whole muscle length, but there is an increase in muscle tension development. When tension equals the load, the subsequent part of the contraction is isotonic, i.e., tone remains constant but shortening now occurs (Fig. 4-4, stage B).

Now the question arises: How does changing the load on the muscle affect the tension developed, the shortening, and the velocity of shortening? The tension or force generated by the muscle is directly proportional to the load placed on

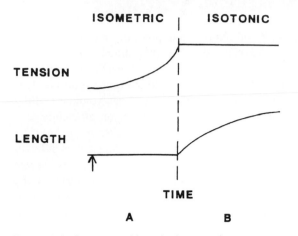

Figure 4-4 Tension and length changes during a contraction. During phase A, tension is developed until the afterload is matched. During phase B, tension remains constant while the muscle shortens (a decrease in length is an upward deflection).

the muscle, i.e., the muscle will generate only enough tension or force to be able to lift the load. For example, if the load is 1g, the muscle will generate 1g of tension and will then shorten. In Fig. 4-5, the effect of increasing load on shortening is depicted. If the load is increased from 1g to 2g, the time until the muscle begins to shorten is prolonged (the muscle is generating two times the tension and this takes a longer time, i.e., the latent period increases). The amount of shortening is decreased and the initial rate or velocity of shortening is decreased. When the load is increased to 3g, the pattern is repeated (i.e., it takes a longer time for shortening to occur) less shortening occurs, and there is a decreased velocity of shortening. Thus increasing load on a muscle increases the force the

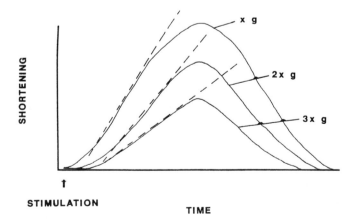

Figure 4-5 Muscle shortening as a function of time. The muscle shortening at three different afterloads, 1, 2, and 3g, shows progressively less shortening and a lower velocity of shortening.

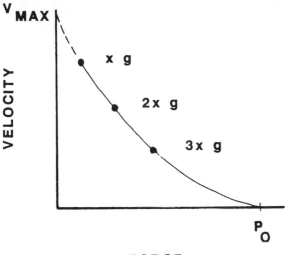

FORCE

Figure 4-6 The velocity of shortening from contractions shown in Fig. 4.5. Velocity of shortening is plotted as a function of the force that must be generated to shorten and to lift the afterload. There is an inverse relation between force and velocity of shortening. At P_0, there is no shortening and the maximum tension that the muscle can generate from that preload is shown. V_{max}, is the theoretical maximum velocity of shortening with 0 afterload (a theoretical point).

muscle generates and results in decreased velocity of shortening. Figure 4-6 shows this relation as a force-velocity curve. The point on the intercept of the x axis (P_0) represents an isometric contraction in which there is no shortening but the maximum amount of force is developed by that muscle from that initial length. Note that the curve connecting the points is continuous until it approaches the ordinate at which point it is dashed. Since the muscle can never be "unloaded," i.e., there is a preload or load used to set the initial length of the muscle, no velocity measurements can be made at loads less than the initial preload. Therefore, the force velocity curve is extrapolated to the y axis. The point of interception is called the *Vmax* or *maximum velocity of shortening.*

The study described earlier was performed with the muscle set at one length or preload prior to stimulation. Recall, however that cardiac muscle has a length-tension relationship. What happens if the study is repeated but the initial length of the muscle is increased ($m + 2$). After this length is set, the muscle will not be allowed to lengthen but will be able to shorten on stimulation. The force-velocity curve generated by the muscle from a greater length or preload is shifted to the right (Fig. 4-7). The P_0, or point at which maximum isometric tension is developed but no shortening occurs, is increased, i.e., from the greater initial length the muscle can generate a greater maximum force. Note also that at load x, $2x$, and $3x$, the muscle shortens with a greater velocity than it did when the initial length was less (m). Thus by increasing muscle *length,* the muscle could develop: a greater maximum tension (P_0), and a greater velocity of shortening for a given load. However, note that V_{max} was not altered by increasing the initial length or preload.

In skeletal muscle, the V_{max} is set by the properties of the myosin ATPase and does not change. However, in cardiac muscle, the V_{max} can be changed by agents such as epinephrine and norepinephrine (NE). The effect of NE, a beta-adrenergic agonist, on the force-velocity curve of cardiac muscle is shown in Fig. 4-8. Norepinephrine causes the force-velocity curve to shift to the right and both the P_0 and the V_{max} are increased. Recall that the initial muscle length is the same for these two curves, so that the length-tension relationship is not used to increase P_0 or V_{max}. The shift in the curve resulting from NE results from a change in *contractility* or *inotropy*. This property of cardiac muscle, i.e., this ability to change the inotropic state or contractility, is dependent on Ca^{2+} availability to the contractile proteins. With increased Ca^{2+} availability there is an increased rate of cross-bridge cycling, which thus results in increased contractile performance.

In summary, the force-velocity curve can be improved in two ways: one by increasing preload and the other by increasing contractility. Both mechanisms will result in an increase in P_0 or the maximum tension that the muscle can produce. However, only an increase in contractility will result in an increase in V_{max} or the maximum velocity of shortening. As discussed later, V_{max} can be used as an index of contractility.

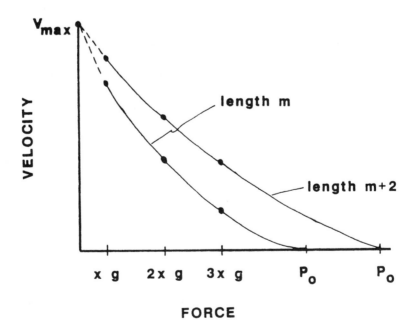

FORCE

Figure 4-7 Force-velocity curves generated on cardiac muscle from two different preloads—(m) and (m + 2). The maximum tension (P_0) is shifted to the right when the muscle is studied from a higher preload or initial muscle length. However, the maximum velocity of shortening, V_{max}, is not altered by changing preload.

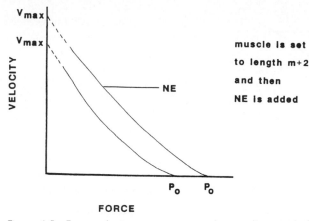

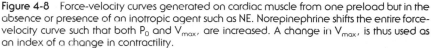

FORCE

Figure 4-8   Force-velocity curves generated on cardiac muscle from one preload but in the absence or presence of an inotropic agent such as NE. Norepinephrine shifts the entire force-velocity curve such that both P_0 and V_{max}, are increased. A change in V_{max}, is thus used as an index of a change in contractility.

If the properties of cardiac muscle are used to assess the performance of the intact heart, we see that cardiac function displays the length-tension relationship or Frank-Starling mechanisms as previously discussed. The length of the muscle fibers is set by the preload or end-diastolic volume. As the action potential is produced in each cell and Ca^{2+} enters the cell via the slow channels, the Ca^{2+} binds to the troponin, the configuration of the contractile proteins changes, and the actin and myosin binding sites are unmasked. Cross-bridge cycling begins. The initial stage of the contraction is comparable to stage A in Fig. 4-4. It is isometric–like or isovolumic or isovolumetric because pressure (tension) increases but there is no shortening or ejection of volume from the ventricle since the AV and semilunar valves are closed. When ventricular tension development matches the afterload, i.e., when ventricular pressure just exceeds aortic diastolic pressure, the aortic valve opens and ejection of blood occurs (comparable to stage B in Fig. 4-4). In this phase of the contraction, shortening of muscle fibers occurs. Although in isolated cardiac muscle studies this shortening phase is isotonic, with the intact heart there is still some increase in pressure development because as the SV is being ejected into the aorta, aortic pressure is progressively increasing. For ejection to continue, ventricular pressure must continue to exceed aortic pressure.

Contractility

As mentioned previously, via the Frank-Starling mechanism, an increase in preload will normally result in an increase in SV. Fig. 4-9 depicts a ventricular function curve, i.e., a curve showing the relation between ventricular filling and some index of ventricular performance. How is a change in contractility manifested in the intact heart? One way to demonstrate changes in contractility is to

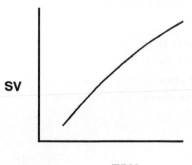

SV

EDV

Figure 4-9 Ventricular function curve showing the relation between end-diastolic volume (preload) and ventricular performance (SV). Other indexes of performance such as stroke work, cardiac output, or minute work could also be used. Other indexes of preload such as left ventricular end-diastolic pressure, left atrial pressure, or pulmonary capillary wedge pressure could also be used.

determine the effects of catecholamines or the sympathetic nervous system on the ventricular function curve. As shown in Fig. 4-10, the degree of sympathetic stimulation to the heart can affect the relation between end-diastolic volume and SV or stroke work.

$$SW = SV \times [MABP - LVEDP]$$

where SW = stroke work

MABP = mean arterial blood pressure

and LVEDP = left ventricular end-diastolic pressure

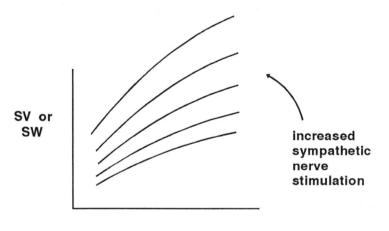

**SV or
SW**

**increased
sympathetic
nerve
stimulation**

EDV

Figure 4-10 Ventricular function curves generated with different levels of sympathetic nerve stimulation. Increased contractility results in an upward and leftward shift in the curve.

(For the right ventricle, the pressure component of the equation is mean pulmo-nary artery pressure minus right ventricular end-diastolic pressure.) Sympathetic stimulation shifts the ventricular function curve upward and to the left. Note, however, that with the different levels of sympathetic stimulation, a family of ventricular function curves is generated suggesting that there is a large reserve in ventricular performance that can be elicited by neurohumoral stimulation of the heart.

Thus far, there have been two variables that vary with changes in inotropic state of the heart: the maximum velocity of shortening and an upward and leftward shift in the ventricular function curve. A third estimator of contractility is the maximum rate of ventricular pressure development.

If ventricular pressure is recorded throughout one cardiac cycle, the tracing shown in Fig. 4-11A is obtained. The dashed line or tangent represents the rate of pressure change measured at one time point. The slope of the dashed line is called dP/dt or the rate of pressure change over a finite time period. The point on the pressure tracing at which the tangent has the greatest slope is the dP/dt_{max}, and this parameter can be used as an estimate of contractility. With decreases in contractility, the rate of pressure development is slowed (as shown in Fig. 4-11B), and therefore the dP/dt_{max} is decreased. For dP/dt_{max} to be a useful estimate of a change in contractility, other factors that influence cardiac muscle contraction (and therefore might influence the rate of pressure development), such as preload, afterload and heart rate, must not have changed. For example, if dP/dt_{max} increases for a contraction but preload also increases, the change in dP/dt_{max} may be due to an increase in contractility or due to the Frank-Starling mechanism. Thus the enhanced function cannot be definitely attributed to a change in inotropic state. In Fig. 4-11, the effects of a negative inotropic agent are shown in panel B. Some

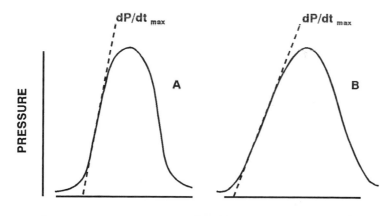

Figure 4-11   Left ventricular pressure as a function of time during a cardiac cycle. The dashed line represents the maximum rate of pressure development. The trace in panel A shows a higher rate of pressure development (dP/dt_{max}) than present in panel B.

agents that are negative inotropes are calcium channel blockers that block calcium entry into the myocyte, some anesthetics such as barbiturates, and beta$_1$-adrenergic blockers that prevent the positive inotropic actions of the sympathetic nervous system neurotransmitter, NE. NE and epinephrine are physiologic positive inotropic agents. There are also pharmacological agents that increase contractility. These include beta$_1$-adrenergic agonists such as isoproterenol (Isoprel), cardiac glycosides such as digitalis, and drugs that inhibit the breakdown of cyclic adenosine monophosphate (cyclic AMP) such as the methylxanthines, caffeine, and theophylline.

The cellular phenomenon that causes a change in contractility or inotropy is dependent on calcium kinetics. The greater amount of calcium available for a contraction (up to some limit since overloading a myocyte with calcium can result in a decreased contractile force), the greater the cycling rate at the cross bridges and the greater the force of contraction. This increase in force of contraction is not dependent on an increase in the number of cross bridges that can interact (Frank-Starling mechanism) but is related to the *velocity* of cross-bridge interaction. Agents mentioned earlier that decrease inotropic state generally do so by inhibiting calcium entry into the cell or inhibiting calcium release from the sarcoplasmic reticulum, or possibly by interfering with the calcium binding to troponin. Agents that increase inotropy do so usually by increasing calcium entry into the cell (NE) or decreasing calcium extrusion from the cell (digitalis). The mechanism by which beta$_1$-adrenergic agonists seem to increase contractility is the following:

1   NE binds to the beta-adrenergic receptor subsequently activating adenylate cyclase, which converts adenosine triphosphate (ATP) to cyclic AMP.

2   cAMP activates protein kinase, which in turn results in phosphorylation of many cellular proteins—a high-energy phosphate is removed from ATP and binds to proteins located in the plasma membrane and the sarcoplasmic reticulum, to troponin and to proteins involved in metabolism.

Phosphorylation of proteins in the plasma membrane allows more calcium to enter the cell and, thus, the cross-bridge cycling rate to increase. Phosphorylation of a sarcoplasmic reticulum protein results in an increased rate of calcium uptake and thus an increased rate of relaxation. Increased uptake of calcium may increase the calcium pool in the sarcoplasmic reticulum and thus allow more calcium to be released with each action potential. Phosphorylation of troponin decreases the affinity of this protein for calcium which probably promotes a more rapid relaxation of heart muscle. Since the cell is flooded with more calcium during phase 2 of the action potential, the decreased affinity of troponin for calcium does not seem to impair the contraction process.

In summary, ventricular performance is affected by preload, afterload, and contractility. Cardiac muscle also has two "reserve" mechanisms on which ventricular performance can depend:

1   The length-tension or Frank-Starling mechanism, i.e., an increase in the number of cross bridges that can form
2   Contractility, i.e., an increase in the cycling rate of cross-bridge turnover

PRESSURE-VOLUME RELATIONSHIP

As a mechanism of relating cardiac muscle properties to cardiac performance, left ventricular pressure and volume changes during a cardiac cycle (Fig. 4-12) will be discussed. Panel A shows a cycle on which changes will be imposed in panels B, C, D, and E. From points A to B, the ventricle is filling during diastole. Since the ventricle is normally very compliant during diastole, volume can triple with very little change in diastolic pressure. Just prior to point B, the cells in the sinoatrial node generate an action potential that travels through the conduction system of the heart, and during the plateau phase of the action potential, calcium enters the cells and initiates contraction. At point B, ventricular pressure exceeds atrial pressure and during the period from B to C pressure increases rapidly but ventricular volume normally remains unchanged (isovolumic phase of contraction). At point C, ventricular pressure exceeds aortic diastolic pressure and the aortic valve opens. Ejection of the SV occurs with the shortening of cardiac muscle cells between points C and D. At the end systolic point (D), cardiac muscle begins to relax since sarcolemmal calcium channels have closed and no more calcium is entering the cell. The sarcoplasmic reticulum is rapidly taking up calcium from the cytosol, and calcium bound to troponin is diffusing away, resulting in the troponin-tropomyosin inhibition of actin-myosin interaction. At point D, the aortic valve closes because ventricular pressure is lower than aortic pressure. From D to A the volume in the ventricle is not changing but the pressure is falling rapidly—isovolumic relaxation—until ventricular pressure is lower than atrial pressure and the AV or bicuspid valve opens. The cycle repeats itself with the passive filling of the compliant ventricle until the next contraction is initiated. Recall that approximately 50 ms prior to ventricular contraction, atrial contraction occurs to assist in filling the ventricle. Note also that in a steady state, the volume of blood ejected is replaced by a similar volume during diastole, i.e., the SV is equal to the venous return for that beat.

In Fig. 4-12B, the normal pressure-volume relation ABCD has been altered by an increase in preload (point E). As described by the Frank-Starling mechanism, contraction will be more forceful. Since the afterload or aortic pressure is not different, the greater energy available for contraction due to interaction of more cross bridges results in greater shortening and thus ejection of a greater SV.

The increase in SV is generally proportional to the increase in end-diastolic volume and therefore the EF (SV/EDV) is not changed very much.

In Fig. 4-12C, the normal pressure-volume relation ABCD has been altered by an increase in afterload or aortic pressure. Thus, more energy for that contraction is expended upon pressure or tension development and less is remaining for shortening. Therefore, SV is decreased and end-systolic volume is increased (point I). If the venous return is similar to that of the first cycle, the resulting end-diastolic volume will be increased to point J. More cross bridges can interact on the third contraction (the dashed lines of Fig. 4-12D), and there is more energy for contraction, i.e., the greater tension is developed to match the elevated afterload but more energy is available such that more shortening can occur and the SV can be normalized. This normalization of the SV may require a few cardiac

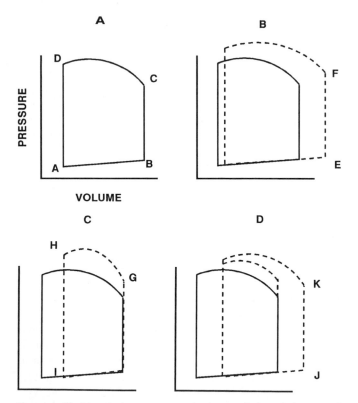

Figure 4-12 Ventricular pressure and volume relations during a cardiac cycle. Panel A shows one contraction under normal conditions. Panel B shows the effects of an increase in preload (to point E) resulting in an increased stroke volume (SV). Point C shows the results of an increase in afterload (to point G) leading to a decrease in SV. Panel D shows the compensatory increase in end-diastolic volume that occurs if venous return remains the same as it was in panel C. From a higher end-diastolic volume (point J), the ventricle can develop greater pressure and return SV to its original level. Panel E shows the effects of a decrease (loop BCNO) in contractility under circumstances in which preload and afterload were not different from the original pressure volume loop (ABCD) in panel A.

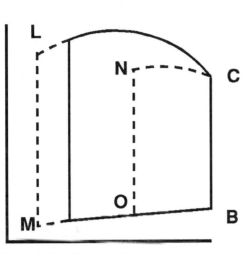

Figure 4-12 (Continued)

cycles to reach some new equilibrium but once the system is in a steady state, the ventricle will be ejecting a normal SV but will be working from a higher end-diastolic volume. If the sympathetic nervous system were to be activated in response to the initial increase in afterload and decrease in SV, an increase in cardiac contractility may also contribute to the recovery of SV. In this case, more calcium would be available for cross-bridge cycling and SV could be maintained from a smaller end-diastolic volume (lower than point J).

In comparing the force-velocity relationship of isolated muscle with the pressure-volume relation of the whole heart, an increase in afterload for both preparations results in, first, an increase in tension, force, or pressure development and, second, a decrease in shortening, velocity of shortening, and ejection of blood. Relying on the length-tension properties of cardiac muscle, an increase in preload or initial length in the muscle will allow for greater shortening and a higher initial velocity of shortening for the increased load. In the whole heart, an increased preload (end-diastolic volume) will allow for a greater shortening (ejection of SV) at the increased afterload.

In Fig. 4-12E, the effects of changes in inotropy are shown as shifts in the pressure-volume loops. An increase in contractility allows the ventricle to eject a greater SV at a given end-diastolic volume or preload and aortic pressure or afterload (loop BCLM). A negative inotropic agent would alter the contractility such that, from a given end-diastolic volume and aortic pressure, a smaller SV would be ejected (loop BCNO). With the positive inotropic agent, the EF (SV/EDV) increases. The heart with decreased contractility has a lower EF.

BIBLIOGRAPHY

Berne RM, Levy MN: *Physiology* 3rd ed., St. Louis, Mosby Year Book, 1993, pp 281–291; 397–410; 417–437.

Guyton AC, Hall JE: *Textbook of Medical Physiology* 9th ed. Philadelphia, W.B. Saunders Company, pp 107–108; 115–118.

Rhoades RA, Tanner GA: *Physiology,* Boston, Little, Brown and Company, 1995, pp 263–269; 272–274.

5

THE PERIPHERAL VASCULAR SYSTEM

The vascular component of the cardiovascular system consists of the arteries and their multiple branches, which carry blood away from the heart; the capillaries, which are one cell layer thick so that exchange can occur between the blood and the interstitial space and tissue cells; and the veins and their multiple branches, which carry blood back to the heart. The functions of the different conduits that carry blood are matched by the anatomy of the vessels.

All blood flow is dependent on a pressure gradient. The pressure in the arteries is greater than the pressure in the capillaries which in turn is greater than the pressure in the veins. Thus in the systemic circulation, blood flows from the aorta to the right atrium along a pressure gradient which is generated by the heart pumping a volume of blood into the aorta from whence the blood moves to the peripheral arteries. The pressure produced in the aorta during ventricular ejection (systole) usually peaks at 120 mmHg. During relaxation of the ventricle (diastole), pressure in the aorta falls to approximately 80 mmHg. Thus blood pressure is generally reported as 120/80. The difference between the systolic pressure and the diastolic pressure is called the pulse pressure. In this example, the pulse pressure is equal to 40 mmHg. The average pressure during a cardiac cycle is the mean arterial blood pressure (MABP). This can be estimated as ($\frac{1}{3}$ × pulse pressure) + diastolic pressure. In this example, this equals 93 mmHg. The regulation of the mean arterial blood pressure is discussed in Chap. 8.

The properties of the vascular wall are important in determining arterial blood pressure. The aorta is a large vessel with a thick wall containing smooth muscle and connective tissue – predominantly elastin and collagen. Elastin confers elastic properties to the wall such that when the aorta is distended from the ejection of blood by the ventricle, the aortic wall returns back to its preejection state. This elastic recoil property of the aorta prevents arterial pressure from falling to 0 during ventricular relaxation. If the aorta were a rigid tube, pressure in the aorta would drop to 0 when the ventricle relaxed. The more elastic the aorta, the better arterial pressure is maintained during diastole. When the aorta is stiff, pressure tends to fall more during diastole. In progressing from the aorta to the large arteries, the small arteries, and the arterioles, the diameter of the vessels decreases, the number of vessels increases (due to branching of the arterial tree), and vessel-wall thickness decreases. However, the change in vessel diameter is much greater than the change in wall thickness. Therefore, in the arterioles the wall thickness to vessel diameter ratio is greater than it is in the arteries and the aorta. This increase in wall thickness per vessel diameter is mainly a function of increasing the relative amount of smooth muscle and decreasing the relative amount of elastic tissue in the vessel wall. The arterioles are the most muscular blood vessels in the peripheral circulation. Due to the contractile properties of vascular smooth muscle, the diameter of the arterioles can be altered by contraction or relaxation of the smooth muscle. The arterioles are thus able to alter vascular resistance since resistance, as defined by Poiseuille's equation, is inversely proportional to radius raised to the fourth power.

$$R = 8nl/\pi r^4$$

where $8/\pi$ is a constant,

l = length of the tube

n = viscosity of the fluid

r = radius of the tube

R = resistance

In addition, resistance is proportional to the length of the vessel and the viscosity of the blood. Of the three parameters that are not constants—length, viscosity, and radius—radius is the variable that can be adjusted instantaneously by contraction or relaxation of vascular smooth muscle. It has been shown empirically that radius raised to the fourth power most closely approximates the effects of changing radius on resistance. Vessel length refers to the total length of the vasculature through which blood flows. Viscosity, a property of the blood, is normally not altered physiologically but can be affected by changes in hematocrit and temperature of the blood. For example, a decrease in blood temperature will cause an increase in viscosity and therefore an increase in resistance. An increase in hematocrit will cause an increase in viscosity and an increase in resistance.

In progressing from the aorta to the large arteries to the small arteries there is only a small drop in MABP mean arterial blood pressure (averaging 93 mmHg in the aorta to approximately 85 mmHg at the beginning of the arterioles). There is a large drop in pressure as blood flows across the high resistance presented by the arterioles. Pressure at the arterial end of the capillaries may average 30 to 40 mmHg. Across the capillaries there is a smaller drop in pressure. At the venous end of the capillaries pressure averages 15 to 20 mmHg. From the small venules back to the right atrium the pressure drops from approximately 15 to 0 mmHg. In addition to the large drop in pressure across the arterioles, there is also a change in the blood flow. Blood flow is pulsatile in vessels proximal to the arterioles but steady or nonpulsatile in vessels distal to the arterioles. Therefore blood flow through the capillaries is relatively constant or steady.

Another property of blood flow through the vasculature is the velocity component. *Velocity* is defined as the flow divided by the cross-sectional area through which the flow occurs (velocity = flow/area). Flow or cardiac output (CO) can be expressed per second as milliliter per second or centimeters cubed per second; cross-sectional area can be expressed as centimeters squared. Therefore, velocity = flow/area = centimeters cubed per second per centimeters squared = centimeters per second. Due to the multiple branching that occurs in the arterial system and the increase in total cross-sectional area that results from the branching, the total cross-sectional area for blood flow is maximal in the capillaries. Therefore the velocity of the blood is the lowest in the capillaries. Since the capillary is the primary site for exchange between the blood and the tissue cells, the low velocity facilitates exchange.

Exchange of materials from the interstitial fluid and the blood occurs in the thin-walled capillaries which are made up of one layer of endothelial cells. The capillaries in different tissues differ anatomically in that some capillaries have a tighter cell-to-cell junction, i.e., are continuous, whereas other capillaries have less tight junctions. Some capillaries have windows or fenestrations in the cells whereas other capillaries have large spaces between cells, i.e., are discontinuous. The anatomy of the endothelium then influences the magnitude of exchange that can occur in a capillary. For example, cardiac muscle has continuous-type capillaries and, therefore, more restricted movement of materials, especially larger molecules, across the capillary wall. The liver, spleen, and gastrointestinal tract tend to have endothelial cells that allow exchange of larger molecules across the capillary wall.

The conduits that carry blood from the capillaries back to the heart are larger in diameter than their corresponding arteries. These vessels also have thinner walls than their corresponding arteries. As the venules combine to form veins, the total cross-sectional area of the venous system decreases and blood flow velocity progressively increases. In the inferior and superior vena-cavae, blood flow velocity is at its highest on the venous side of the circulation. Due to the relative composition of smooth muscle and connective tissue in the venous walls, veins are very distensible or compliant, i.e., veins can contain a large volume of blood but do so at a low intravascular pressure. For example, it has been estimated that under resting conditions approximately 65 percent of the total blood volume (which is approximately 80 ml/kg of body weight) is in the venules, veins, and venae cavae. For a 70-kg human, blood volume would be 5600 ml so 3360 ml of blood would be present in the venous side of the circulation returning to the heart at any one time. That volume of blood is present in a vascular network in which pressures range from approximately 15 to 0 mmHg.

The role of the venous circulation in altering venous return is discussed in Chap. 6.

The pulmonary circulation is estimated to contain approximately 12 percent of the blood volume under resting conditions. The blood pressure in the pulmonary circulation is much lower than is the blood pressure in the systemic circulation. Pulmonary artery systolic and diastolic pressures are approximately 20 and 12 mmHg, respectively, and mean pulmonary artery pressure is approximately 15 mmHg. Although the CO of the right ventricle is equal to the CO of the left ventricle, pressures are lower in the pulmonary circulation than they are in the systemic circulation because the pulmonary vessels are more distensible. The blood vessel walls are thinner than comparable vessel walls in the systemic circulation and contain much less vascular smooth muscle.

HEMODYNAMICS

The kinetics of blood movement through the vasculature is called *hemodynamics*. The properties of the blood vessels and the blood and the interaction of the two in addition to the constant input from the heart determine the ultimate distribution of blood throughout the body. The three components to be discussed in this Section are pressure, flow, and resistance.

Resistance

Resistance can be defined as the ratio of the pressure drop across the system to the blood flow through the system. This is analogous to an electrical circuit in which resistance is defined as the ratio of the voltage drop to the current flow.

In the cardiovascular system, the systemic vascular resistance (SVR) can be calculated from the flow through the systemic circulation (the CO) and the pressure drop across the systemic circulation (mean arterial blood pressure minus right atrial pressure). The actual value for the SVR is calculated because the derivation of the total SVR would be complex since the systemic circulation has such a vast combination of branches and the circuitry consists of vessels that are in series and vessels that are in parallel. For example, the aorta to the coronary artery to the coronary arterioles, capillaries, venules, veins, and coronary sinus represents a series of resistances. However, as the coronary artery branches, parallel resistances are set up. With each set of branches, more parallel resistances occur. This same combination of series and parallel resistances occurs throughout the cardiovascular system.

In a simple circuit in which all resistances are in series, the total resistance (R) of the circuit is equal to the sum of the individual resistances.

$$R_{\text{Total}} = R_1 + R_2 + R_3$$

Note from Fig. 5-1 that flow into the tube (Q_{in}) equals flow out of the tube (Q_{out}) (P = pressure):

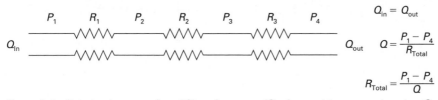

Figure 5-1 Relation between flow (Q) and pressure (P) when resistances are in series. Q_{in} equals Q_{out} and the pressure drop over the entire circuit is $P_1 - P_4$. The total resistance of the circuit is equal to the sum of the three individual resistances, i.e., $R_T = R_1 + R_2 + R_3$.

$$Q = (P_1 - P_4)/R_T$$

therefore

$$R_{Total} = (P_1 - P_4)/Q$$

$$P_1 - P_4 = (P_1 - P_2) + (P_2 - P_3) + (P_3 - P_4)$$

therefore

$$R_{Total} = ((P_1 - P_2) + (P_2 - P_3) + (P_3 - P_4))/Q$$

and

$$R_{Total} = (P_1 - P_2)/Q + (P_2 \quad P_3)/Q + (P_3 - P_4)/Q$$

since

$$(P_1 - P_2)/Q = R_1, \text{ etc.}$$

$$R_{Total} = R_1 + R_2 + R_3$$

Thus the total resistance due to multiple resistances in series is simply the sum of those resistances. An increase (or decrease) in resistance in one component will directly affect the total resistance by that exact increment. For example, if $R_1 = 2$, $R_2 = 4$, and $R_3 = 5$; $R_{Total} = 11$. If R_1 increases by two units, i.e., $R_1 = 4$, R_{Total} increases by two units also and the new $R_{Total} = 13$.

Resistances in parallel contribute to the total resistance by a different formulation as shown in Fig. 5-2.

$$Q_{Total} = (P_1 - P_2)/R_T$$

$$Q_{Total} = Q_1 + Q_2 + Q_3$$

$$Q_1 = (P_1 - P_2)/R_1, Q_2 = (P_1 - P_2)/R_2,$$

$$Q_3 = (P_1 - P_2)/R_3$$

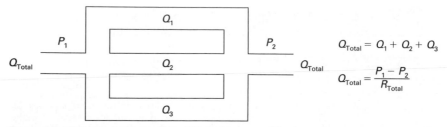

Figure 5-2 Relation between flow (Q) and pressure (P) when resistances are in parallel. Total flow (Q_T) equals the sum of flows through each of the three parallel circuits. The pressure drop over the circuit is $P_1 - P_2$.

therefore,

$$Q_{Total} = (P_1 - P_2)/R_1 + (P_1 - P_2)/R_2 + (P_1 - P_2)/R_3$$
$$= (P_1 - P_2)(1/R_1 + 1/R_2 + 1/R_3)$$

$$Q_{Total}/(P_1 - P_2) = 1/R_1 + 1/R_2 + 1/R_3 = 1/R_{Total}$$

Therefore, the inverse of the total resistance is equal to the sum of the inverse of the individual resistances. With resistances in parallel, the total resistance is less than each individual resistance and a change in the resistance of one of the components has a small effect on the total resistance. For example, if $R_1 = 2$, $R_2 = 4$, and $R_3 = 5$, $1/R_{Total} = \frac{1}{2} + \frac{1}{4} + \frac{1}{5}$; $1/R_{Total} = 19/20$ and $R_{Total} = 20/19 = 1.05$. If R_1 increases by 2, $1/R_{Total} = \frac{1}{4} + \frac{1}{4} + \frac{1}{5} = 14/20$ and $R_{Total} = 20/14 = 1.43$. Thus for an increase in resistance of one of the components (e.g., R_1) by two units, R_{Total} changes by only 0.38 resistance units. In both cases, R_{Total} is less than the smallest resistance.

The systemic circulation is a complex set of resistances in series and parallel. Therefore the only way to determine SVR is to calculate it. The mean arterial blood pressure minus the right atrial pressure divided by CO is the SVR. Pulmonary vascular resistance (PVR) equals mean pulmonary artery pressure minus left atrial pressure divided by CO. Resistance is usually expressed in peripheral resistance units (PRU), i.e., 1 mmHg/ml/min = 1 PRU. For the systemic circulation, if CO = 5600 ml/min, mean arterial blood pressure = 95 mmHg, and right atrial pressure = 0 mmHg, SVR = (95 − 0)/5600 = .017 PRU. If mean pulmonary artery pressure = 15 mmHg and left atrial pressure = 5 mmHg, PVR = (15 − 5)/5600, PVR = 0.002 PRU.

Resistance of the various organs can be estimated if organ blood flow through that organ is known. For example, if blood flow through one kidney is measured as 550 ml/min, renal vascular resistance (RVR) can be estimated as: (mean arterial blood pressure minus right atrial pressure/renal blood flow) or 95/550, and RVR = .173 PRU. To be more accurate in the calculation of RVR, renal venous pressure could be used instead of right atrial pressure. Notice that the SVR is less than the RVR (and all other individual tissue vascular resistances).

Note that in each of the examples for estimating vascular resistance, a pressure gradient is part of the equation, i.e., the difference between an upstream pressure or input pressure, mean pulmonary artery pressure or mean arterial blood pressure, and a downstream pressure, left atrial or right atrial pressure. A pressure gradient is required as the net driving force for blood flow. The downstream pressure becomes a more prominent component in determining resistance in some organ beds in which central venous pressure or right atrial pressure is less than that tissue pressure. For example, in cardiac muscle, blood vessels are compressed during ventricular contraction such that intravascular pressure is greater than right atrial pressure and the gradient for blood flow is less than that which would be predicted by the (mean arterial blood pressure minus right atrial pressure) term.

Recall that resistance can be described as a relation between length (l), radius (r) and viscosity (n): $R = 8nl/\pi r^4$. Length is set primarily by body size and as such changes with growth but is constant when a stable body size is achieved. Radius of the vasculature can be adjusted by vascular smooth muscle contraction, particularly at the level of the arterioles. Temperature and hematocrit may affect viscosity.

Viscosity

Viscosity can be explained in terms of a fluid separating two parallel plates. One plate is stationary and the other plate is moved across the fluid. If the fluid is thought of as consisting of layers, the layer touching the top plate is moving at the same velocity as is the plate. The layer of fluid adjacent to the bottom plate is not moving, i.e., velocity is 0. Between the top layer of fluid moving at a velocity of v_1 and the bottom layer, there are an infinite number of layers of fluid moving at progressively lower velocities than v_1. The shear rate of the fluid is equal to the rate of velocity change (across the layers of fluid)—dv—divided by the distance (d) between the two plates or the depth of the fluid—dd. Shear rate = dv/dd.

The shear stress is the force (F) that must be applied to the top plate, which has a contact area (A), in order to move that plate with the velocity (v_1). Shear stress equals force per area (F/A). Viscosity was defined by Newton as shear stress per shear rate or as the ratio of the force applied to cause movement of the upper plate to the gradient of velocities that occurs across the depth of the fluid. For viscous liquids, the gradient of velocities will be low. For less viscous liquids, the gradient of velocities will be higher. Viscosity is reported in units called poise and is usually expressed relative to the viscosity of H_2O at 20°C. For water and other homogeneous fluids the ratio of the shear stress to shear rate is constant, and the fluid is said to be a Newtonian fluid. Blood is non-Newtonian because it consists of formed elements (cells) and plasma, and the ratio of shear stress to shear rate (viscosity) is not constant. Since resistance is directly proportional to viscosity, any change in viscosity will induce a similar change in resistance.

Since blood is not a homogeneous fluid, changes in viscosity can occur in the circulation and thus the terms *apparent viscosity* or *anomalous viscosity* are used to describe blood. For example, the apparent viscosity of blood is dependent on the size of the tube through which it is flowing. In tubes of less than 0.3 mm, the apparent viscosity of blood decreases (relative to that of water). Of significance is the fact that the arterioles are generally smaller in diameter than 0.3 mm. Therefore, in the smaller vessels of the circulation, the decrease in apparent viscosity offers less resistance for blood flow. This has been termed the *Fahraeus-Lindquist effect.*

The explanation for changes in viscosity that occur relate to the properties of red blood cells which tend to travel at the center of the lumen. This phenomenon has been termed *axial streaming*. That red blood cells are deformable seems to facilitate axial streaming. The plasma tends to move at the periphery of the vessel wall. The red blood cells tend to travel "faster" than the plasma. Related to axial streaming of the red blood cells is the phenomenon in which apparent viscosity of blood decreases at high shear rates (shear rate referring to the velocity of one layer of fluid in relation to the next layer of fluid). High shear rates facilitate the red blood cell movement along the center of the vessel lumen. In contrast, at low shear rates, more interaction between red blood cells (and white blood cells) can occur thus increasing viscosity and affecting vascular resistance. The viscosity properties of blood in the circulation are more complex than flow through rigid tubes since blood is nonhomogeneous and blood vessel walls are not rigid.

Flow

Laminar and Turbulent Flow   Another aspect of blood flow through blood vessels is whether the flow is turbulent or streamlined (also called laminar). As blood travels down a long tube, layers of fluid are set up in the tube. The layer at the center moves at the greatest velocity, and a gradient of lower velocities develops out toward the wall of the vessel. The layer at the vessel wall has the lowest velocity due to interaction with the blood vessel wall. These lamina, or layers, are produced, and the resultant flow is called *laminar flow*. Recall that the formed elements will tend to travel in the center most layer (axial streaming). If any impediment to flow occurs in the vessel, irregular motion can occur in the fluid. Flow becomes nonlaminar, and mixing of the different layers of fluid occurs. This is termed *turbulent flow*. When flow is turbulent, a greater pressure gradient is necessary to generate the same amount of flow than when flow is laminar. Factors that favor turbulent flow are large tube diameter (D), high velocity of flow (v), and high density of the fluid (p). Viscosity is inversely related to turbulence so that a high viscosity tends to decrease the tendency for turbulence. Reynold's number defines the relation between density, diameter, velocity, and viscosity pDv/n. When Reynold's number exceeds 2000, as in the ascending aorta, turbulent flow usually exists. Other factors that can cause turbulence are irregularities of the blood vessel wall which would impede the establishment of laminar flow. Abrupt variations in tube size such as a stenotic lesion of the vessel wall can also result in turbulence. Turbulent flow is generally associated with sound that can be heard with a stethoscope. Clinically, turbulence is used for measuring blood pressure. A cuff is used to impede flow, and a stethoscope is placed over the artery. Sound occurs when the cuff pressure is released enough to allow some flow (which is turbulent) to occur. When all restriction to flow is removed, laminar flow is reinstated, and the sound disappears. The pressure at which the first sound is heard through the stethoscope is the systolic pressure. The pressure at which all sound disappears is the diastolic pressure.

Murmurs or abnormal sounds can occur in the circulation as a result of abnormal flow patterns that induce turbulent flow. Cardiac murmurs are generated particularly when the atrioventricular or semilunar valves are not functioning properly. For instance, a stenotic valve will result in an increased amount of turbulence as blood is pumped across its surface. Abnormal sounds related to cardiac pathophysiology are discussed with "Heart Sounds."

Pressure

Pressure in a blood vessel is caused by the force of the blood exerted on the wall of the vessel and is defined as *force per area*. In the measurement of arterial pressure via a catheter inserted into an artery, the level of pressure that is measured will be determined by the site of the opening on the catheter, i.e., whether the opening is at the tip of the catheter facing blood flow or on the side of the catheter with blood flowing across the opening. The opening at the side measures only static or lateral pressure since it is perpendicular to the direction of flow. The opening at the tip measures lateral pressure plus pressure related to kinetic energy At the tip of the catheter, blood flow is impeded (does not enter the catheter) so that the kinetic energy component ($1/2pv^2$; where p = density and v = velocity) is 0. The resultant measured pressure is greater than that measured at a side opening by that increment which converts kinetic energy to pressure. The site of the opening on the catheter for pressure measurement is most significant in the vasculature where blood flow velocity is high. Thus in the ascending aorta, pressure measured in an opened tip catheter might be 10 to 15 mmHg greater that the pressure that would be measured from a side opening. For example, if blood flow velocity is 200 cm/sec in the ascending aorta, kinetic energy (KE) will be the following:

$$(\text{KE}) = \tfrac{1}{2}pv^2$$
$$= \tfrac{1}{2}(1 \text{ g/cm}^3) (200 \text{ cm/s})^2$$
$$= 20,000 \ (\text{g/cm}^3) \ (\text{cm}^2/\text{s}^2)$$

In the centimeter-gram-second system:

$$1 \text{ g cm/s}^2 = 1 \text{ dyn}$$

therefore,

$$KE = 20{,}000 \text{ dyn/cm}^2$$

$$1 \text{ mmHg} = 1330 \text{ dyn/cm}^2$$

therefore,

$$KE = 20{,}000/1330 = 15 \text{ mmHg}.$$

The difference in pressure measured in the ascending aorta can be 15 mmHg when measured in an opened tip catheter versus a side-opened catheter. Since blood flow velocity decreases as blood travels away from the aorta into the multiple series of branches of the arterial tree (recall that velocity = flow per cross-sectional area), the kinetic energy component of measured pressure becomes less significant. The difference between total pressure and lateral pressure becomes smaller.

BIBLIOGRAPHY
Berne RM, Levy MN: *Physiology* 3rd ed., St. Louis, Mosby Year Book, 1993, pp 361–363; 438–452; 453–464.

Guyton AC, Hall JE: *Textbook of Medical Physiology* 9th ed. Philadelphia, W.B. Saunders Company, pp 161–179.

Rhoades RA, Tanner GA: *Physiology,* Boston, Little, Brown and Company, 1995, pp 278–287.

6

VENOUS RETURN & CARDIAC OUTPUT

For the heart to pump a cardiac output (CO) that is adequate to supply the oxygen and nutrient requirements of the tissues, blood must return to the heart at the appropriate rate; that is, for CO to be increased, venous return must increase.

Venous return, like all blood flow, is determined by a pressure gradient. Since in a steady state, CO and venous return are the same, the pressure gradient for venous return is mean arterial blood pressure−right atrial pressure and the following:

$$CO = VR - (MABP - RAP)/SVR$$

where VR = venous return

$MABP$ = mean arterial blood pressure

RAP = right atrial pressure

SVR = systemic vascular resistance

In analyzing blood flow from the venules to the right atrium, one can isolate the venous system and analyze the effective pressure gradient for venous return, which is venous pressure minus right atrial pressure:

$$VR = (VP - RAP)/VVR$$

where VP = venous pressure

VVR = venous vascular resistance

Since venous vascular resistance is generally thought to be very low, venous return is mainly affected by changes in venous pressure and right atrial pressure.

Venous pressure is actually the passive result of the presence of a certain volume of blood in the venous vasculature and the properties (compliance) of the vascular wall. Venous pressure is proportional to venous volume and inversely proportional to venous compliance. Since the systemic veins have thin walls and only a small amount of vascular smooth muscle, the most apparent property of the venous circulation is its compliance or capacitance characteristics. Veins are approximately 24 times more compliant than arteries. Veins can contain large volumes of blood (up to 60 percent of the blood volume under resting conditions) at low pressures. Venous pressure varies from the highest value of approximately 15 to 20 mmHg (ignoring the effects of gravity) at the venous end of a systemic capillary bed to approximately 0 in the venae cavae at the entrance to the right atrium. Since venous pressure is "downstream" from the capillaries and arterioles in any organ, venous pressure is usually less than capillary pressure. For any individual organ, capillary pressure is mainly determined by the level of vaso-constriction of the arterioles of that organ. With greater vasoconstriction, capillary pressure decreases as does capillary blood flow and thus pressure at the venous end of that capillary bed also decreases relative to the pressure there prior to the increased vasoconstriction. Generally venous pressure is estimated by measuring central venous pressure in the thoracic region. Since venous pressures are very low (0 to 5 mmHg), central venous pressure often is measured in centimeters of water since water is less dense and 1 mmHg equals 13.6 mmH_2O.

Venous pressure is altered by two factors: changes in the volume of blood in the venous system and changes in the compliance of the venous walls. The total blood volume does not normally change but the distribution of the blood volume (and CO) can be varied by sympathetic nervous system effects on vascular smooth muscle. Sympathetic stimulation to smooth muscle in the venous system results in a change in venous compliance. With decreased compliance, the pressure in the veins containing a certain volume of blood will increase. This higher venous pressure will increase the effective driving force for venous return: More blood will be forced back to the heart. As more of that blood is mobilized from the venous system (particularly the venous vasculature of the gastrointestinal tract), the venous blood volume will decrease and venous pressure may tend to decrease toward the levels found during resting conditions. Importantly, the per-centage of the blood volume present in the veins will be decreased and the ef-fective pressure gradient for improving venous return will be enhanced.

Several other factors are important in maintaining or enhancing venous re-turn. Skeletal muscle contraction compresses the veins and helps to drive blood back to the right atrium. The presence of one-way valves in many of the systemic veins prevents the backward flow of venous blood. This is especially important in the standing position in which gravity effects can be significant in altering the distribution of the blood volume. Contraction of skeletal muscle surrounding veins can force blood back to the heart with the valves preventing the reverse flow.

The thoracoabdominal pump, i.e., the effects of inspiratory and expiratory movements on thoracic (and thus venae cavae) pressures and abdominal pressure, can result in increases in venous return during inspiration and decreases in venous return during expiration. With the lowering of the diaphragm, thoracic pressure decreases whereas abdominal pressure increases, thereby increasing venous pressure by compression of the venous vasculature in the abdomen. In contrast, the great veins in the thoracic cavity are exposed to a more negative intrathoracic pressure on contraction of the diaphragm and thus tend to have a lowering of intravascular pressure. A greater abdominal to thoracic pressure gradient yields a greater venous return. These effects on venous return can be measured as oscillations in mean arterial blood pressure as the changes in venous return to the right atrium and ventricle result in increased right ventricular stroke volume (Frank-Starling mechanism). This increased volume passes through the pulmonary circulation to finally result in increased venous return to the left atrium and ventricle. Increased filling of the left ventricle results in increased left ventricular output and increased arterial pressure. With relaxation of the diaphragm, the increased pressure gradient for venous return is lost and venous return is restored to a lower level until the next inspiratory activity. Note that during positive pressure ventilation or a forced expiration, thoracic pressure becomes positive, impeding venous return.

Since the venous system is very compliant, the effects of going from a supine position to a standing position are much more evident on the veins. In changing to a standing position, gravity causes intravascular pressure to increase in proportion to the height of the column of blood existing between the heart and the feet. The immediate effect is an increase in venous volume in the dependent parts of the body, a decrease in venous return and stroke volume, and ultimately a decrease in blood pressure, which is sensed by the arterial baroreceptors (see Chap. 8). Activation of the sympathetic nervous system then results in decreased venous compliance which would tend to increase venous pressure and push more blood back to the heart. In addition, arteriolar constriction decreases blood flow to the tissues in the dependent parts of the body thus impeding inflow of blood and minimizing the effects of gravity. However, transmural pressure does increase and filtration can increase. One other mechanism assists in preventing excessive fluid accumulation. Skeletal muscle contraction increases both venous return and also lymphatic flow, both of which will prevent excessive fluid accumulation in the interstitial space in the dependent parts of the body.

BIBLIOGRAPHY

Berne RM, Levy MN: *Physiology* 3rd ed., St. Louis, Mosby Year Book, 1993, pp 494–500; 505–509.

Guyton AC, Hall JE: *Textbook of Medical Physiology* 9th ed. Philadelphia, W.B. Saunders Company, pp 245–250.

Rhoades RA, Tanner GA: *Physiology,* Boston, Little, Brown and Company, 1995, pp 333–336.

7

CAPILLARY FUNCTION

The main function of the cardiovascular system occurs at the capillaries. Exchange of metabolic substrates and waste products occurs across the thin-walled capillary endothelium. This function is well suited to the capillaries not only because of the low diffusion distances across the capillary (most cells are only 20 to 30μ from a capillary), but also because blood flow velocity is lowest in the capillaries and the capillaries present a very large surface area for exchange. As discussed previously, different capillary beds have different types of endothelium, i.e., continuous endothelium with tight junctions between cells; fenestrated endothelium with openings within the cells; and discontinuous endothelium with large openings between cells. Therefore the structure of the capillary wall will affect transport across the walls, especially transport of large molecules.

The main mechanisms by which materials cross the capillary wall are diffusion, bulk flow, and pinocytosis. Diffusion is the process by which most materials cross the endothelium. Diffusion of a material depends on a concentration gradient and the properties of the material that is diffusing. Lipid soluble materials can pass through endothelial cells as well as between cells. Therefore substances such as carbon dioxide, oxygen, and lipid soluble drugs, such as anesthetics, can diffuse readily across the capillary wall. Substances that are water soluble such as glucose, ions, and amino acids can diffuse through pores or fenestrations of the capillary wall. In addition, the size of water soluble materials affects diffusion; molecules such as glucose with a molecular weight of 180 can diffuse readily whereas molecules such as albumin which has a molecular weight of approximately 69,000 diffuses very little. Globulin, with a molecular weight of approximately 120,000, essentially does not diffuse.

Diffusion, therefore, is directly proportional to the diffusion properties of the substance that is moving, the area available for diffusion, and the concentration gradient of the substance; and inversely proportional to the thickness of the membrane across which diffusion is occurring. In studying diffusion across the capillary wall, diffusion is determined by the concentration of the substance, the surface area available for diffusion, and the permeability properties of the solute and the capillary wall. The surface area available for diffusion can be greatly increased by augmenting blood flow through a tissue because normally not all of the capillaries in a tissue are perfused under resting conditions. Dilation of arterioles in that tissue would increase capillary blood flow and thus increase the surface area for diffusion.

Bulk flow is the process by which water and water soluble substances cross the endothelium. The forces that determine movement of water across the endothelium are called the *Starling forces,* named for Ernest Starling, who first described them. Two forces determine the movement of water across the capillary wall: hydrostatic forces and oncotic or colloid osmotic forces. The hydrostatic forces tend to "push" water across the endothelium, whereas the oncotic forces tend to "pull" water across the endothelium. The hydrostatic force in the capillary is the blood pressure which causes fluid to move out of the capillary. The capillary oncotic pressure is exerted by the plasma proteins, albumin and globulin, with albumin exerting the major component of the oncotic pressure. Capillary oncotic pressure causes fluid to move from the interstitial space into the vascular space. Hydrostatic force in the tissue or interstitial space is generally very low and sometimes even estimated to be negative. A positive hydrostatic pressure would tend to cause water to move from the interstitial space into the vascular space. Tissue oncotic pressure is exerted by any plasma proteins, primarily albumin, that cross the endothelium into the interstitium. This force will vary depending on the structure of the endothelium and how much albumin moves into the interstitial space. Tissue or interstitial oncotic pressure tends to cause water to move from the vascular space into the interstitial space. The movement of fluid from vascular space into interstitial space is termed *filtration,* whereas the movement of fluid from the interstitial space into the vascular space is termed *reabsorption.* Generally, filtration tends to occur at the arterial end of the capillary, whereas reabsorption tends to occur at the venous end of the capillary. If filtration exceeds reabsorption, excess interstitial fluid is removed by way of the lymphatic circulation. The lymphatic circulation is also the major way by which albumin is returned to the vasculature.

An ideal capillary can be used to analyze the balance of the Starling forces across the capillary (Fig. 7-1). Forces at the arterial end of the capillary are approximated as follows: capillary hydrostatic pressure is 30 mmHg and tissue oncotic pressure is approximately 5 mmHg. These forces for filtration equal 35 mmHg. Reabsorptive forces are capillary oncotic pressure, which equals approximately 25 mmHg, and tissue hydrostatic pressure, which we will approximate as 0 mmHg. The reabsorptive forces at the arterial end of the capillary equal 25 mmHg. The filtration forces exceed the reabsorptive forces by 10 mmHg, and net filtration of fluid occurs. The major change in Starling forces that occurs between the arterial and venous ends of the capillary is that capillary hydrostatic pressure decreases to approximately 15 mmHg at the venous end. Therefore, the filtration forces equal 20 mmHg (tissue oncotic pressure remains at approximately 5 mmHg), whereas the reabsorptive forces equal 25 mmHg. Thus, the net forces

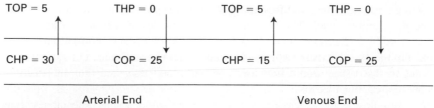

	Arterial End	Venous End
	Net Force = Filtration	Net Force = Reabsorption

Figure 7-1 Starling forces in an ideal capillary bed showing the difference in those forces on the arterial and venous ends of the capillary bed. Arrows show the direction of fluid movement resulting from the hydrostatic or oncotic forces. CHP = capillary hydrostatic pressure, TOP = tissue oncotic pressure, COP = capillary oncotic pressure, and THP = tissue hydrostatic pressure.

favor reabsorption. The magnitude of movement of water across the capillary wall is influenced by the area available for filtration and the anatomical properties of the capillary wall, i.e., whether the endothelium is continuous, fenestrated, or discontinuous. The filtration and reabsorption equation is therefore multiplied by a coefficient that is determined by surface area and permeability properties of the capillary wall. This coefficient is termed the K_f. Therefore net fluid movement equals the following:

$$\text{Fluid movement} = K_f \left[(\text{CHP} + \text{TOP}) - (\text{COP} + \text{THP}) \right]$$

where CHP = capillary hydrostatic pressure, also termed P_c

TOP = interstitial or tissue oncotic pressure, also termed π_i

COP = capillary oncotic pressure, also termed π_c

THP = interstitial or tissue hydrostatic pressure, also termed P_i

Although the Starling forces are fairly stable, they can be changed either physiologically or pathophysiologically. Physiologic alterations of the Starling forces can occur by changes in arteriolar resistance in the arterioles supplying the capillary bed. Vasoconstriction causes a decrease in capillary blood flow and capillary hydrostatic pressure and therefore tends to decrease filtration and favor reabsorption. There are estimates that under conditions of severe blood loss, reabsorption of interstitial fluid can be as great as 1 liter/h in a 70-kg man. With an estimated blood volume of 5 to 5.6 liters, this reabsorption of interstitial fluid is an effective compensatory mechanism. Vasodilation of arterioles increases capillary blood flow and capillary hydrostatic pressure and thus favors filtration. Other factors that can alter capillary hydrostatic pressure are changes in venous pressure. Since venous pressure must be lower than capillary pressure in order for blood to flow from capillaries to veins, any increase in venous pressure such as that caused by a decrease in venous compliance or an increase in venous volume (e.g., a transfusion) will

also result in an increase in capillary hydrostatic pressure and tend to favor filtration.

Other pathologic changes that can alter the Starling forces at the capillary
are changes in plasma protein concentrations such as might occur with liver dysfunction or malnutrition. Decreased plasma protein concentration will decrease
capillary oncotic force and thus decrease the reabsorption of interstitial fluid into
the vascular space. Increase in endothelial permeability will also result in greater
filtration forces since plasma proteins will cross the capillary wall more easily
and thus exert a greater oncotic pressure in the interstitial space.

The final process by which material moves across the endothelium is pinocytosis. Generally only large substances move by pinocytosis which occurs when
the cell membrane pinches off to form a vesicle that may contain a large particle.
The vesicle moves through the cell and empties its contents on the other surface
of the cell. Pinocytosis does not represent a major mechanism for movement of
materials across the endothelium, but probably represents the major way that large
materials can be moved across the capillary wall.

BIBLIOGRAPHY

Berne RM, Levy MN: *Physiology* 3rd ed., St. Louis, Mosby Year Book, 1993, pp 465–
    477.
Guyton AC, Hall JE: *Textbook of Medical Physiology* 9th ed. Philadelphia, W.B. Saunders
    Company, pp 183–196.
Rhoades RA, Tanner GA: *Physiology,* Boston, Little, Brown and Company, 1995, pp 289–
    303.

8

REGULATION OF ARTERIAL BLOOD PRESSURE

Mean arterial blood pressure is the average pressure measured in the aorta or a large artery during a cardiac cycle. Mean arterial blood pressure can be estimated from the systolic and diastolic arterial pressures:

$$MABP = (\tfrac{1}{3}PP) + DP$$

where MABP = mean arterial blood pressure

PP = pulse pressure or systolic pressure − diastolic pressure

DP = diastolic pressure

If systolic pressure is 120 mmHg and diastolic pressure is 80 mmHg, then the following is true:

$$PP = 40$$
$$MABP = (40/3) + 80 = 93$$

or

$$MABP = [2(DP) + SP]/3$$

where DP = diastolic pressure

SP = systolic pressure

If SP = 120 and DP = 80, then

$$MABP = [2(80) + 120]/3 = 93$$

The mean arterial blood pressure is the driving force for blood flow to the systemic vasculature. The counterpart to mean arterial blood pressure for the pulmonary circulation is the mean pulmonary artery pressure. All flow is dependent on a pressure gradient, P. Therefore cardiac output (CO) = ΔP/systemic vascular resistance (SVR). The actual pressure gradient for systemic blood flow is the following:

$$MABP - RAP$$

where RAP = right atrial pressure

Since right atrial pressure is approximately 0, we often express the pressure gradient, ΔP, as simply the mean arterial blood pressure.

The pressure gradient for pulmonary blood flow is actually the following:

$$PAP - LAP$$

where PAP = mean pulmonary artery pressure

LAP = left atrial pressure

Left atrial pressure is generally greater than 0 and therefore flow to the pulmonary circulation is expressed as the following:

$$CO = (PAP - LAP)/PVR$$

where PVR = pulmonary vascular resistance

Since mean arterial blood pressure is the driving force for blood flow to all organs except the lungs, it is essential that it be regulated within a fairly limited range. Regulation of mean arterial blood pressure is the result of both short-term mechanisms (the baroreceptor reflex) and long-term mechanisms (blood volume and blood composition—osmolarity and sodium concentration—as regulated by the kidney).

The baroreceptor reflex consists of four components: a sensor or detector (the baraoreceptors); afferent pathways: a comparator or controller (the central nervous system); and efferents to the effector systems—the heart, arterioles, and veins.

The baroreceptors for mean arterial blood pressure regulation are located in the carotid sinus and the aortic arch. The baroreceptors are mechanoreceptors or stretch receptors that increase their nerve firing rate with increases in stretch induced by increases in mean arterial blood pressure. The maximum sensitivity, i.e., the maximum change in nerve firing rate for a given change in mean arterial blood pressure, occurs at the normal operating range for mean arterial blood pressure (85 to 95 mmHg). The minimum mean arterial blood pressure that will stimulate the baroreceptors is approximately 50 to 60 mmHg. The maximum firing rate occurs at approximately 200 mmHg and above this mean arterial blood pressure, the firing rate cannot increase further. With the pressure changes recorded during a cardiac cycle, there is a variation in the firing rate of the baroreceptors. Firing rate is high as pressure is increasing, less if it is unchanging, and lower as it is declining. In addition, the baroreceptors can adapt to chronic changes in mean arterial blood pressure. For example, with chronic hypertension, receptor sensitivity will be shifted to the right such that the maximum sensitivity of the receptors will be at the new operating mean arterial blood pressure. The maximum firing rate will occur at a greater than normal mean arterial blood pressure, and the initial stimulation of the baroreceptors will occur at a higher than normal mean arterial blood pressure, i.e., greater than 50 to 60 mmHg.

The afferent pathways consist of fibers traveling in the vagus nerve (X) from the aortic arch and via Hering's nerve from the carotid sinus. Hering's nerve joins the glossopharyngeal nerve (IX) to enter the central nervous system.

The comparators or control systems that process afferent information and modulate efferent output are in the medulla. Although there are no discreet "centers" in the medulla, there are regions in the medulla that affect sympathetic and parasympathetic nervous system activity to the periphery. It has been suggested that cardioinhibitory regions and cardioaccelerator regions affect myocardial rate, while vasomotor regions alter vascular smooth muscle tone, primarily in the arterioles and veins. Although no discreet centers can be distinguished in the medulla, the tendency for sympathetic- and parasympathetic-predominant areas seems to exist. Lateral regions tend to modulate sympathetic output, whereas medial regions of the medulla tend to modulate parasympathetic output.

The efferents from the central nervous system innervate the effector organs. Heart function is modulated by both branches of the autonomic nervous system. The parasympathetic system causes a decrease in heart rate and, possibly, a decrease in myocardial force of contraction or contractility. The sympathetic nervous system induces an increased heart rate and an increased contractility (primarily of the ventricles). Increased heart rate and contractility can increase the CO (heart rate × stroke volume). Increasing CO causes a proportional increase in mean arterial blood pressure (CO × SVR).

The other two effectors of the baroreceptor reflex are innervated primarily by the sympathetic nervous system. The arterioles and veins in most vascular beds have some innervation from the sympathetic nervous system. Few vascular beds have innervation from the parasympathetic nervous system. Most of the alterations in vascular tone that can occur within the baroreceptor reflex occur via increased sympathetic nervous system discharge or withdrawal of sympathetic drive.

The primary effect of sympathetic nervous system discharge to vascular smooth muscle in the arterioles is to stimulate smooth muscle contraction, which causes a decreased radius of the vessel thereby increasing its resistance. Sympathetic nervous system vasoconstriction is mediated by stimulation of alpha receptors on the vascular smooth muscle cells by the sympathetic nervous system neurotransmitter, norepinephrine. Circulating epinephrine and norepinephrine can also interact with vascular smooth muscles, but the endothelial barrier may modulate the effects of circulating catecholamines on arteriolar resistance. The general effect of sympathetic nervous system stimulation of the arterioles is an increase in SVR, which is directly related to mean arterial blood pressure (CO × SVR).

Sympathetic nervous system discharge to the vascular smooth muscle of veins causes a decreased compliance of the veins. If venous blood volume is not changed, then venous pressure must increase when compliance is decreased. Thus, venoconstriction results in an initial increase in venous pressure, which favors an increase in venous return. The decreased compliance can also effect a decrease in the percent of the blood volume that is located in the venous system. Normally under basal conditions, approximately 60 percent of the blood volume is present in the venous system. By decreasing compliance, the venous volume can be decreased. The main effect of decreased venous compliance is to increase venous return which can, via the Frank-Starling mechanism, increase CO and thus mean arterial blood pressure (CO × SVR).

Figure 8-1 shows the interactions of the different components of the baroreceptor reflex. For a fall in mean arterial blood pressure (e.g., transferring from the supine to the standing position and the resultant gravitational effects on peripheral venous blood volume) the following changes will occur in sequence as depicted in Fig. 8 1:

1. Decreased mean arterial blood pressure will result in decreased baroreceptor nerve firing rate.

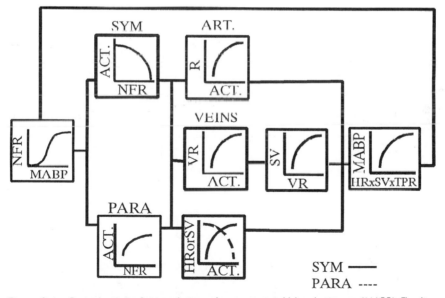

Figure 8-1 Control system for regulation of mean arterial blood pressure (MABP). The line going into the box is represented on the abscissa, whereas the line going out of the box is represented on the ordinate. NFR = baroreceptor nerve firing rate; SYM ACT = sympathetic nervous system activity; PARA ACT = parasympathetic nervous system activity; ART = arterioles; R = total peripheral resistance; VR = venous return; HR = heart rate; SV = stroke volume; TPR = total peripheral resistance (or systemic vascular resistance)

2. Decreased nerve firing rate to the parasympathetic region of the medulla will result in decreased parasympathetic nervous system activity. Decreased parasympathetic nervous system activity leads to an increased heart rate, which leads to an increased CO and thus to an increased mean arterial blood pressure (back toward normal).

3. Decreased nerve firing rate to the sympathetic regions of the medulla will result in increased sympathetic nervous system activity. Increased sympathetic activity leads to the following:
    a. Increased arteriolar resistance, which leads to increased SVR and thus mean arterial blood pressure;
    b. Decreased venous compliance, which leads to an increased venous pressure and an increased pressure gradient for venous return and thus to increased CO and mean arterial blood pressure;
    c. Increased heart rate, which leads to increased CO and thus mean arterial blood pressure;
    d. Increased ventricular contractility, which leads to increased stroke volume and CO and thus mean arterial blood pressure.

In summary, via decreased parasympathetic activity and increased sympathetic activity, CO (stroke volume and heart rate) and SVR have been increased in order to bring mean arterial blood pressure back toward normal.

Using the flow chart in Fig. 8-1, follow the sequence of events that would occur to compensate for an acute increase in mean arterial blood pressure.

BIBLIOGRAPHY

Berne RM, Levy MN: *Physiology* 3rd ed., St. Louis, Mosby Year Book, 1993, pp 289–303.

Guyton AC, Hall JE: *Textbook of Medical Physiology* 9th ed. Philadelphia, W.B. Saunders Company, pp 209–218.

Rhoades RA, Tanner GA: *Physiology,* Boston, Little, Brown and Company, 1995, pp 321–336.

9

CARDIAC OUTPUT
AND ITS DISTRIBUTION

The two variables within the cardiovascular system that are well controlled are the mean arterial blood pressure and the cardiac output (CO). As discussed in Chap. 8, mean arterial blood pressure is controlled within a fairly limited range by the baroreceptor reflex. Cardiac output, however, is not controlled within a limited range but rather is linked to the workload of the body and the metabolism or oxygen consumption of the body (see Fig. 3.1). Cardiac output can therefore vary from a resting level that is approximately 8 percent of the body weight (kg) to a level that is four- to sixfold higher. There is no one sensor for CO as there is for mean arterial blood pressure. The CO is the result of an interaction between the pump and the vasculature into which it ejects blood. For a normal cardiovascular system, the pump has little control over the magnitude of the CO. The heart's two properties of contractility (as altered by the sympathetic nervous system) and length-tension (as altered by venous return) allow the heart to pump various stroke volumes. The metabolic needs of the peripheral tissues more directly determine the absolute level of CO since it is the sum of the blood flow to all of the tissues. The distribution of the CO is independent of pump function but is dependent on the interaction of the central nervous system, via the sympathetic nervous system, with the local control of blood flow by individual organs. The balance between central control and local control of tissue blood flow is tailored to each tissue. For example, blood flow to some tissues, such as the brain and heart, is regulated primarily by local mechanisms. Blood flow to other tissues, such as the gastro-intestinal tract, may be more influenced by the central nervous system than by local mechanisms. Local mechanisms predominate when sympathetic nervous system activity is low; however, sympathetic nervous system activity predominates over local mechanisms in many tissues when sympathetic nervous system activity is high.

The two control mechanisms for regulating tissue blood flow then consist of the autonomic nervous system and locally mediated effects. As discussed previously, the sympathetic nervous system is the major component of the central nervous system to affect the vasculature. Its effect is primarily mediated by the transmitter norepinephrine released from the sympathetic postganglionic fibers. Norepinephrine binds to alpha receptors and, via stimulation of phosphatidy-linositol turnover, initiates smooth muscle contraction. In venous blood vessels, smooth muscle contraction results in a decrease in compliance. In arteriolar vessels, contraction results in decreased vessel radius, increased resistance, and decreased blood flow. A tissue's response or sensitivity to autonomic control is dependent on:

1. The type of receptors present on the vascular smooth muscle cells, i.e., alpha receptors mediate vasoconstriction whereas $beta_2$ receptors mediate vasodilation
2. The density of alpha and/or $beta_2$ receptors—the more alpha receptors present in an arteriolar bed, the greater the likelihood of central control of local blood flow
3. The type of smooth muscle that predominates in the blood vessel wall —the greater the contribution of smooth muscle to the vessel wall, the greater the central control that can be exerted

Unitary-type smooth muscle is not innervated, has spontaneous contractile activity, and responds to stretch by contracting. These latter two features of smooth muscle represent its myogenic properties. Unitary-type smooth muscle does not respond to the autonomic nervous system to any extent and, therefore, is important in contributing to the local mechanisms for controlling tissue blood flow.

To understand the local mechanisms that contribute to the regulation of a tissue's blood flow, an understanding of three conditions is useful: autoregulation, active hyperemia, and reactive hyperemia. Autoregulation is the property of many tissues to maintain a relatively constant blood flow over a certain range of perfusion pressures (Fig. 9-1). For example, as shown in Fig. 9-1, tissue blood flow is maintained at approximately 50 ml/min at perfusion pressures ranging from 60 to 180 mmHg. Over this range of pressures, the tissue is regulating its blood flow. Since blood flow = pressure/resistance; if pressure increases but blood flow remains constant, resistance must have increased. If pressure decreases but blood flow remains relatively constant, resistance must have decreased. Tissues exhibit the property of autoregulation even when removed from the body, i.e., autoregulation is not dependent on innervation of the vascular smooth muscle. Autoregulation is intrinsic to the tissue—the tissue cells and the vasculature in the tissue.

Several theories have been proposed to explain autoregulation. The two most prominent theories are the *myogenic theory* and the *vasodilator theory*. The myogenic theory uses the property of smooth muscle whereby the muscle contracts in response to stretch to explain the changes in resistance that occur with changing perfusion pressure. With increased perfusion pressure there is initially an increased blood flow which stretches the blood vessel wall. This stretch induces a contraction of the vascular smooth muscle thus decreasing vessel radius and increasing resistance to flow. The initial increase in blood flow returns to the orig-

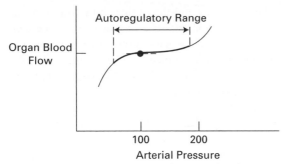

Figure 9-1 Tissue blood flow as a function of perfusion pressure. Tissue blood flow is relatively constant over a range of perfusion pressures due to autoregulation of vascular resistance. At pressures less than about 50 mmHg, tissue blood flow decreases because arterioles cannot dilate further. At pressures greater than approximately 180 mmHg, tissue blood flow increases because arterioles cannot constrict further.

inal blood flow. The opposite sequence occurs when the perfusion pressure is decreased within the autoregulatory range. When pressure decreases, the initial response is a decrease in blood flow. This results in less stretch on the vessel wall, and the vessel relaxes and increases radius. Resistance decreases and blood flow increases toward the original level.

The vasodilator theory explains autoregulation on the basis of an interaction between tissue cells and their metabolic rate and the level of arteriolar smooth muscle contraction. The tissue or parenchymal cells produce certain metabolites such as adenosine (from utilization of adenosine triphosphate, or ATP), CO_2, K^+, H^+, and lactate that can leave the cell, diffuse through the interstitial space, and alter vascular tone. The more metabolically active the tissue is, the more vasodilator material is produced. In the study shown in Fig 9-1, the metabolic rate of the tissue is kept constant and presumably the production of vasodilator substances is constant. The changes in vascular resistance that occur over the autoregulatory range result from the accumulation or washout of vasodilator materials. For example, when pressure is increased, the initial effect is an increase in blood flow which in turn leads to washout of the vasodilators and a decrease in their concentration. Vascular resistance thus increases and blood flow decreases toward the original level. With a decrease in pressure, blood flow initially falls and the vasodilator concentration increases. Vascular resistance decreases and blood flow increases toward the original level.

Above the autoregulatory range, increases in pressure are accompanied by increases in blood flow because vasoconstriction is maximum and cannot further increase. Below the autoregulatory range, the opposite is true, a decrease in pressure results in a decreased blood flow. The vasculature cannot dilate any further.

The phenomenon of active hyperemia seems also to be well explained by the vasodilator hypothesis. As a tissue becomes more active in performing whatever its primary function is, it produces more metabolites that can affect vascular tone. With the production of more vasodilators and the increase in concentration of these substances, vascular tone decreases and thus blood flow to that tissue increases. Since physiologically the perfusion pressure for each tissue is essentially the mean arterial blood pressure, which is well controlled by the baroreceptor reflex, an organ's blood flow is primarily adjusted by changes in arteriolar tone or vascular resistance within that organ. These changes in vascular tone are modulated by the metabolic activity of the tissue.

The third phenomenon that occurs by local control of blood flow is reactive hyperemia. Reactive hyperemia is an increase in blood flow (above control) that occurs after a temporary occlusion of an artery. During occlusion of an artery and the subsequent decrease in blood flow that follows, vasodilator materials accumulate in the tissue. With the release of the occlusion, blood flow is reinstated. Since the arterioles have responded to metabolites by vasodilating and decreasing vascular resistance, the resultant blood flow is greater than the control blood flow. As the increased blood flow washes out the vasodilator metabolites, the tissue returns to the control equilibrium in which metabolic activity was matched by the control blood flow. The amount of overshoot in blood flow following the occlusion of an artery is proportional, to some extent, to the length of the occlusion. With longer periods of occlusion, more vasodilator metabolites are produced and accumulate and a greater change in vascular resistance occurs. Thus the reactive hyperemic flow is greater. Also the time to recovery of control blood flow after release of the occlusion is extended. Of course there is some point at which increasing the length of the occlusion does not result in a proportionally greater reactive hyperemia. If the metabolic rate of the tissue decreases as a result of the ischemia or occlusion of the artery, then further accumulation of metabolites may not occur. In addition, as the period of occlusion reaches some critical point, tissue or cell damage can occur such that even with release of the occlusion, blood flow cannot completely reverse the consequences of the ischemia and tissue death can occur.

The magnitude and the distribution of CO are thus the result of the interaction of the heart and the vasculature. The balance between central control mechanisms and local control mechanisms in modulating vascular resistance in the various tissues of the body is the primary determinant of the distribution of the CO. To illustrate the interaction of the central and local mechanisms in regulating CO and its distribution, the following discussion illustrates two physiological states in which the sympathetic nervous system is very active but in which the outcome of high sympathetic nervous system activity is dependent on many contributing factors. One state in which the sympathetic nervous system activity is elevated is exercise, which is characterized by a high CO. Another state in which the sympathetic nervous system is active is blood loss or hemorrhage in which CO is normal or depressed depending on the severity of the blood loss. Not only is the magnitude of the CO different in these two states, but also the distribution of the CO is different. In both states the blood flow to the brain and the myocardium is preserved (as long as the organism can maintain compensatory processes in the hemorrhagic condition) because local mechanisms are most effective in maintaining cerebral and coronary blood flow. In both states, blood flow to tissues that are highly innervated by the sympathetic nervous system will be restricted. These tissues are primarily organs of the gastrointestinal tract. The decrease in blood flow to the kidney following hemorrhage will depend on the severity of the blood loss; renal blood flow during exercise may only decrease at the more strenuous levels of exercise. Blood flow to the skin will be severely compromised under conditions of hemorrhage, whereas in exercise cutaneous blood flow will be modulated by the temperature control mechanisms initiated in the hypothalamus. Thus the central nervous system will be primarily responsible for changes in cutaneous blood flow that occur under both conditions of exercise and blood loss. The blood flow to skeletal muscle will show the greatest diversity in these two states of high sympathetic tone, and the distribution of the CO to skeletal muscle will depend on the level of activity by the individual muscles. The muscles that are active in the exercise state will have a significant increase in blood flow, whereas the muscles that are not involved in the exercise regime will have a minimal decrease or no change in their blood flow. The vasodilator theory can explain the control of muscle blood flow under exercise conditions. For example, if an arm exercise is performed, the metabolic rate in the arm skeletal muscle will increase to supply the greater amount of ATP required for muscle contraction. With this increased utilization of ATP and O_2 and increased production of vasodilator materials, such as adenosine, the arterioles of the active skeletal muscle dilate and blood flow increases. Local mechanisms will override central (sympathetic nervous system) mechanisms. Skeletal muscle blood vessels in nonactive muscles are contricted under the influence of the sympathetic nervous system. Since very little vasodilator material is produced, central mechanisms predominantly regulate tissue blood flow. Thus the distribution of the CO under exercise conditions is a balance between the sympathetic nervous system effects on vascular resistance and the active tissue's modulation of vascular resistance.

Table 9-1 gives an approximation of organ blood flow under three conditions. Cardiac output under resting conditions in a 70-kg individual is approximately 5800 ml/min. During an exercise bout, CO may increase four- to sixfold. For the example, CO is increased approximately fourfold to 25,500 ml/min. As an example of blood loss, CO has dropped by one-half to 2700 ml/min.

The following points should be noted:

1. Systemic vascular resistance is very low in the exercise state because of skeletal muscle vasodilation. This drop in vascular resistance in one organ system is balanced by increased vascular resistance in other organs (note the decrease in blood flow to gastrointestinal and kidney areas) and the CO that is so greatly increased that mean arterial blood pressure is maintained (or possibly even increased).

2. Systemic vascular resistance is very high in the hemorrhage state: although CO may be decreased by 40 to 50 percent, mean arterial blood pressure may be maintained or slightly decreased because of the high degree of sympathetic nervous system influence on vascular smooth muscle. If blood loss continues, compensatory mechanisms may not be

Table 9-1   Distribution of Organ Blood Flow and Other Cardiovascular
Variables in Rest, Exercise, and Hemorrhage

Variable	Rest	Exercise	Hemorrhage
Cerebral	750	750	750
Coronary	250	1000	250
Skeletal	1200	22,000	600
Renal	1100	250	250
Gastrointestinal	1400	300	250
Skin	500	600	100
Other	600	600	500
Cardiac output	5800	25,500	2700
Heart rate	70	180	180
Stroke volume	83	142	15
End-diastolic volume	124	167	18
Mean Arterial blood pressure	93	110	70
Systemic Vascular Resistance	16	4	26

able to maintain mean arterial blood pressure at this level and it may
fall progressively.

3. Cerebral blood flow is maintained constant to support tissue metabolic
    activity. Thus, it represents approximately 13 percent of the CO under
    resting conditions, 3 percent with maximum exercise, and 20 to 30 per-
    cent during blood loss.

4. Coronary blood flow is approximately 4 to 5 percent of the CO. With
    the increase in cardiac work that occurs with exercise, coronary blood
    flow increases to meet the increased O_2 demand. With hemorrhage, it is
    more difficult to predict an absolute level of coronary flow since the
    work demands are drastically changed. Contractility and heart rate are
    both increased by the sympathetic nervous system; they increase myo-
    cardial O_2 use. However, mean arterial blood pressure or afterload and
    volume work (CO) are both decreased and result in lower O_2 use by the
    heart. The absolute coronary blood flow (assuming normal coronary
    arteries) would probably be adequate for O_2 delivery until mean arterial
    blood pressure fell to 40 to 50 mmHg.

5. Under both conditions of high sympathetic nervous system activity, the
    venous compliance, especially in the splanchnic circulation, would be
    low, such that less of the blood volume would be in the venous system
    and mechanisms to enhance venous return would be elicited. Venous
    return (or CO) in the exercise state may be four- to sixfold greater than
    it was during resting conditions. In the hemorrhage state, however, ve-
    nous return is lower than it is during resting conditions (exactly how
    much lower will be determined by the extent of blood loss and capacity
    to compensate). In our example, venous return and CO would be 50
    percent of the resting level.

6. The effects of sympathetic nervous system stimulation on the heart are similar in exercise and hemorrhage in that both chronotropy and inotropy will be enhanced. However, due to the difference in blood volume, venous return is very different and therefore the loading conditions on the heart are very different. Although the ejection fraction (stroke volume/end-diastolic volume) may be increased above resting levels (67 percent) and similar in the two states, in hemorrhage the end-diastolic volume will be very low. With an ejection fraction of 85 percent in the example, end-diastolic volume would be 18 ml. During exercise, heart rate might be 180 beats per minute as in hemorrhage and the ejection fraction might be 85 percent, but the heart would be working from a higher end-diastolic volume. If the stroke volume is 142 ml and the ejection fraction is 85 percent, the end-diastolic volume would be approximately 167 ml. High levels of sympathetic nervous system stimulation of the heart under two different conditions can result in very different COs and in a very different distribution of the COs depending on the coupling between the heart, the vasculature, and the blood volume.

Thus, not only can CO vary depending on the work demands of the body, but also the distribution of the CO can be altered to promote (facilitate) the delivery of O_2 and nutrients to the most active tissues.

BIBLIOGRAPHY

Berne RM, Levy MN: *Physiology* 3rd ed., St. Louis, Mosby Year Book, 1993, pp 478–486; 491–493; 532–543.

Guyton AC, Hall JE: *Textbook of Medical Physiology* 9th ed. Philadelphia, W.B. Saunders Company, pp 199–205, 253–254, 286–290.

Rhoades RA, Tanner GA: *Physiology*, Boston, Little, Brown and Company, 1995, pp 616–618.

10

CARDIOVASCULAR FUNCTION IN PATHOLOGIC SITUATIONS

Heart diseases are either congenital or acquired. The principal pathology can involve the heart valves, myocardial cells, gross anatomic defects, and coronary arteries, as well as the conducting system. Valvular heart disease produces its circulatory effects by either regurgitant or stenotic lesions. A regurgitant valve produces a relative volume overload, while a stenotic valve causes a pressure overload of the involved cardiac chambers. The contractile function of the myocardial cells can be diminished by inborn errors of metabolism, infections, or other toxicities such as alcoholic cardiomyopathy. Gross anatomic defects frequently result from congenital cardiac anomalies but can develop later in life (e.g., idiopathic hypertrophic subaortic stenosis or avulsion of a papillary muscle following myocardial infarction). Coronary artery disease is a frequent cause of heart disease in adults but is uncommon in pediatric patients. Diseases of the conducting system can be congenital, such as the presence of accessory conducting pathways (including Kent's bundle which causes Wolff-Parkinson-White syndrome), or acquired, such as the dysrhythmias associated with myocardial infarction. Pericardial abnormalities can also interfere with cardiac function.

VALVULAR HEART DISEASE

Abnormalities of the cardiac valves are either congenital or acquired. The etiology of the defect is probably less important than its location, the extent of the defect, and the rapidity of its onset. Lesions are functionally classified as stenotic, regurgitant, or both. Additionally, more than one valve can be affected at a time. Defects with a more gradual onset (e.g., rheumatic valvulitis) are better tolerated due to the development of compensatory mechanisms, while lesions of sudden onset (e.g., traumatic aortic incompetence) are not as well tolerated.

Valvular disease causes impairment of cardiac function, frequently with subsequent development of secondary myocardial failure. The two ways that valvular problems impede the heart's ability to function as a pump are the following:

1   Interference with ventricular filling during diastole (as in mitral or tricuspid stenosis).
2   Ventricular overloading with either excessive pressure (as in aortic or pulmonic stenosis) or excessive volume (such as caused by any valvular incompetence).

Aortic Regurgitation

With aortic regurgitation, the left ventricle must eject both the effective forward stroke volume as well as the regurgitant volume. Although the left ventricle must eject into the relatively high pressure aorta, the low aortic diastolic pressure facilitates early ventricular emptying. Characteristically, the left ventricle becomes markedly dilated and eccentrically hypertrophic. Compensatory mechanisms include elevated preload, tachycardia, and increased sympathetic tone. Although tachycardia and low aortic diastolic pressure reduce diastolic coronary perfusion to the hypertrophic left ventricle, coronary ischemia is uncommon because the oxygen demand for volume overload is less than that for pressure overload (e.g., as in aortic stenosis). Anesthetic considerations include maintenance of preload, slight afterload reduction (which helps reduce regurgitation), and tachycardia.

Acute aortic regurgitation is most commonly caused by trauma (e.g., chest-to-steering-wheel injury) and aortic dissection (secondary to conditions such as thoracic aortic aneurysm, syphilis, and Marfan syndrome). Left ventricular end-diastolic pressure rapidly increases due to inadequate time for left ventricular dilation and hypertrophy. Pulmonary edema is a frequent finding. The back flow of blood into the left ventricle causes premature closing of the mitral valve thus pulmonary artery pressure monitoring is no longer reliable in representing left ventricular diastolic pressure. Anesthetic considerations are similar to those during chronic aortic regurgitation, including aggressive vasodilator therapy and maintenance of tachycardia. The presence of aortic dissection increases the risk of inotropic therapy because increasing contractility can produce greater shearing forces to the weakened aortic wall.

Aortic Stenosis

Narrowing of the aortic valve causes obstruction to left ventricular ejection. To maintain forward flow, greater intraventricular systolic pressure is required. Conforming to Laplace's law (pressure = tension/radius), the increased intraventricular pressure proportionately increases wall tension even if the chamber radius remains relatively unchanged. In order to compensate, concentric left ventricular hypertrophy increases wall thickness normalizing wall tension and contractility. The cost of the thickened wall is decreased systolic compliance. Large changes in diastolic pressure produce small changes in left ventricular end diastolic volume. Due to the decreased ventricular compliance, normal or greater than normal sinus atrial contraction is necessary to maintain ventricular filling and stroke volume. The exceedingly high intraventricular systolic pressure precludes coronary perfusion during systole, while the combination of decreased aortic diastolic pressure and increased ventricular filling pressures can impair diastolic coronary perfusion, especially in the presence of coronary artery disease.

In summary, aortic stenosis causes obstruction to left ventricular ejection. The increased intraventricular pressure stimulates hypertrophy of the left ventricular wall. As an early response, the left ventricular compliance decreases while contractility is maintained. Increased ventricular filling pressure combined with the "atrial kick" maintains normal stroke volume. Later fibrosis and progressive myocardial disfunction decrease ventricular contractility producing chamber dilation, decreased stroke volume, and reduced ejection fraction.

Mitral Regurgitation

Mitral regurgitation reduces the net movement of blood from the left atrium into the left ventricle. The resultant build-up of blood in the left atrium progressively increases left atrial pressure and can result in pulmonary edema. The elevated left atrial pressures distend the thin chamber wall and increase the distance that cardiac impulses must travel during atrial depolarization. When the pathway becomes long enough, due to atrial dilation, impulses spreading progressively around the chamber can continue to travel around the circle causing "reentry" of the impulse into muscle that has already been excited (also called a *circus movement*). Thus, dilation of a heart chamber favors progression to relative refractoriness or even out of the refractory phase by the time the impulse arrives back to cells originally depolarized. In a dilated atrium, the originally stimulated muscle may no longer be refractory by the time the impulse arrives from the other side of the chamber and so the impulse will continue to circle again and again. Decreased conduction velocity (due to blockage of the conducting system, myocardial ischemia, or electrolyte abnormalities) also favors circus movement. Additionally, shortening of the refractory period, which occurs in response to catecholamines (e.g., due to increased sympathetic tone commonly present in patients with valvular heart disease), predisposes to reentry as well. Reentry (Table 10-1) can result in the development of flutter or fibrillation.

The dilated atrium usually is in fibrillation, which further reduces the effectiveness of cardiac function. Compensation for mitral valvular disease results in increased blood volume mainly due to fluid retention by the kidneys. By increasing venous return cardiac output is maintained until late stages of the disease.

Table 10-1   Factors Contributing to Reentry (Circus Movement)

Dilated chamber lengthens pathway for the impulse
Decreased conduction velocity
Shortened refractory period

The backup of blood into the pulmonary circulation raises pulmonary artery pressure causing right ventricular hypertrophy.

During exercise, fatigue rapidly develops because the diminished cardiac reserve does not allow cardiac output to increase as it should. The decrease in cardiac reserve is proportional to the severity of the valvular dysfunction. Exercise can cause acute left ventricular failure and severe pulmonary edema due to great increases in blood returning from the peripheral circulation.

Rupture of the papillary muscle due to trauma or necrosis (e.g., secondary to myocardial infarction) can produce acute mitral regurgitation, left heart failure, and acute pulmonary edema. The highly compliant left atrium markedly enlarges, resulting in normal or only slightly elevated left atrial pressure even with long-standing regurgitation. Pulmonary hypertension is late in development unless there is a significant degree of left ventricular dysfunction.

Anesthetic considerations are summarized as "fast, full, and vasodilated." An enlarged V wave on the left atrial pressure tracing is related to left atrial compliance and extent of regurgitation. The presence of the V wave on the pulmonary artery catheter tracing can be misinterpreted as a ventricular pressure tracing when the tip of the catheter is already in the pulmonary artery. This can result in advancing the catheter too far distally, increasing the risk of pulmonary arterial rupture.

Mitral Stenosis

Rheumatic heart disease, while decreasing in frequency, is still the most common cause of mitral valve stenosis. The combination of volume underload of the left ventricle and pressure overload of the left atrium predisposes to pulmonary edema and low cardiac output. Tachycardia reduces diastolic time for left ventricular filling, frequently precipitating acute pulmonary edema. The high left atrial pressure leads to pulmonary hypertension and right heart failure. Diastolic filling time is probably more important than atrial contractions for left ventricular filling. Atrial fibrillation does not cause acute decompensation unless there is a rapid ventricular rate that reduces diastolic ventricular filling time.

Anesthetic considerations include maintenance of a low-to-moderate heart rate with mild afterload reduction. Pulmonary hypertension should be minimized by reducing the stimulants for hypoxic pulmonary vasoconstriction: hypoxia, hypercarbia, acidosis, and atelectasis.

Pulmonic Stenosis

Congenital valvular stenosis most commonly involves the pulmonary valve, usually associated with a ventricular septal defect or the tetralogy of Fallot. When pulmonic or subpulmonic stenosis (which occurs in the pulmonary ventricular infundibulum below the pulmonary valve) is severe, survival is possible only if an adequate volume of blood flows through the ductus arteriosus. Patency of the

Table 10-2   Surgical Palliative Proedures to Increase Pulmonary Blood Flow

Classic Blalock-Taussig shunt	Right subclavian artery to right pulmonary artery
Modified Blalock-Taussig shunt	Left subclavian artery to left pulmonary artery (using synthetic graft)
Glenn shunt	Superior vena cava to right pulmonary artery
Pott's shunt	Descending aorta to left pulmonary artery
Waterston's shunt	Ascending aorta to right pulmonary artery
Fontan operation	Right atrium to pulmonary artery

ductus arteriosus is essential to allow blood to go from the aorta to the pulmonary artery and be oxygenated. Spontaneous closure of the ductus arteriosus can be inhibited by infusions of prostaglandin E_1. Surgical anastomoses (Table 10-2) must be created when there is inadequate pulmonary blood flow.

Successful repair of the tetralogy of Fallot opens the pulmonary stenosis and closes the septal defect, increasing average life expectancy from only 3 to 4 years to 50 or more years. With tetralogy of Fallot, up to 75 percent of the venous blood entering the right atrium can bypass the pulmonary circulation and enter the aorta, producing severe cyanosis. Other associated findings include polycythemia, clubbing of the finger tips, systolic murmurs [caused by the pulmonary stenosis and ventricular septal defects (VSD)], systolic thrills, and a characteristic x-ray silhouette of the heart. Complications include gross retardation, failure of the right side of the heart, bacterial endocarditis, brain abscess, and frequent pulmonary infections usually causing death before adolescence in the untreated patient.

Rheumatic Valvulitis

Rheumatic heart disease can involve any valve, but the mitral valve alone is affected in nearly 50 percent of the cases. Both the mitral and aortic valves are involved in about 50 percent of the cases. Involvement of the aortic valve alone, or of the pulmonic or tricuspid alone or in combination with other valves, is rare. A development of thickening on the free margins of the cusps produces irregular warty vegetation (verrucae). Adhesions across the valvular commissures produces "fish mouth" or "button hole stenosis" of the involved valves. Relatively deficient coronary vasculature to the hypertrophic left ventricular wall predisposes the patient to coronary ischemia and angina.

Cardiomyopathy

Cardiomyopathy implies decreased myocardial contractile force. The decreased amount of functioning heart muscle frequently results in depressed QRS voltage. The most common cause of cardiomyopathy is ischemia. Both idiopathic and viral cardiomyopathy are also common diagnoses, in addition to end-stage congenital heart disease. The progressive reduction in ejection fraction leads to severe congestive heart failure refractory to conventional drug therapy. Low cardiac output may lead to decreased renal function and chronic passive congestion of the liver with hepatomegaly and ascites. Additionally, pulmonary venous congestion and interstitial edema may occur. Other types of cardiomyopathy include alcoholic cardiomyopathy, catecholamine myocarditis, and cardiomyopathy resulting from daunorubicin or doxorubicin (cancer chemotherapy drugs) toxicity. Other causes include systemic lupus erythematosus, hypertension, anemia, uremia, and coronary artery disease.

GROSS CARDIAC DEFECTS

Structural abnormalities interfere with the normal function of the heart by reducing its efficiency as a pump. Gross anatomic defects are either congenital or acquired and can involve any of the heart's chambers, valves, or the vessels leading to or from the heart. Embryonic defects in development during the period when the heart and great vessels are formed from the primitive vascular tube are responsible for congenital cardiac anomalies. They can be lethal *in utero* or can exert their effect during the transition from the fetal to the mature circulation. Their incidence is less than 1 percent of all births and their etiology is frequently unknown. Maternal infections such as German measles or nutritional disorders particularly during the first trimester of pregnancy are associated with an increased incidence of congenital heart anomalies. A simple classification of the more common congenital heart abnormalities is shown on Table 10-3.

About 80 percent of all congenital heart disease is caused by the eight most common lesions:

1 VSD
2 Atrial septal defect (ASD)
3 Pulmonary stenosis

Table 10-3 Common Congenital Cardiac Abnormalities

Without Shunt
Right-sided pulmonic stenosis
Left-sided coarctation of the aorta
Aortic (valvular) stenosis
With Shunt
Acyanotic
Atrial septal defect
Patent ductus arteriosus
Ventricular septal defect
Cyanotic
Tetralogy of Fallot
Pulmonic stenosis with reversed interatrial shunt
Eisenmenger syndrome
Tricuspid atresia (with arterial septal defect)

    4   Patent ductus arteriosus (PDA)
    5   Tetralogy of Fallot
    6   Aortic stenosis
    7   Coarctation of the aorta
    8   Transposition of the great vessels

Pathophysiology of Congenital Heart Disease

Normal development of the cardiovascular and pulmonary system depends on the presence of normal blood flows and pressures. Congenital heart disease produces abnormal systemic and pulmonary blood flow and resistance impairing cardiovascular development and decreasing cardiovascular reserve.

Pathophysiology of the Pulmonary Circulation

Excessive pulmonary blood flow (which can result from several causes including PDA, VSD, and ASD) produces hypertrophy of pulmonary vascular muscle, increased pulmonary vascular resistance, and elevated pulmonary artery and right ventricular pressures. If this condition persists for an extended period of time, *cor pulmonale* (right ventricular failure) frequently ensues. Conversely, pulmonary stenosis, whether valvular or involving all or part of the pulmonary artery, can cause right ventricular failure, while the reduced pulmonary artery blood flow produces ventilation-perfusion mismatching—predominately alveolar dead space.

Increased Pulmonary Blood Flow   The normal reduction in pulmonary vascular resistance (PVR) that occurs in the postnatal period is due to the expansion of the lungs with air. This expansion of the alveoli likewise expands the pulmonary vessels and reduces their resistance to blood flow. Additionally, inflation of the previously uninflated (atelectatic) alveoli releases hypoxic pulmonary vasoconstriction (HPV). The HPV is triggered not only by hypoxia but also hypercarbia, acidosis, and atelectasis.

The postnatal decrease in PVR results in left to right shunting from congenital heart defects such as VSD, ASD, and PDA. The increased pulmonary blood flow and pressure impede normal development of the pulmonary arterial system. Progressive hypertrophy of the medial (predominately smooth muscle) layer of the pulmonary arteries and thickening of the intima cause increased PVR. Later, changes include dilatation of the pulmonary vascular tree and pulmonary vascular sclerosis. If the excessive pulmonary blood flow persists, the anatomic changes in the pulmonary arteries become permanent, resulting in irreversible pulmonary hypertension. Severe increases in pulmonary blood flow can produce pulmonary hypertension in infancy, while lesser increases can be associated with onset of pulmonary hypertension delayed for several decades.

Decreased Pulmonary Blood Flow   Congenital heart defects associated with decreased pulmonary blood flow result in pulmonary arteries that are small and have decreased muscularity. Tetralogy of Fallot has been associated with a decrease in the number of alveoli and in the number of pulmonary arteries.

Pathophysiology of the Ventricles

Volume and pressure overload of the ventricles due to congenital heart disease produces degeneration of the cardiac muscle fibers and decreased cardiac reserve.

Patent Ductus Arteriosus   Persistent PDA can occur as an isolated lesion but more commonly can be associated with other congenital anomalies. Certain congenital heart defects such as transposition of the great arteries, tetralogy of Fallot, or severe pulmonary stenosis depend on the persistence of PDA to insure adequate oxygenation of blood. Other associated congenital anomalies include coarctation (narrowing) of the aorta, pulmonary stenosis, tetralogy of Fallot, and tricuspid stenosis or atresia. The ductus arteriosus arises from the left sixth aortic arch. The ductus connects the main or left pulmonary artery with the aorta distal to the take-off of the left subclavian artery. The ductus normally closes in the first 3 months of life but may persist as long as 1 or 2 years. Beyond this time, it is considered abnormal. PDA is about three times more common in females.

Characteristic clinical features include a pronounced systolic and diastolic murmur, characterized as machinery-like, usually with a systolic thrill. The systemic blood pressure is frequently reduced especially if the communication is large. An even greater reduction in diastolic blood pressure causes a wide pulse pressure similar to that found in aortic regurgitation.

The severity of complications associated with this condition depends on the size of the defect. Large defects are associated with heart failure, bacterial endarteritis of the ductus, and shortened life span. A small defect can be asymptomatic, with a normal life expectancy even if left untreated.

Mitral Stenosis with Atrial Septal Defect (Lutembacher's Disease)
Mitral stenosis may be caused by either a congenital valvular anomaly or acquired heart disease. The ASD would be relatively insignificant but for the high left atrial pressure due to mitral stenosis. The increased volume load to the right side of the heart causes right ventricular hypertrophy. Excessive pulmonary blood flow produces pulmonary vascular congestion, sclerosis, and pulmonary hypertension. Blood flow persists as a left to right shunt because the mitral stenosis raises the left-sided pressures and inhibits reversal of the shunt. Complications are the same as for simple ASD and include the following: 1. heart failure; 2. paradoxical embolism (a venous embolus into the systemic circulation via a right to left shunt), which can give rise to brain abscesses; 3. bacterial endocarditis with vegetations on the defect margins; and 4. pulmonary hemorrhages secondary to the pulmonary hypertension.

Coronary Artery Disease

Coronary artery disease is uncommon in pediatric patients except in the presence of certain congenital abnormalities such as hyperlipidemia or progeria. The usual progression of coronary artery disease is due to atherosclerosis starting with the development of a "fatty streak" in the lumen of the vessels. This is followed by organization, fibrosis, and calcification, which act to reduce the area of the lumen and restrict blood flow. Breakdown of the calcified plaque exposes a roughened area of intima which is prone to thrombosis (clot formation following platelet adherence and activation of the clotting cascade).

Focal reduction in coronary blood flow distal to obstructed vessels produces myocardial ischemia. This reduces the contractility of the affected cells and increases their dysrhythmogenicity. Additionally, ischemic cells are unable to sustain depolarization for as long as normal cells so repolarization occurs early in the affected area (which can produce S-T abnormalities and inverted T-waves, as discussed in Chap. 2).

Coronary ischemia results from an imbalance in myocardial oxygen supply and demand. Coronary oxygen supply is reduced by hypoxemia, anemia (although the decreased viscosity tends to increase flow), decreased diastolic blood pressure, and coronary obstruction. Myocardial oxygen demand is increased by elevations in heart rate and chamber wall tension (which is determined by contractility, afterload, and preload). The balance between supply and demand is the basis of complex clinical interactions involving myocardial ischemia and infarction. For example, digitalis increases contractility but can decrease ventricular rate, reduce wall tension, and improve diastolic pressure, usually resulting in improvement in myocardial oxygenation.

Conducting System Defects   Abnormalities in the heart's conducting system can produce heart block or hemiblock, reducing the effectiveness of cardiac contraction. Loss of atrial "kick" at a proper interval before ventricular systole can reduce ventricular filling and decrease stroke volume up to 30 percent. Conduction abnormalities are discussed in more detail in Chap. 2. As discussed earlier in this chapter, chamber dilation favors the development of reentry currents and related dysrhythmias.

Pericardial Abnormalities   The tough inelastic fibrous sac that encloses the heart can be associated with life-threatening abnormalities. Accumulation of fluid in the pericardial sac can lead to cardiac tamponade. Although chronic dilation of the heart can stretch the pericardium, acute increases in the volume of the pericardial contents (usually only a few milliliters of pericardial fluid) can cause a sharp increase in the extracardiac pressure of this poorly compliant compartment. As extracardiac pressure increases, diastolic filling of the atria and ventricles is impeded, resulting in elevated filling pressures (central venous pressure and pulmonary capillary wedge pressure) but low chamber volumes. Perioperative events that decrease preload or contractility can dangerously decrease cardiac output and blood pressure. Initiation of positive pressure ventilation, loss of negative intrathoracic pressure (such as caused by a thoracotomy), venodilation, and reduction of sympathetic tone all act to diminish preload. Reduced sympathetic tone, increased parasympathetic tone (reduces contractility up to 30 percent in addition to reducing heart rate), and cardiac depressant action of anesthetic drugs such as halothane all produce negative inotropic effects. Effective resuscitation of a patient decompensating from cardiac tamponade can be performed by pericardiocentesis with ketamine and/or local anesthesia. In this way, sympathetic tone, spontaneous ventilation, and negative intrathoracic pressure are maintained. Extracardiac tumors, such as pericardial cysts, can also interfere with chamber filling in a similar manner and additionally can compress and restrict venous inflow.

Constrictive pericarditis usually results from pericardial inflammation and subsequent adhesion of the fibrous pericardium to the epicardium, resulting in diminished cardiac compliance. Pericarditis can cause electrocardiogram changes—initially, ST elevation and PR depression, and later, T-wave inversion. Symptoms of pericarditis also include deep, constant, or pleuritic pain mimicking that of myocardial infarction in quality and location and frequently a pericardial friction rub (although this does not coexist with a pericardial effusion).

Diseases of the heart and pericardium reduce the effectiveness of the heart as a pump. Blood vessel disease affects the distribution of blood to the tissues and by altering the heart's afterload can affect cardiac output. Additionally, conditions such as Padgett's disease, hyperthyroidism, and arteriovenous malformations can reduce vascular resistance to the point that preload is so increased that heart failure ensues.

BIBLIOGRAPHY

Braunwald E: *A Textbook of Cardiovascular Medicine*, 3/e, Philadelphia, Saunders, 1980.

Guyton A: *Human Physiology and Mechanics of Disease*, 5/e, Philadelphia, Saunders, 1992.

Hollinger IB: Diseases of the cardiovascular system, in Katz J, Steward DJ (eds): *Anesthesia and Uncommon Pediatric Diseases*, Philadelphia, Saunders, 1987, pp. 93–151.

Stoelting RK: *Pharmacology and Physiology in Anesthesia Practice*, 2/e, Philadelphia, Lippincott, 1991, pp. 703–706.

Part Two

RESPIRATORY PHYSIOLOGY

11

FUNCTION AND STRUCTURE OF THE RESPIRATORY SYSTEM

OBJECTIVE

The reader should bo able to describe the function and structure of the respiratory system.

PERSPECTIVE

Oxygen must be available to most of the cells of the body in order for them to produce energy and function normally. Carbon dioxide, a by product of this aerobic metabolism, must be removed from these cells. Hydrogen ions are also produced as a result of several metabolic pathways, and the respiratory system assists in their removal. The respiratory system therefore takes oxygen from the atmosphere, supplies it to the cells, and removes from the body most of the carbon dioxide and hydrogen ions produced by cellular metabolism. Other functions of the respiratory system include acid-base balance, phonation, pulmonary defense and metabolism, and the handling of bioactive materials.

Gas exchange occurs in the lungs, which are ventilated by the action of the respiratory muscles under the control of the respiratory center in the brain. At the same time, the right ventricle pumps venous blood through the lungs via the pulmonary circulation. In the pulmonary capillaries, carbon dioxide is exchanged for oxygen.

STRUCTURE OF THE RESPIRATORY SYSTEM

The respiratory system consists of the lungs, conducting airways, the parts of the central nervous system concerned with the control of the muscles of respiration, and the chest wall. The chest wall is formed of the rib cage and the muscles of respiration, including the diaphragm and intercostal muscles. The abdominal muscles also function as part of the respiratory system, as discussed later.

Upper Airways

Air enters the respiratory system either through the nose, via the *nasopharynx* or through the mouth, via the *oropharynx*. It passes through the glottis and larynx to enter the *tracheobronchial tree*.

111

Tracheobronchial Tree

To reach the alveoli, inspired air usually passes through 23 *generations,* or branchings, of the tracheobronchial tree. The first 16 generations of airways, the *conducting zone,* do not bring inspired air in contact with mixed venous blood and thus are incapable of gas exchange. They constitute the *anatomic dead space.* Alveoli start to appear at the seventeenth through nineteenth generations, in the respiratory bronchioles, which are called the *transitional zone.* The twentieth to twenty-second generations are lined with alveoli. The alveolar ducts and alveolar sacs, referred to as the *respiratory zone,* terminate the tracheobronchial tree.

The many branchings of the airways result in a great total cross-sectional area of the distal portions of the tracheobronchial tree, even though the diameters of the individual airways are quite small.

Alveolar-Capillary Unit

The functional unit of the lung is the alveolus and its capillaries. The alveolus is the site of gas exchange between air and the blood. There are approximately 300 million alveoli in the normal adult lung. Each alveolus is literally enveloped in pulmonary capillaries. Estimates of the number of pulmonary capillaries are on the order of 280 *billion,* which works out to about 1000 capillaries per alveolus. Although not all of the capillaries of the lung are perfused when a person is at rest, estimates of the potential surface area of contact between the alveolar air and pulmonary capillary blood in an adult range from 50 to 100 m². This huge surface area combined with a small distance for gases to travel (normally about ½ μm from alveolus into blood vessel) makes the lung well suited for gas diffusion.

ANATOMY OF THE RESPIRATORY SYSTEM

Introduction

Anesthesiologists must be airway experts. A knowledge of airway anatomy is not only necessary for understanding respiratory physiology but essential for anesthesiological practice. The airway consists of the nose, pharynx, larynx, trachea, and lower airways.

Nose, Nasal Fossae, Paranasal Sinuses

The external nose (Fig. 11-1) is pyramidal in shape, with the bridge running from the forehead to the apex (tip). The external lateral walls are also called nasal alae. Skeletal structures of the nose include the lateral, greater, and lesser alar cartilages, the septal cartilage, and the nasal bone, which articulates with the frontal bone of the skull.

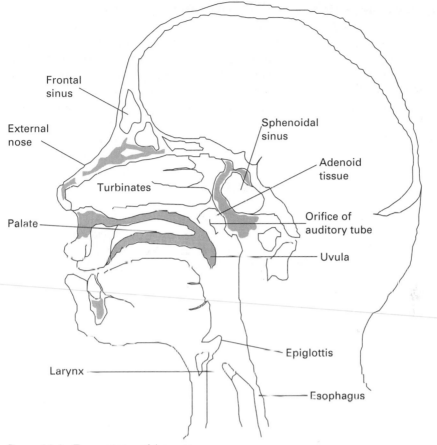

Figure 11-1 The anatomy of the nose.

    Each nostril or anterior naris opens directly into the vestibule, which is the slightly expanded forward portion of the nasal cavity. This vestibule is lined with cutaneous epithelium and in the lower half has hairs and sebaceous glands. The floor of the nose is at a higher level than the opening of the nostril, so when an anesthesiologist is performing nasal intubation, the apex should be pulled superiorly rather than directing the tube upward. The pathway of the tube is parallel to the roof of the mouth. Prolonged nasotracheal intubation is associated with obstruction of the nasal sinuses, sinus infection, and fever. Intranasal infections can produce intracranial infection via vascular connections, as noted later.

    The anterior portion of the external nose, the vestibule, expands above and behind into triangular spaces, or fossae, which are separated from each other by the nasal septum, which also separates the two nostrils. These fossae usually communicate freely with the paranasal air sinuses. They open into the pharynx by the posterior nares (also known as *choanae*) and are bordered medially by the nasal septum and laterally by three turbinate scrolls (*nasal conchae*) arranged one above the other. *Choanal atresia* is a birth defect that obstructs the airway of the obligate nose-breathing newborn.

The conchae project as more or less horizontally placed ledges from the lateral walls and have their free margins directed downward and inward. The spaces that these conchae overlie and partly shut off from the nasal cavity are the superior, middle, and inferior meatus (openings to the paranasal sinuses).

The superior concha is by far the smallest of the three, and the middle extends forward much farther than the superior. The inferior concha, which lies along the lower part of the lateral wall of the nasal cavity, is in the pathway of airflow in the nose. It reaches within about 2 cm of the middle of the anterior naris and its posterior tip lies approximately 1 cm in front of the pharyngeal orifice of the eustachian tube. Eustachian drainage can become obstructed when it becomes inflamed, which may lead to middle ear disease.

The nasal cavities are lined with mucous membranes continuous with those of the pharynx. The mucosa can be divided into respiratory and olfactory areas because it not only lines the tracts followed by respired air but also covers the cells that act as the receptors for smell. The respiratory mucosal tract lines the lower two-thirds of the nose, most of the pharynx, and the rest of the airways down to the level of the terminal bronchioles. It consists of ciliated epithelial cells and mucous glands. The motion of the cilia is toward the exterior, and the amount of mucus produced can often be copious. Thus, dust and other particles, as well as the mucus produced, are carried toward the naso- and oropharynx. The olfactory epithelium occupies the apical one-third of the nasal cavity and consists of specialized cells. The principal arterial supply of the nasal fossae comes from the ophthalmic arteries via the anterior and posterior ethmoid branches and from the internal maxillary artery through the sphenopalatine arteries. The veins accompany the arteries; the ethmoid veins open into the superior sagittal sinus while the nasal veins drain into the ophthalmic veins and then into the cavernous sinuses (see Fig. 11-2). Infections in the nose (such as sinusitis caused by prolonged intubation) can result in meningitis, owing to these venous communications between the intracranial and intranasal circulations. The lymphatic drainage from the cavities of the nose is by way of the deep cervical lymph nodes along the internal jugular vein.

The afferent fibers from the olfactory nerves (cranial nerve I) pierce the openings of the cribriform plate of the ethmoid bone, then reach the rhinencephalon of the brain. The sensory nerves from the upper respiratory tract come from the ophthalmic (a branch of V) and the maxillary (another branch of V) nerves.

Functions of the nose include heating, humidification, and filtration of inspired air and olfaction. The inspired air is warmed very efficiently because of the rich vascular supply of the nasal mucosa. As long as the incoming air is not extremely cold, the nose itself can warm the inspired air to nearly body temperature. Inspired air is moistened to nearly 100 percent relative humidity.

The heating and humidifying functions of the nose are affected by general anesthesia. The inspiration of cold, dry gas often dries the nasal and pharyngeal passageways, causing sore throat even if no manipulation of the airway takes place. The hairs at the entrance to the nostrils are of minor importance to filtra-

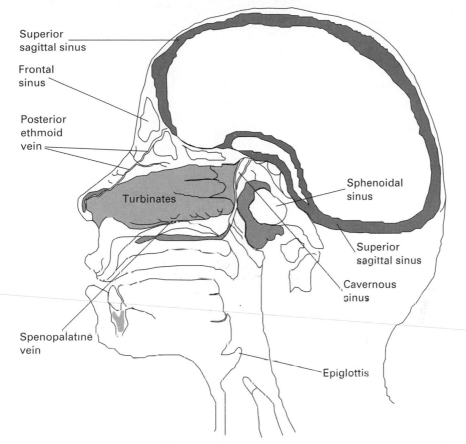

Superior
sagittal sinus

Frontal
sinus

Posterior
ethmoid
vein

Turbinates

Sphenoidal
sinus

Superior
sagittal sinus

Cavernous
sinus

Spenopalatine
vein

Epiglottis

Figure 11-2 Communications between the nasal and intracranial vessels. The posterior ethmoid vein drains the superior aspects of the nasal fossa into the superior sagittal sinus. The sphenopalatine vein drains the lower part of the nose into the cavernous sinus.

tion —they remove only large particles. Much more important is the removal of particles by turbulent precipitation. Air passing through the nasal passageways hits many obstructions—the septum, the turbinates, and the pharyngeal wall. When the air is forced to change direction the inhaled particles cannot change course as rapidly and embed in the sticky mucus-covered surfaces of these processes. The particles trapped in the mucus are moved by the cilia either to the nostril or posteriorly to the pharynx to be either expectorated or swallowed. This nasal mechanism for removing particles from the air is so effective that almost no particle greater than 4 to 6 μm is allowed to enter the trachea.

Pharynx

The pharynx (Fig. 11-3) is a wide muscular tube that is a part of both the respiratory tract and the alimentary tract. Its upper border is the base of the skull, and it extends downward to the level of the C6 vertebra, where it becomes continuous

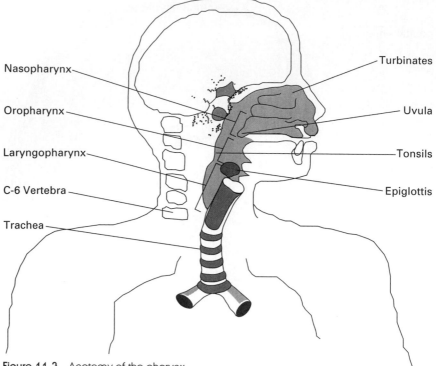

Figure 11-3 Anatomy of the pharynx.

with the esophagus. It is lined by a musculomembranous coat and is divided into three parts: (1) the nasopharynx, extending from the posterior nares (choanae) to the end of the soft palate; (2) the oropharynx, which is bounded superiorly by the soft palate, anteriorly by the tonsilar pillars, and inferiorly to the tip of the epiglottis; (3) the laryngopharynx, which extends from the tip of the epiglottis to C6.

The pharyngeal region includes the tonsils, which comprise three aggregations of lymphoid tissue: (1) the *palatine* tonsils (major tonsils), which lie in the tonsillar fossae; (2) the *lingual* tonsils, which extend across the tongue from the base of each palatine tonsil; and (3) the *pharyngeal* tonsils (adenoids), which lie on the lateral wall of the nasopharynx. The lymphoid tissue of the tonsils forms *Waldeyer's ring,* which acts as a first line of defense against bacterial invasion of the nasal and buccal passages.

Blood supply to the entire mouth and pharyngeal region is from branches of the *external carotid artery.* Venous drainage is via the facial vein and the external jugular vein. The nerve supply to the inner mouth is from cranial nerves VII, IX, X, and XII. The lymphatic drainage is abundant, draining into the cervical lymph nodes located under and anterior to the sternocleidomastoid muscle (explaining why lumps in the neck accompany a sore throat).

Important anesthesiologic considerations concerning the pharynx include peritonsillar abscess and hemorrhage following tonsillectomy. A peritonsillar abscess is a collection of pus in the tonsil region. It can easily be ruptured during intubation, and aspiration of the bacteria-laden material can produce a fulminant pneumonia. Therefore, intubation is usually performed when the patient is awake, so that the airway reflexes will protect against aspiration if the abscess ruptures. Posttonsillectomy hemorrhage is associated with multiple problems: hypovolemia, aspiration of blood, nausea, and vomiting of swallowed blood. During anesthetic induction the anesthesiologist may experience an obstructed field of vision during laryngoscopy because of the blood in the pharynx. Rapid sequence induction with *Sellick's maneuver* (cricoid pressure) is carried out with the patient supine and level. The Trendelenberg position may decrease the likelihood of aspiration but predisposes to regurgitation and thus makes laryngoscopy more difficult. The reverse Trendelenberg position, on the other hand, can decrease bleeding but increase the likelihood of aspiration during induction, so the optimal position for induction in this case is with the patient supine.

Larynx

The larynx (Fig. 11-4) lies at the level of the third to sixth cervical vertebrae. It is a protective structure that prevents aspiration during swallowing; vocalization evolved secondarily. Its structure consists of one bone, nine cartilages (Table 11-1), ligaments, muscles, and membranes.

The hyoid bone is the chief support for the larynx. Its anterior aspect can be easily palpated. The thyroid cartilage and the cricoid cartilage make up the principal part of the framework of the larynx while the epiglottis guards its entrance.

In the adult, the narrowest portion of the laryngeal cavity is the area between the vocal cords, whereas in children less than 10 years old, it is just below the cords at the cricoid cartilage. The clinical significance of this anatomic difference is that when small children are intubated, a tube may pass through the cords but be unable to pass through the cricoid ring.

The Laryngeal Cartilages

The epiglottic cartilage lies closest to the root of the tongue and is vertical to the opening of the larynx. It is attached by the thyroepiglottic ligament to the body of the thyroid cartilage just above the vocal cords, and is connected to the base of the tongue by the glossoepiglottic folds. The thyroid cartilage is the largest cartilage of the larynx, formed by two quadrangular plates or laminae (wings) fused near the midline anteriorly. It has great strength and affords a great deal of protection to the larynx. It is the cartilage of the Adam's apple.

The cricoid cartilage is palpable just below the thyroid and its level corresponds to the beginning of the trachea and the esophagus. It is the only true ring of cartilage encircling the airway. Anteriorly, the cricoid lies below the thyroid cartilage. The arytenoid cartilages articulate on the superior posterior aspect of

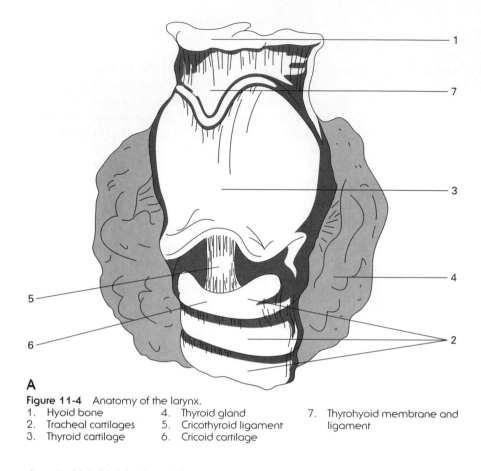

A

Figure 11-4   Anatomy of the larynx.
1.   Hyoid bone   4.   Thyroid gland   7.   Thyrohyoid membrane and
2.   Tracheal cartilages   5.   Cricothyroid ligament   ligament
3.   Thyroid cartilage   6.   Cricoid cartilage

the cricoid (which is slanted forward). The paired arytenoid cartilages are attached
to the posterior ends of the vocal cords. The paired corniculate and cuneiform
cartilages are embedded in the aryepiglottic folds and give support to these structures.

   Membranes of the Larynx   The thyrohyoid membrane suspends the larynx from the hyoid bone. The conus elasticus or cricothyroid membrane lies
between the cricoid and the thyroid cartilages. The easiest and most rapid lar-
yngotomy can be performed through it.

   Interior of the Larynx   The cavity of the larynx is divided into three compartments by the false vocal cords and the true vocal cords. The supraglottic area
extends from the false cords to the tip of the epiglottis. On either side of this area
is located a pharyngeal sinus (pyriform sinus). This recess or sinus is important
because it is likely to be the lodging place of foreign bodies entering the pharynx.
The second component of the larynx is that area between the false cords and the

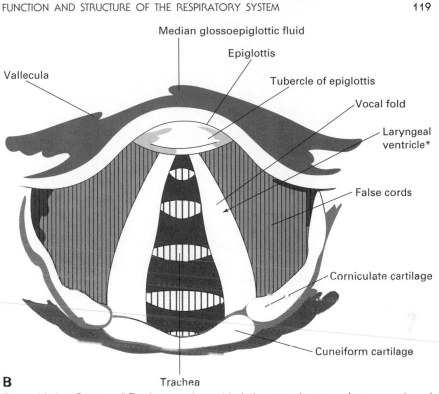

B

Figure 11-4   *(Continued)* The laryngeal ventricle is the space between the true cords and false cords

true cords called the laryngeal ventricles. The third area is the infraglottic region below the true cords and above the beginning of the trachea. The rima glottidis (glottic slit) is the space between the true cords.

Movements of the Vocal Cords   The true vocal cords are fibromembranous folds attached anteriorly to the thyroid cartilage and posteriorly to the arytenoids. The focal points of movement are the arytenoid cartilages which rotate

Table 11-1   The Nine Cartilages of the Larynx

Unpaired cartilages
1. Epiglottis
2. Thyroid
3. Cricoid

Paired cartilages
4 and 5.   Arytenoids
6 and 7.   Corniculates
8 and 9.   Cuneiforms

Table 11-2   The Intrinsic Muscles of the Larynx

A. Laryngeal inlet:
    Closed by the aryepiglottic muscle
    Opened by the thyroepiglottic muscle

B. The glottic slit
    Dilated by the posterior cricoarytenoid muscles
    Closed by the interarytenoid muscles and lateral cricoarytenoid muscles

C. True vocal cords
    Lengthened by the cricothyroid muscles
    Shortened by the thyroarytenoid muscles

and slide up and down on the sloping cricoid cartilage. The muscles controlling laryngeal movement (Table 11-2) are most conveniently thought of as pairs having opposing action. The laryngeal inlet is closed by the aryepiglottic muscle and opened by the thyroepiglottic muscle. The glottic slit is dilated by the posterior cricoarytenoid muscles and is closed by the interarytenoid muscles assisted by the lateral cricoarytenoid muscles. The cricothyroid muscles lengthen the true cords and the thyroarytenoid muscles shorten them. Both sets of muscles can alter the tension on the vocal cords.

Nerve Supply to the Larynx   Both the superior and inferior laryngeal nerves are branches of the vagus. The superior laryngeal nerve arises from the ganglion nodosum of the vagus and divides into two branches, the internal and external. The external gives a branch to the inferior constrictor muscle of the pharynx and also to the cricothyroid. These muscles change the position of the cricoid and thyroid cartilages and by doing so lengthen or increase the tension of the vocal cords. If these membranes are paralyzed, the voice becomes weak, rough, and easily fatigued. The internal branch enters the larynx and then the thyrohyoid membrane and is distributed to the mucous membranes of the larynx and epiglottis. The internal branch also innervates the interarytenoid muscles which are important in phonation.

The inferior or recurrent laryngeal nerves arise from the two vagus nerves at different levels. The left descends with the vagus and then loops around the aorta to come back up to the neck. The right travels with the vagus as far as the subclavian artery, around which it loops, then comes back up the neck. The recurrent laryngeal nerve supplies sensation to the larynx below the level of the vocal cords and innervates all the muscles of the larynx except the cricothyroid and part of the interarytenoid muscles.

The blood supply to the larynx arises from the thyrocervical trunk, which is a branch of the subclavian artery and comes via the superior and inferior thyroid arteries.

Trachea

The trachea (Fig. 11-5) is lined by ciliated columnar epithelium and extends from the inferior larynx to the carina, where the trachea bifurcates into the two main stem bronchi. In normal-sized adults the distances are fairly constant in that the distance from the incisors to the larynx is about 13 cm and from the larynx to the carina about 13 cm, so from the incisors to the carina is about 26 cm (note distance marks on endotracheal tubes). The trachea is formed of rings of cartilage that are open posteriorly, extending down to the level of T_{4-5} where the carina is located. This posterior T_{4-5} level corresponds anteriorly to the angle of Louis on the sternum which is the articulation of the second rib. The trachea is not a

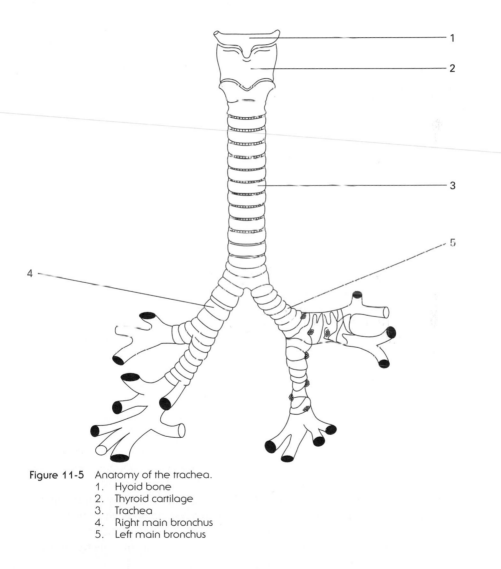

Figure 11-5   Anatomy of the trachea.
  1. Hyoid bone
  2. Thyroid cartilage
  3. Trachea
  4. Right main bronchus
  5. Left main bronchus

"fixed" structure; i.e, it will move with head or neck movement. If the patient flexes the neck, the trachea will move up (and an endotracheal tube will move down, possibly resulting in endobronchial intubation). Likewise, the trachea will move up if the patient turns his head to the left or the right. During extension of the head and neck, the trachea moves down and the endotracheal tube will move up (possibly resulting in extubation).

The blood supply to the trachea is via the inferior thyroid artery, which comes from the thyrocervical branch of the subclavian artery. The innervation is carried by the vagus.

The diameter of the trachea is about as big as the index finger. The main stem bronchi do not branch off at the same angle, the right being more nearly in line with the trachea (see Fig. 11-5).

The right main stem bronchus is wider and shorter than the left. In the adult the right main stem bronchus is only 2.5 cm long while the left is 4 cm long. As the right is more nearly vertical than the left, there is much greater tendency for either endotracheal tubes, suction catheters, or aspirated foreign materials to enter the right side. Additionally, if an endotracheal tube is inserted too far, its beveled tip also makes right-sided intubation more likely. The hole (Murphy's eye) on the nonbeveled edge of the tube is to deliver gas to the left main stem bronchus if the tip of the tube is on the carina.

The right main stem bronchus ends only 1.5 cm from the carina before giving rise to the right upper lobe bronchus. The other divisions of the right main stem bronchus are the right middle lobe bronchus and right lower lobe bronchus. The left main stem bronchus is narrower than the right and nearly 5 cm long. It terminates by bifurcating into the left upper lobe bronchus and the left lower lobe bronchus. The left upper lobe bronchus divides into two, an upper half and a lower (the lingular branch).

Each main stem bronchus divides into segmental bronchi that deliver ventilation to the various bronchopulmonary segments of the lung. Each subsegmental bronchus divides many times, giving rise to many bronchioles that still possess cartilaginous support. These bronchioles divide two or more times before losing their cartilaginous support and are then called terminal bronchioles. The terminal bronchioles are the last structures perfused by the bronchial circulation. The terminal bronchioles divide into the respiratory bronchioles, which are perfused by the pulmonary circulation and are the first place in the airway that alveoli appear. The respiratory bronchioles divide into several alveolar ducts that lead to circular spaces called atria. Each atrium opens into two to five alveolar sacs, which are spaces lined by alveoli or air sacs.

The lungs have a dual blood supply: (1) the bronchial arteries (usually one on the right and two on the left) arise from the descending aorta and in general serve a nutrient function to the lungs and the bronchi and (2) the pulmonary arteries, which bring mixed venous blood to the lungs. The flow through the pulmonary artery is the entire output of the right ventricle, while the flow through the bronchial artery is only about 2 to 3 percent of the output of the left ventricle. Bronchial venous drainage is either via the azygous vein or directly into the pulmonary veins. The pulmonary vessels meet and anastomose with the bronchial vessels at the junction of the terminal and respiratory bronchioles. The venous bronchopulmonary anatomoses are an important part of the normal anatomic shunt (see Chap. 14). During cardiac surgery when the patient is on complete bypass, blood will enter the left atrium even though all blood is shunted from the right ventricle by the venous cannula. This is because blood flow continues through the bronchial vessels that anastomose with the pulmonary veins and ultimately drain into the left atrium. This is one reason why a ventricular drain may be inserted during surgery to prevent overdistention of the heart.

The lungs are divided into lobes and segments. As stated earlier, the right lung is subdivided into the right upper lobe, right middle lobe, and right lower lobe. The left lung has only upper and lower lobes. The right lung has 10 bronchopulmonary segments while the left has 8. Segments containing the word "basal" in their name are located adjacent to the diaphragm. The lobes of the lungs are further subdivided into segments as follows (Fig. 11-6):

Right upper lobe: apical, posterior, and anterior segments
Right middle lobe: lateral and medial segments
Right lower lobe: superior, medial basal, anterior basal, lateral basal,
and posterior basal
Left upper lobe: apical, posterior, anterior, superior lingular and
inferior lingular segments
Left lower lobe: superior, anterior medial basal, lateral basal, and posterior
basal

The nerve supply to the bronchi and lungs arises chiefly from sympathetics and the vagus (which supplies sensation and parasympathetics). All conduits to the lung pass through the hilum, which is the connection of the mediastinum to the pedicle of each lung. The structures included in each hilum are the main stem bronchus, pulmonary artery and vein, bronchial arteries and veins, the lymphatics, lymph nodes, pulmonary nerve plexuses, and the pulmonary ligament. All this is surrounded by connective tissue. The covering of the lung, called the pleura, is a double-walled serous membrane. The two layers are the visceral pleura, which is tightly adherent to the lung surface, and the parietal pleura, which lines the interior of the chest wall and the diaphragm. These two layers meet at the hilum. Between these two layers is a potential space called the pleural cavity. The touching surfaces of the two layers of pleura are kept slippery by a small amount of serous fluid.

Mediastinum

The mediastinum (Fig. 11-7) is the region between the two pleural sacs. It is roughly in the center of the thoracic cavity but is slightly displaced to the left. It is divided into four sections: (1) The superior section is the space above a line from the angle of Louis to the body of T_4. Its contents are the thymus, lymph

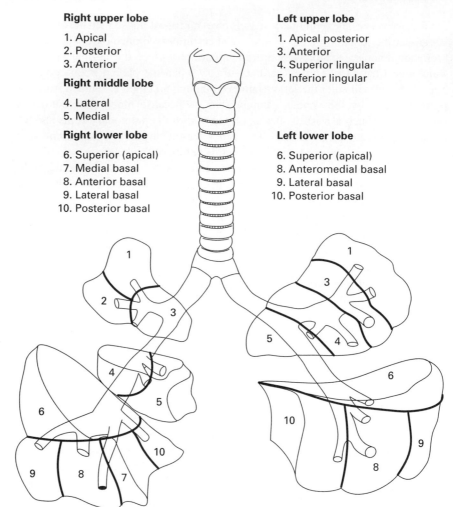

Right upper lobe

1. Apical
2. Posterior
3. Anterior

Right middle lobe

4. Lateral
5. Medial

Right lower lobe

6. Superior (apical)
7. Medial basal
8. Anterior basal
9. Lateral basal
10. Posterior basal

Left upper lobe

1. Apical posterior
3. Anterior
4. Superior lingular
5. Inferior lingular

Left lower lobe

6. Superior (apical)
8. Anteromedial basal
9. Lateral basal
10. Posterior basal

Figure 11-6   Lobes and bronchopulmonary segments.

nodes, the great vessels, left and right brachiocephalic veins (from the head, neck, and upper extremities), superior vena cava, aortic arch, trachea, esophagus, thoracic duct, vagus nerves, phrenic nerves, left recurrent laryngeal nerve, and parts of the roots of the lungs. (2) The anterior section is located between the anterior pericardium and the sternum. Its contents are inferior thymus, lymph nodes, fatty tissue, and internal thoracic blood vessels. (3) The middle section includes the pericardium, heart, ascending aorta, trunk of the pulmonary arteries, cardiac portion of the inferior vena cava and superior vena cava, azygous vein, phrenic nerves, lymph nodes, and part of the roots of the lungs. (4) The posterior section includes the bifurcation of the trachea, bronchi, esophagus, descending aorta,

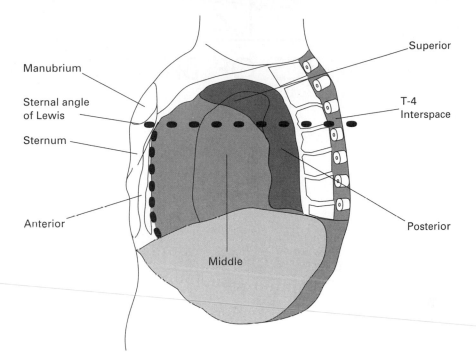

Figure 11-7 Compartments of the mediastinum.

thoracic duct, azygous and hemiazygous veins, vagus, sympathetic nerves, and lymph nodes.

BIBLIOGRAPHY

Levitzky MG, Cairo JM, Hall SM: *Introduction to Respiratory Care*. Philadelphia, Saunders, 1990, pp 88–99.

Netter FH: *The Ciba Collection of Medical Illustration*. Summit, NJ, Ciba, 1979, vol 7.

Netter FH: *Atlas of Human Anatomy*. Summit, NJ, Ciba-Geigy, 1989.

Nunn JF: *Nunn's Applied Respiratory Physiology*, 4th ed. Oxford, Butterworth-Heinemann, 1993, pp 13–35.

Proctor DF: The upper airways. *Am Rev Resp Dis* 115:97–129, 315–342, 1977.

Proctor DF, Andersen I (eds): *The Nose: Upper Airway Physiology and the Atmospheric Environment*. Amsterdam, Elsevier Biomedical, 1982.

Staub NC, Albertine KH: Anatomy of the lungs, in Murray JF, Nadel JA (eds): *Textbook of Respiratory Medicine*, 2d ed. Philadelphia, Saunders, 1994, pp 3–35.

Weibel ER: *The Pathway for Oxygen: Structure and Function in the Mammalian Respiratory System*. Cambridge, MA, Harvard University Press, 1984.

Williams PL, Warwick R (eds): *Gray's Anatomy*, 36th ed. Philadelphia, Saunders, 1980.

12

MECHANICS OF BREATHING

OBJECTIVES
The reader should be able to:

1 Describe the generation of a pressure gradient between the atmosphere and the alveoli.
2 Describe the passive expansion and recoil of the alveoli and the mechanical interaction of the lung and chest wall.
3 Describe the pressure-volume characteristics of the lung and chest wall and state the roles of pulmonary surfactant and alveolar interdependence in the recoil and expansion of the lung.
4 Define airways resistance and list the factors that contribute to or alter the resistance to airflow.
5 Describe the dynamic compression of airways during a forced expiration.

PERSPECTIVE
Air, like other fluids, moves from a region of higher pressure to one of lower pressure. Therefore, for air to be moved into or out of the lungs, a pressure difference between the atmosphere and the alveoli must be established. If there is no pressure gradient, no airflow occurs.

Air is normally moved from the atmosphere into the alveoli by causing alveolar pressure to fall sufficiently below atmospheric pressure to overcome the resistance to airflow offered by the airways. Because atmospheric pressure is conventionally referred to as 0 cmH_2O in discussions of pulmonary physiology (measurements in cmH_2O are used instead of mmHg because the pressures are generally lower than those encountered in cardiovascular physiology), lowering alveolar pressure below atmospheric pressure is referred to as *negative-pressure breathing*. In clinical practice it is frequently necessary to deliver air or other gas mixtures to the alveoli by raising the pressure at the nose and mouth above alveolar pressure. Such *positive-pressure breathing* is used on patients unable to generate a sufficient pressure gradient between the atmosphere and alveoli to move air through the airways. Expiration occurs when alveolar pressure exceeds atmospheric pressure by an amount sufficient to overcome the resistance to airflow offered by the conducting airways.

PRESSURE-FLOW RELATIONSHIPS IN BREATHING

The alveoli are not capable of expanding themselves. They expand passively in response to an increased distending pressure (that is, an increased transmural pressure gradient). This is usually explained by saying that contraction of the muscles of inspiration increases the volume of the sealed thoracic cavity, which, according to Boyle's law, decreases the pressure in the pleural space (the intrapleural pressure or, more correctly, *pleural surface pressure*), which pulls open the very distensible or *compliant* alveoli (Fig. 12-1).

The intrapleural pressure is normally slightly negative with respect to atmospheric pressure, even when no respiratory muscles are contracting. This pressure is usually about -3 to -5 cmH$_2$O at the end of a normal expiration (when all of the respiratory muscles are relaxed), because of the mechanical interaction between the lung and chest wall. The lung and chest wall are recoiling in opposite directions at the end of a normal expiration. The lung is tending to *decrease* its volume because of the *inward* elastic recoil of its distended alveoli; the chest wall is tending to *increase* its volume because of its *outward* elastic recoil. These two opposing forces are responsible for the negative intrapleural pressure. The intrapleural space is about 5 to 10 μm across and is filled with a *total* volume of lining liquid estimated to be only 7 to 15 ml. Thus the outside of the lung is virtually sealed to the inside of the chest wall by the pleural liquid. In certain pathologic conditions, material can accumulate in the pleural space (Table 12-1).

The events involved in breathing are summarized in Table 12-2. The diaphragm is the primary muscle of inspiration and is usually said to be responsible for about two-thirds of the air that enters the lungs during normal quiet breathing. It is innervated by the two phrenic nerves, which leave the spinal cord at the third through the fifth cervical segments. When the diaphragm contracts, its dome descends into the abdominal cavity, elongating the thorax. Because it is inserted into the lower rib margins, the lower ribs are also elevated during deep inspirations. The external intercostal muscles (and parasternal intercartilaginous muscles) raise and rotate the ribs, increasing the diameter of the chest and the transverse dimension of the lower portion of the chest. These muscles are innervated by the intercostal nerves, leaving the spinal cord at the first through the eleventh thoracic segments.

Initially, before any airflow occurs, the pressure inside the alveoli is the same as atmospheric pressure, that is, 0 cmH$_2$O, as shown in Fig. 12-1. *Note that the alveolar pressure is equal to the sum of the intrapleural pressure and the alveolar elastic recoil pressure.* As the inspiratory muscles contract, expanding the tho-

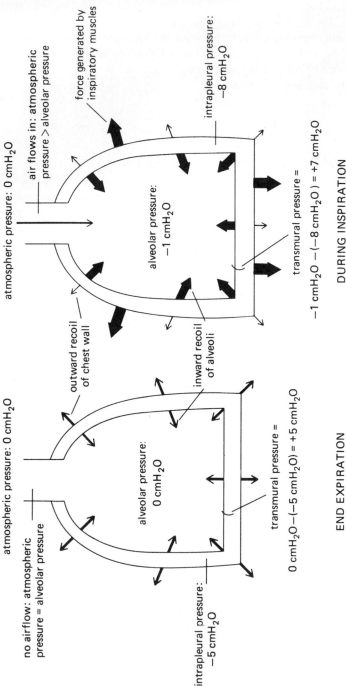

atmospheric pressure: 0 cmH₂O

no airflow: atmospheric pressure = alveolar pressure

intrapleural pressure: −5 cmH₂O

alveolar pressure: 0 cmH₂O

outward recoil of chest wall

inward recoil of alveoli

transmural pressure = 0 cmH₂O − (−5 cmH₂O) = +5 cmH₂O

END EXPIRATION

atmospheric pressure: 0 cmH₂O

air flows in: atmospheric pressure > alveolar pressure

force generated by inspiratory muscles

intrapleural pressure: −8 cmH₂O

alveolar pressure: −1 cmH₂O

transmural pressure = −1 cmH₂O − (−8 cmH₂O) = +7 cmH₂O

DURING INSPIRATION

Figure 12-1 The interaction of the lung and chest wall: A. At end expiration the muscles of respiration are relaxed. The inward elastic recoil of the lung is balanced by the outward elastic recoil of the chest wall. Intrapleural pressure is −5 cmH₂O; alveolar pressure is 0. The transmural pressure gradient across the alveolus is therefore 0 cmH₂O − (−5 cmH₂O) or 5 cmH₂O. Since alveolar pressure is equal to atmospheric pressure, no airflow occurs. B. During inspiration, contraction of the muscles of inspiration causes intrapleural pressure to become more negative. The transmural pressure gradient increases, and the alveoli are distended, decreasing alveolar pressure below atmospheric pressure, which causes air to flow into the alveoli. (*From Levitzky MG: Pulmonary Physiology, 4th ed. New York, McGraw-Hill, 1995, with permission.*)

Table 12-1   Abnormal Accumulations in the Pleural Space

Material	Name of condition
Air	Pneumothorax
Air under pressure	Tension pneumothorax*
Blood	Hemothorax
Pus	Empyema
Lymph	Chylothorax
Watery fluid (i.e., inflammatory exudate)	Hydrothorax (pleural effusion)

*A life-threatening emergency.

racic volume and increasing the outward stress on the lung, the intrapleural pressure becomes more *negative,* the transmural pressure gradient tending to distend the alveolar wall increases, and the alveoli enlarge passively. This lowers alveolar pressure below atmospheric, and air flows into the lung. Only a small number of alveoli are directly exposed to the intrapleural surface pressure; the distending pressure of the alveoli at the pleural surface is transmitted to more centrally located alveoli through the mechanically linked alveolar walls.

When alveolar pressure returns to 0 cmH$_2$O, airflow into the lung stops. When the inspiratory muscles relax, the intrapleural pressure becomes less negative, and the elastic recoil of the alveolar walls, which is higher at higher lung

Table 12-2   Events Involved In a Normal Tidal Breath

Inspiration

1. Brain initiates inspiratory effort.
2. Nerves carry the inspiratory command to the inspiratory muscles.
3. Diaphragm (and/or external intercostal muscles) contracts.
4. Thoracic volume increases as the chest wall expands.*
5. Intrapleural pressure becomes more negative.
6. Alveolar transmural pressure gradient increases.
7. Alveoli expand (according to their individual compliance curves) in response to the increased transmural pressure gradient. This increases alveolar elastic recoil.
8. Alveolar pressure falls below atmospheric pressure as the alveolar volume increases, thus establishing a pressure gradient for airflow.
9. Air flows into the alveoli until alveolar pressure equilibrates with atmospheric pressure.

Expiration (passive)

1. Brain ceases inspiratory command.
2. Inspiratory muscles relax.
3. Thoracic volume decreases, causing intrapleural pressure to become less negative and decreasing the alveolar transmural pressure gradient.†
4. Decreased alveolar transmural pressure gradient allows the increased alveolar elastic recoil to return to the alveoli to their preinspiratory volumes.
5. Decreased alveolar volume increases alveolar pressure above atmospheric pressure, thus establishing a pressure gradient for airflow.
6. Air flows out of the alveoli until alveolar pressure equilibrates with atomospheric pressure.

*Note that Nos. 4 to 8 occur simultaneously.
†Note that Nos. 3 to 5 occur simultaneously.
From Levitzky MG, Cairo JM, Hall SM: *Introduction to Respiratory Care.* Philadelphia, Saunders, 1990, with permission.

volumes, forces air out of the lung until an alveolar pressure of 0 cmH$_2$O is restored. Thus, during normal quiet breathing, expiration is *passive* and does not involve respiratory muscles.

   Active expiration occurs during exercise, speech, singing, and the expiratory phase of coughing or sneezing, and in pathologic states such as chronic bronchitis. The muscles of expiration are the muscles of the abdominal wall, including the rectus abdominus, external and internal oblique muscles, and transversus abdominus, and the internal intercostal muscles. Contraction of the abdominal muscles presses the abdominal contents against the relaxed diaphragm, forcing it upward into the thoracic cavity. They also depress the lower ribs and pull down the anterior part of the lower chest. The abdominal muscles are innervated by the lower six thoracic and first lumbar spinal nerves. Contraction of the internal intercostal muscles depresses the rib cage downward in a manner opposite to the actions of the external intercostals.

PRESSURE-VOLUME RELATIONSHIPS AND COMPLIANCE

One way to study the pressure-volume relationships of the lung is to remove the lungs from an animal and graph the changes in volume that occur as the transpulmonary pressure is changed. That is how Fig. 12-2 was obtained. The *trans-*

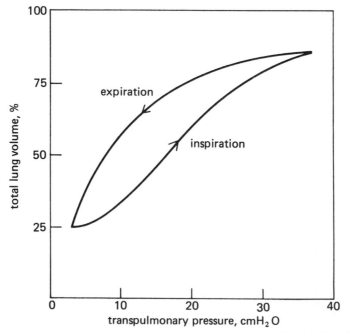

Figure 12-2 Pressure-volume curve for isolated lungs. *(From Levitzky MG: Pulmonary Physiology, 4th ed. New York, McGraw-Hill, 1995, with permission.)*

pulmonary pressure is equal to the pressure in the trachea minus the intra-pleural pressure; thus, it is the pressure difference across the whole lung. Under static conditions the pressure in the alveoli is the same as the pressure in the airways, so the transpulmonary pressure is equal to the *alveolar transmural pressure* or *alveolar distending pressure* when no air is flowing. Figure 12-2 shows that as the transpulmonary pressure increases, the lung volume increases. Note that at low lung volumes the lung distends easily, but at high lung volumes the elastic tissue components of alveolar walls have already been stretched and large increases in transpulmonary pressure yield only small increases in volume.

Elastic Recoil of the Lung

The slope between two points on a pressure-volume curve, like the one in Fig. 12-2, is called the *compliance*. Compliance is therefore defined as the change in volume divided by the change in pressure. Compliance is the *inverse* of elasticity or elastic recoil. *Compliance* denotes the ease with which something can be stretched or distorted; *elasticity* refers to the tendency for something to oppose stretch or distortion, as well as its ability to return to its original configuration after the distorting force is removed. As noted in the previous paragraph, the lungs are more compliant at lower volumes and less compliant at higher volumes. Note that the pressure-volume curves for inflation and deflation differ in Fig. 12-2. Such a difference is called *hysteresis*. Each alveolus can be thought of as having its own pressure-volume curve like the one in Fig. 12-2.

The compliances of the lung and chest wall can provide important clinical information, because many diseases affect the compliance of the lung and/or chest wall (Fig. 12-3). Pathologic conditions that decrease lung compliance, such as pulmonary fibrosis, pneumothorax, abnormally high alveolar surface tension, or lung collapse, shift the pulmonary pressure-volume curve to the right so that greater transpulmonary pressures must be generated to inhale the same volume of air. Decreased compliance of the chest wall may be caused by obesity or musculoskeletal deformities, and that also increases the work of breathing. Note that while total compliance for the emphysema patient is increased owing to loss of elastic fibers, breathing is usually carried out at very high lung volumes (barrel-chest) at which compliance is greatly decreased.

Compliances in series add as reciprocals; compliances in parallel add directly. The compliances of the lungs and the chest wall are in series, so

$$\frac{1}{C_T} = \frac{1}{C_L} + \frac{1}{C_W}$$

where C_T is the total compliance, C_L is the lung compliance, and C_W is chest wall compliance. The two lungs are in parallel, so their compliances add directly.

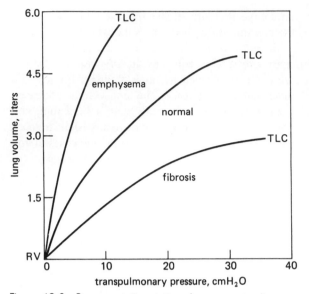

Figure 12-3 Representative static pulmonary compliance curves for normal lungs, fibrotic lungs, and emphysematous lungs. (*From Murray JF: The Normal Lung, 2nd ed., Philadelphia, Saunders, 1986, with permission.*)

Surface Tension in Alveoli

There is another component of the elastic recoil of the lung tissue besides the constituents of the lung tissue. That is the *surface tension* at the air-liquid interface in the alveoli.

The role of surface tension forces in the elastic recoil of the lung can be investigated using an excised lung, as shown in Fig. 12-4. At the right side of the figure, the lung was inflated with air and surface tension forces contributed to the elastic recoil of the lung. Then, all of the gas was removed from the lung, and it was inflated again, this time with saline instead of air, as shown at the left. In this situation of no gas-liquid interface, surface tension forces are absent. The elastic recoil resulted only from the elastic recoil of the lung tissue itself, and the lung was more compliant. Note that there is no hysteresis with saline inflation. Whatever causes the hysteresis appears to be related to surface tension in the lung.

The large role of surface tension forces in the recoil pressure of the lung could potentially make the alveoli unstable. If the alveolus is considered to be a sphere, then the relationship between the pressure inside the alveolus and the wall tension of the alveolus is given by Laplace's law:

$$T \propto \frac{Pr}{2}$$

where T is the tension in dynes/cm, P is the pressure in dynes/cm2, and r is the radius of the sphere in cm.

The surface tension of most liquids (such as water) is constant and not dependent on the surface area of the air-liquid interface. If we imagine two alveoli of different sizes connected by a common airway, then according to Laplace's law the pressure in the smaller alveolus must be greater than that in the larger alveolus if the surface tension is the same in both alveoli. Therefore, the smaller alveolus would empty into the larger alveolus.

Thus, if the lung were composed of interconnected alveoli of different sizes (which it is) with a *constant surface tension* at the air-liquid interface, it would be inherently unstable, with a tendency for smaller alveoli to collapse into larger ones. Normally, this does not occur, which is fortunate because collapsed alveoli require very high distending pressures to reopen. At least two factors contribute to the stability of the alveoli: *pulmonary surfactant* and the *structural interdependence of the alveoli*.

Pulmonary surfactant appears to be continuously produced by type II alveolar epithelial cells and is in some way destroyed or used up in the lung. Pulmonary surfactant lowers the work of inspiration by *lowering the surface tension of the alveoli*, thus making the lung more compliant. Surfactant also helps stabilize the alveoli by *decreasing the surface tension of smaller alveoli*, thus equalizing the pressure inside alveoli of different sizes. Thus, a relative lack of functional pulmonary surfactant decreases lung compliance and increases lung elastic recoil and the inspiratory work of breathing. It also leads to collapse of alveoli (*atelectasis*), which may result in an increased shunt (defined in Chap. 13) and decreased arterial PO_2.

The second factor helping to stabilize alveoli is their *mechanical interdependence*. An alveolus that begins to collapse increases the mechanical stresses on the walls of the adjacent alveoli, which then tend to hold it open. Conversely,

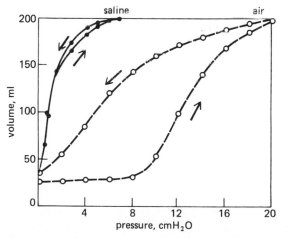

Figure 12-4   Pressure-volume curves for excised cat lungs inflated with air or saline. *(From Clements JA, Tierney DF: Alveolar instability associated with altered surface tension, in Fenn WO, Rahn H (eds): Handbook of Physiology, vol 2. Washington, DC, American Physiological Society, 1965, with permission.)*

if a whole subdivision of the lung (such as a lobule) collapses, the first alveolus to reinflate helps pull the other alveoli open.

Mechanical Interdependence of the Lung and Chest Wall

If the integrity of the lung–chest wall system is disrupted, as by a surgical incision or a knife wound, the inward elastic recoil of the lung is no longer opposed by the outward recoil of the chest wall; they are no longer interdependent. Lung volume decreases and alveoli begin to collapse. Air is sucked into the wound, causing a pneumothorax, until intrapleural pressure equals atmospheric pressure and the transpulmonary pressure gradient is abolished. At this point, nothing holds the alveoli open in opposition to their elastic recoil and they collapse. At the same time, the chest wall tends to expand because its outward recoil is no longer opposed by the inward recoil of the lung.

When the lung–chest wall system is intact and the respiratory muscles are relaxed, the volume of gas left in the lungs is determined by the balance of forces between lung and chest wall. The volume of gas in the lungs at the end of a normal expiration is known as the *functional residual capacity* (FRC); that is, the FRC is the lung volume at which the outward recoil of the chest wall balances the inward recoil of the lungs. At chest wall volumes below about 75 percent of the total lung capacity (TLC)—the volume of air in the lungs after a maximal inspiratory effort—the chest wall elastic recoil is outward; at chest wall volumes above 75 percent of the TLC, the recoil is inward. The higher the lung volume, the greater the inward elastic recoil of the lungs. Therefore, at high lung volumes, both lung and chest wall elastic recoil is inward and the total system recoil pressure measured at the mouth is positive. At low lung volumes (below the FRC), the system recoil pressure measured at the mouth is negative because the outward recoil of the chest wall is now greater than the reduced inward recoil of the lungs.

The lung volume at which the outward recoil of the chest wall is equal to the inward recoil of the lung (FRC) is much lower when a person is lying down than in the upright position. This is largely because gravity pushes the abdominal contents against the diaphragm, whereas when a person is standing or sitting gravity pulls it away. Studies have shown that the FRC decreases by about 1 liter (or about one-third) when a person lies down (see Chap. 21).

AIRWAYS RESISTANCE

We have seen that a major portion of the work of breathing is to overcome the elastic recoil of the lungs and chest wall; the other major component of the work of breathing is to overcome the resistance to airflow offered by the conducting airways. A few other factors are involved in the work of breathing, including the inertia of the system, which is usually negligible, and the pulmonary tissue resistance caused friction as lung tissues move against each other. The airways resistance plus pulmonary tissue resistance is often referred to as *pulmonary resistance*. Pulmonary tissue resistance normally contributes about 20 percent of the pulmonary resistance, with airways resistance responsible for the other 80 percent.

Laminar and Turbulent Flow

The relationship for pressure, flow, and resistance is

Pressure difference = flow × resistance

The symbol $\dot{V}$ is used to denote airflow, so

$$\Delta P = \dot{V} \times R$$

or

$$R = \frac{\Delta P}{\dot{V}}$$

The units of airways resistance are usually cmH$_2$O/liter/s. Recall that resistances in series add directly; resistances in parallel add as reciprocals ($1/R_T = 1/R_1 + 1/R_2 + 1/R_3 + \cdots$).

Airflow, like blood flow (see Chap. 5), can be laminar, turbulent, or transitional (a mixture of laminar and turbulent). During laminar flow:

$$\Delta P \propto \dot{V} \times R_1$$

and follows Poiseuille's law ($R = 8\eta l/\pi r^4$), but during turbulent flow:

$$\Delta P \propto \dot{V}^2 \times R_2$$

Flow changes from laminar to turbulent flow when a Reynolds number of about 2000 is exceeded. Reynolds number $= \dfrac{\rho \times Ve \times D}{\eta}$. One important difference between laminar and turbulent airflow is that during turbulent flow, the resistance term R_2 is influenced more by the gas density ρ; during laminar flow, the resistance term R_1 is influenced more by the gas viscosity η.

According to the formula for Reynolds number, turbulent flow tends to occur if the linear velocity Ve of airflow is high, if gas density ρ is high, and/or if the tube diameter D radius is large. True laminar flow probably occurs only in the smallest airways, where the linear velocity of airflows is extremely low. Linear velocity (cm/s) is equal to the flow (cm^3/s) divided by the cross-sectional area. The total cross-sectional area of the smallest airways is very large, so the linear velocity of airflow is very low. The airflow in the trachea and larger airways is either turbulent or transitional.

Airways resistance can be assessed with a *forced vital capacity* (FVC) maneuver. The subject makes a maximal forced expiration after a maximal inspiration, and the volume (in liters) exhaled is plotted versus time (in seconds). Normal subjects exhale more than 80 percent of the total volume in the first second; that is, the FEV_1/FVC is greater than 80 percent (Fig. 12-5). The FEV_1 is the forced expiratory volume in 1 s. The slope of a line drawn between the points at which 25 and 75 percent of the FVC has been exhaled (the $FEF_{25-75\%}$) is also useful.

Determinants of Airways Resistance

About 25 to 40 percent of the total resistance to airflow is located in the upper airways: the nose, nasal turbinates, oropharynx, nasopharynx, and larynx. Resistance is greater when one breathes through the nose rather than the mouth. Loss of pharyngeal tone during general anesthesia or endotracheal intubation can greatly affect airways resistance as discussed in Chap. 21.

In the tracheobronchial tree, the component with the highest individual resistance would obviously be the smallest airway, which would have the smallest radius. However, because the smallest airways are all arranged in parallel, their resistances add as reciprocals. Thus, during normal, quiet breathing the total resistance to airflow offered by the millions of small airways is extremely low, and the greatest resistance to airflow occurs in the medium-sized bronchi.

Bronchial Tone

The smooth muscle of the airways from the trachea down to the alveolar ducts is under the control of efferent fibers of the autonomic nervous system. Stimulation of the cholinergic *parasympathetic* postganglionic fibers causes constriction of bronchial smooth muscles (as well as increased mucus secretion). The preganglionic fibers travel in the vagus. Stimulation of the adrenergic *sympathetic* fibers causes dilation of bronchial and bronchiolar smooth muscle (and inhibits mucus secretion). This dilation of the airway smooth muscle is mediated by β_2-adrenergic receptors, which predominate in the airways. Selective stimulation of the alpha receptors with pharmacologic agents causes bronchoconstriction.

Inhalation of chemical irritants, smoke, or dust, as well as stimulation of the arterial chemoreceptors and other stimuli such as histamine, causes *reflex constriction of the airways*. Decreased CO_2 in the small branches of the conducting system causes a *local* constriction of the smooth muscle of the nearby airways.

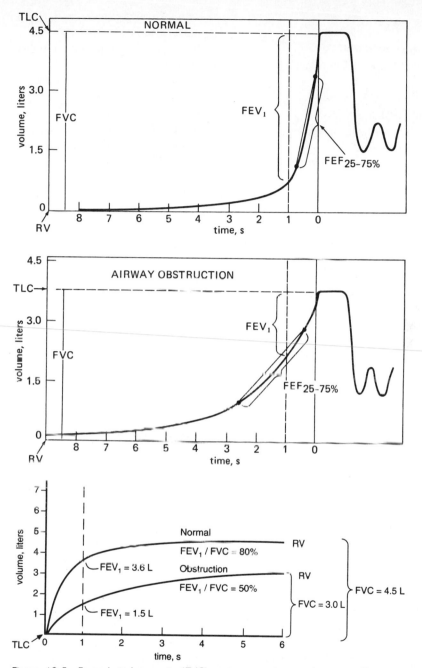

Figure 12-5 Forced vital capacity (FVC) maneuver using a spirometer. *Upper trace:* FVC from a normal subject. *Middle trace:* FVC from a patient with obstructive disease. FEV$_1$ = forced expiratory volume in the first second; FEF$_{25-75\%}$ = forced expiratory flow between 25 and 75 percent of the FVC. *Bottom traces:* Similar curves obtained from a more commonly used rolling seal spirometer. Note that the TLC is at the bottom and the RV's are at the top. The time scale is from left to right. *(From Levitzky MG: Pulmonary Physiology, 4th ed. New York, McGraw-Hill, 1995, with permission.)*

This may help to balance ventilation and perfusion after a pulmonary embolus. Increased CO_2 causes a local dilation of the small airways.

Lung Volume

Airways resistance decreases at higher lung volumes, and increases dramatically at low lung volumes (Fig. 12-6). Two factors explain this relationship between lung volume and airways resistance, both involving the distensibility and com- pressibility of the smaller airways, which have little or no cartilaginous support. The first involves the transmural pressure gradient. When a person breathing normally takes a deep breath to expand the lungs to a high volume, the intrapleural pressure becomes very negative. The transmural pressure gradient across the wall of the airways exposed to intrapleural pressure therefore becomes much more positive, and the small airways are distended. The second reason for the decreased airways resistance seen at higher lung volumes is the *traction* exerted on the small airways by attached alveolar septa (Fig. 12-7). As the alveoli expand during a deep inspiration, the increasing elastic recoil in their walls is transmitted to the attached airways, pulling them open.

Airways resistance is extremely high at low lung volumes. A forced expi- ratory effort to achieve low lung volumes generates *positive* intrapleural pressure, which can be as high as 120 cmH_2O during a maximal forced expiratory effort. (Maximal inspiratory intrapleural pressures can be as low as -80 cmH_2O.) This high positive intrapleural pressure generates a negative transmural pressure gra- dient that compresses and may even collapse small airways. The resulting in- creased resistance to airflow during a forced expiration is called *dynamic com- pression* of airways.

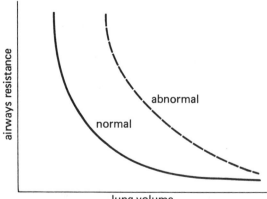

Figure 12-6 Relationship between lung volume and airways resistance. Total lung capacity is at right; residual volume is at left. *(Reproduced by permission of The Western Journal of Medicine (formerly California Medicine), Murray JF, Greenspan RH, Gold WM, Cohen AB: Early diagnosis of chronic obstructive lung disease, West J Med 116:43, 1972.)* (Reprinted by permission of The Western Journal of Medicine.)

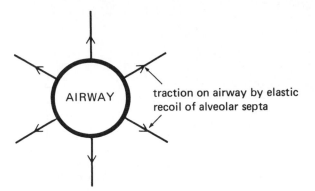

traction on airway by elastic
recoil of alveolar septa

Figure 12-7   Representation of "traction" of the alveolar septa on small distensible airways. *(From Levitzky MG: Pulmonary Physiology, 4th ed. New York, McGraw-Hill, 1995, with permission.)*

One way of looking at dynamic compression is the *equal pressure point hypothesis.* According to this hypothesis, at any instant during a forced expiration, there must be a point where the pressure inside the airway is just equal to the pressure outside the airway and the transmural pressure gradient is zero. Above that point, the pressure outside the airway is greater than the pressure inside it, and the airway is compressed and may even collapse if cartilaginous support or alveolar septal traction is insufficient to keep it open. As the forced expiratory effort continues, the equal pressure point is likely to *move down the airway* from larger to smaller airways because, as the muscular effort of expiration increases, intrapleural pressure increases and because, as lung volume decreases, the alveolar elastic recoil pressure tending to hold the airways open decreases. As the equal pressure point moves down the airway, dynamic compression increases and airways begin to collapse. This airway closure can only be demonstrated at especially low lung volumes in healthy subjects, but the *closing volume* may occur at higher lung volumes in patients with emphysema or in elderly subjects. Increased closing volumes result in increased shuntlike alveolar-capillary units, as discussed later.

Consider the pressure gradient for airflow during dynamic compression. During a passive expiration, the pressure gradient for airflow (the ΔP in $\Delta P = \dot{V}R$) is simply alveolar pressure minus atmospheric pressure. But if dynamic compression occurs, the effective pressure gradient is alveolar pressure minus *intrapleural pressure,* because intrapleural pressure is greater than atmospheric pressure and because intrapleural pressure can exert its effect on the compressible portion of the airways. Because the alveolar pressure minus the intrapleural pressure is equal to the alveolar elastic recoil pressure, *the effective driving pressure is the alveolar elastic recoil pressure.* Thus, as lung volume decreases, alveolar elastic recoil decreases, and the driving pressure for forced expiratory airflow decreases.

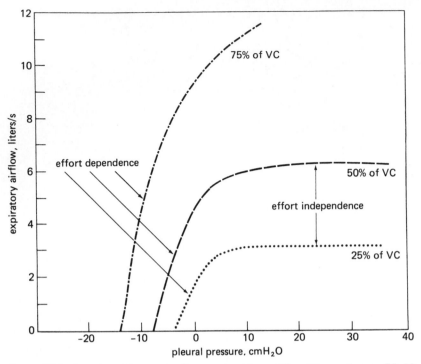

Figure 12-8 Isovolumetric pressure-flow curves at three different lung volumes: 75, 50, and 25 percent of the vital capacity. *(From Hyatt RE: Dynamic lung volumes, in Fenn WO, Rahn H (eds): Handbook of Physiology, vol 2. Washington, DC, American Physiological Society, 1965, with permission.)*

One way to demonstrate the interaction of the dynamic compression of the airways and the lung volume is the *isovolumetric pressure-flow curve*. These curves are obtained by having a subject make repeated forced expiratory maneuvers with different degrees of effort and plotting the pressure-flow relationship at a *particular lung volume*. For example, the middle curve of Fig. 12-8 was constructed by determining the intrapleural pressure and airflow for each expiratory manuever at the instant the subject's lung volume passed through 50 percent of vital capacity. (Vital capacity is defined as the maximum volume of air that can be exhaled following a maximal inspiratory effort.) The alveolar elastic recoil is constant for the curve because all points were obtained at the same lung volume. Increasing the expiratory effort increases airflow up to a point, beyond which further increases in intrapleural pressure do not increase airflow: Airflow becomes *effort-independent* because airways resistance increases with increasing expiratory effort. The equal pressure point has moved to compressible small airways and is fixed there. At very low lung volumes (25 percent of the vital capacity), at which there is less alveolar elastic recoil, this occurs with lower maximal airflow rates. At high lung volumes (75 percent of the vital capacity), airflow increases steadily with increasing effort and is entirely *effort-dependent* because

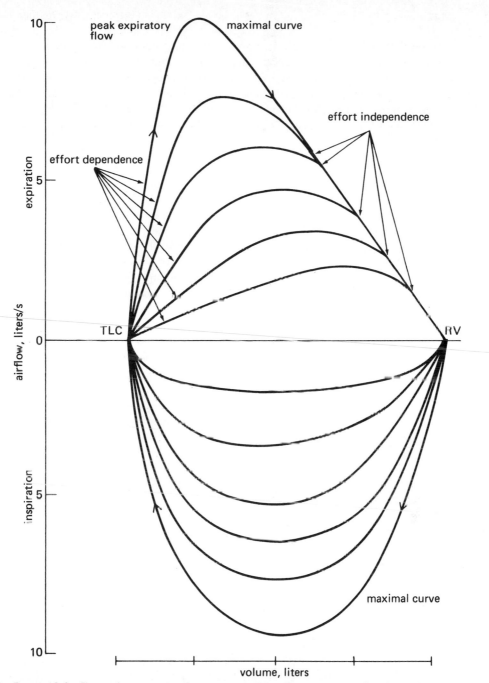

Figure 12-9 Flow-volume curves of varying intensities, demonstrating effort dependence at high lung volumes and effort independence at low lung volumes. Note that there is no effort independence in inspiration. *(From Levitzky MG, Pulmonary Physiology, 4th ed. New York, McGraw-Hill, 1995, with permission.)*

alveolar elastic recoil pressure is high and because highly positive intrapleural pressures cannot be attained at such high lung volumes (if the glottis is open). The concepts of dynamic compression and effort independence can also be seen in *flow-volume curves* (Fig. 12-9) that plot lung volume versus airflow for expiratory and inspiratory efforts of varying intensities. Note the effort independence at low lung volumes in the expiratory curves. There is no effort independence in the inspiratory curves.

THE WORK OF BREATHING

We can summarize the main points of the mechanics of breathing by considering the *work of breathing*. This can be defined as the pressure change times the volume change. The volume change is the volume of air moved into and out of the lung during breathing, the *tidal volume*. The pressure change is the change in transpulmonary pressure necessary to overcome the *elastic* work of breathing and the *resistive* work of breathing.

The elastic work of breathing is the work done to overcome the elastic recoil of the chest wall and the pulmonary parenchyma and to overcome the surface tension of the alveoli. The resistive work of breathing is the work done to overcome the tissue resistance and airways resistance. Normally, most of the resistive work is that done to overcome airways resistance, which is great during a forced expiration, particularly in patients who already have elevated resistance during normal quiet breathing. The work of breathing is increased in patients with restrictive lung diseases who have to expend much effort to inhale deeply. As a result, they usually breathe at higher rates with smaller tidal volumes. Patients with obstructive lung diseases usually breathe at lower rates and deeper tidal volumes. The mechanisms by which the respiratory centers in the brain make these adjustments are not completely understood.

BIBLIOGRAPHY

Barnes PJ: Neural control of human airways in health and disease. *Am Rev Resp Dis* 134: 1289–1314, 1986.

Barnes PJ: Airway pharmacology, in Murray JF, Nadel JA (eds): *Textbook of Respiratory Medicine,* 2d ed. Philadelphia, Saunders, 1994, pp 285–311.

Clements JA, Tierney DF: Alveolar instability associated with altered surface tension, in Fenn WO, Rahn H (eds): *Handbook of Physiology,* vol 2. Washington, DC, American Physiological Society, 1965, pp 1567–1568.

Gross NJ: Pulmonary surfactant: unanswered questions. *Thorax* 50:325–327, 1995.

Hyatt RE: Dynamic lung volumes, in Fenn WO, Rahn H (eds): *Handbook of Physiology,* vol 2. Washington, DC, American Physiological Society, 1965, pp 1381–1398.

Hyatt RE: Expiratory flow limitation. *J Appl Physiol* 55:1–8, 1983.

Levitzky MG: *Pulmonary Physiology,* 4th ed. New York, McGraw-Hill, 1995, pp 12–54.

Levitzky MG, Cairo JM, Hall SM: *Introduction to Respiratory Care.* Philadelphia, Saunders, 1990, pp 99–111.

Milic-Emili J: Pulmonary statics, in Widdicombe JG (ed): *MTP International Review of Science: Respiratory Physiology.* London, Butterworth, 1974, pp 105–137.

Murray JF: *The Normal Lung,* 2d ed. Philadelphia, Saunders, 1986, pp 83–138.

Murray JF, Greenspan RH, Gold WM, Cohn AB: Early diagnosis of chronic obstructive lung disease. *West J Med* 116:37–55, 1972.

Nunn JF: *Nunn's Applied Respiratory Physiology,* 4th ed. Oxford, Butterworth-Heinemann, 1993, pp 36–89, 117–128.

Ward ME, Roussos C, Macklem PT: Respiratory mechanics, in Murray JF, Nadel JA (eds): *Textbook of Respiratory Medicine,* 2d ed. Philadelphia, Saunders, 1994, pp 90–138.

Weibel ER: *The Pathway for Oxygen: Structure and Function in the Mammalian Respiratory System.* Cambridge, MA, Harvard University Press, 1984, pp 302–338.

13

ALVEOLAR VENTILATION

OBJECTIVES

The reader should be able to:

1 Define alveolar ventilation and the standard lung volumes and capacities.
2 Define physiologic, anatomic, and alveolar dead space.
3 Predict the effects of alterations of alveolar ventilation on alveolar carbon dioxide and oxygen levels.
4 Describe the regional differences in alveolar ventilation found in the normal lung and explain these differences.

PERSPECTIVE

Alveolar ventilation is defined as the volume of fresh air entering and alveolar air leaving the alveoli per minute. The two volumes are not usually exactly equal because not every molecule of oxygen used by the body results in a molecule of CO_2 released by the body, and also because of the heating and humidification of inspired air. Alveolar ventilation is not the same as the ventilation per minute measured at the nose or mouth because not all of the air entering the body per breath reaches the alveoli. A substantial portion of each inspired breath remains in the conducting airways and does not enter the alveoli.

LUNG VOLUMES

The volume of gas in the lungs at any instant depends on the mechanics of the lungs and chest wall and the activity of the respiratory muscles. Standardization of the conditions under which lung volumes are measured allows comparisons to be made between normal subjects and patients. Because the size of a person's lungs depends on their height and weight or body surface area, as well as age and sex, the lung volumes for a patient are usually compared with data from a table of predicted lung volumes matched to age, sex, and body size. The lung volumes are normally expressed at body temperature, ambient pressure, and saturated with water vapor (BTPS). Note that to obtain most of the standard lung volumes and capacities, the subject must be conscious and cooperative. Subjects or patients unwilling or unable to fully comply with the instructions they are given for these tests will give erroneous data.

There are four standard lung *volumes* and four standard lung *capacities,* which are combinations of the standard lung volumes. These are shown in Fig. 13-1.

Tidal Volume   The tidal volume (TV, or V_T) is the volume of air coming into or out of the nose or mouth per breath. It is determined by the activity of the respiratory control centers in the brain, the contraction of respiratory muscles, and the mechanics of the lung and chest wall. During normal quiet breathing (eupnea), the tidal volume of a 70-kg adult is about 500 ml per breath, but this can be greatly increased, as in exercise.

Residual Volume   The residual volume (RV) is the volume of gas left in the lungs after a maximal forced expiration. It is determined by the force generated by the muscles of expiration acting in concert with the inward elastic recoil of the lungs, in opposition to the outward elastic recoil of the chest wall. Dynamic compression of the airways during the forced expiratory effort may also be an important determinant of the residual volume as airway collapse occurs, trapping gas in the alveoli. The residual volume of a healthy 70-kg adult is about 1.5 liters, but it can be much greater in obstructive lung diseases such as emphysema.

Expiratory Reserve Volume   The expiratory reserve volume (ERV) is the volume of gas expelled from the lungs during a maximal forced expiration that *starts* at the end of a normal tidal expiration. It is therefore determined by the difference between the functional residual capacity and the residual volume. The expiratory reserve volume is about 1.5 liters in a healthy 70-kg adult.

Inspiratory Reserve Volume   The inspiratory reserve volume (IRV) is the volume of gas inhaled into the lungs during a maximal forced inspiration that starts at the end of a normal tidal inspiration. It is determined by the strength of contraction of the inspiratory muscles, the inward elastic recoil of the lungs and chest wall, and the starting point, which is the functional residual capacity plus the tidal volume. The inspiratory reserve volume of a normal 70-kg adult is about 2.5 liters.

Functional Residual Capacity   The functional residual capacity (FRC) is the volume of gas remaining in the lungs at the end of a normal tidal expiration. Because no respiratory muscles are contacting at this time, it represents the balance point between the inward elastic recoil of the lungs and the outward elastic recoil of the chest wall, as discussed earlier. The FRC, as seen in Fig. 13-1, consists of the residual volume plus the expiratory reserve volume. It is therefore about 3 liters in a healthy 70-kg adult.

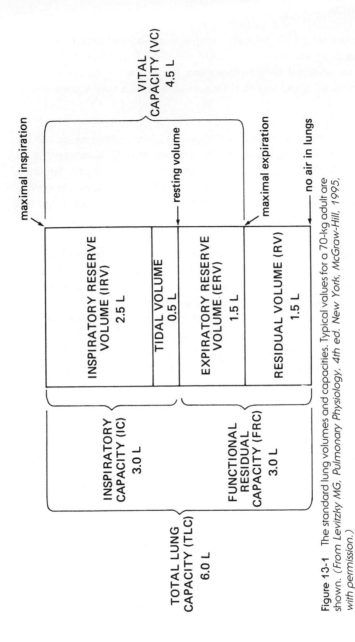

Figure 13-1 The standard lung volumes and capacities. Typical values for a 70-kg adult are shown. (*From Levitzky MG, Pulmonary Physiology, 4th ed. New York, McGraw-Hill, 1995, with permission.*)

Inspiratory Capacity   The inspiratory capacity (IC) is the volume of air inhaled into the lungs during a maximal inspiratory effort that begins at the end of a normal tidal expiration (the FRC). It is therefore equal to the tidal volume plus the inspiratory reserve volume. The inspiratory capacity of a normal 70-kg adult is about 3 liters.

Total Lung Capacity   The total lung capacity (TLC) is the volume of air in the lungs after a maximal inspiratory effort. It is determined by the strength of contraction of the inspiratory muscles and the inward elastic recoil of the lungs and chest wall. The total lung capacity consists of all four lung volumes: the residual volume plus the tidal volume plus the inspiratory and expiratory reserve volumes. It is about 6 liters in the healthy 70-kg adult.

Vital Capacity   The vital capacity (VC) is the volume of air expelled from the lungs during a maximal forced expiration starting after a maximal forced inspiration. The vital capacity is therefore equal to the total lung capacity minus the residual volume, or about 4.5 liters in a healthy 70-kg adult. The vital capacity is also equal to the sum of the tidal volume and the inspiratory and expiratory reserve volumes. It is determined by the same factors that determine total lung capacity and residual volume.

Measurement of the lung volumes is important because many pathologic states can alter specific lung volumes or their relationships to each other. *Restrictive diseases* (those decreasing lung and/or chest wall compliance) generally decrease the lung volumes and capacities; *obstructive diseases* generally increase the lung volumes and capacities, especially the TLC, FRC, and RV. Lung volumes can also change for normal physiologic reasons. Lying down decreases the functional residual capacity because gravity is no longer pulling the abdominal contents away from the diaphragm. If the functional residual capacity is decreased, then the expiratory reserve volume also decreases, and the inspiratory reserve volume increases. The vital capacity may also decrease slightly when a person lies down because some of the venous blood that collected in the lower extremities and abdomen returns to the thoracic cavity.

Standard spirometry can be used for the determination of many of the standard lung volumes and capacities but cannot measure the RV, FRC, or TLC, which must be determined by other techniques.

ANATOMIC DEAD SPACE

The volume of air entering and leaving the nose or mouth per minute, the *minute volume,* is not equal to the volume of air entering and leaving the alveoli per minute. *Alveolar ventilation* is less than the minute volume because the last part of each inspiration and each expiration remains in the conducting airways. No gas exchange occurs in the conducting airways, which constitute the *anatomic dead space*.

The relationship between the tidal volume V_T, the dead space volume V_D, and the volume of gas entering and leaving the alveoli per breath V_A is

$$V_T = V_D + V_A$$

or

$$V_A = V_T - V_D$$

Thus, if a person with an anatomic dead space of 150 ml has a tidal volume of 500 ml per breath, only 350 ml of gas enters and leaves the alveoli per breath.

Multiplying both sides of the above equation by the breathing frequency n in breaths per minute:

$$n(V_A) = n(V_T) - n(V_D)$$
$$\dot{V}_A = \dot{V}_E - \dot{V}_D$$

The alveolar ventilation $\dot{V}_A$ in liters per minute is equal to the minute volume $\dot{V}_E$ minus the volume wasted ventilating the dead space per minute $\dot{V}_D$.

The dots over the V's indicate *per minute*. The symbol $\dot{V}_E$ is used because expired gas is usually collected.

Alveolar ventilation cannot be measured directly but must be determined from the tidal volume, breathing frequency, and dead space ventilation. The anatomic dead space is normally about 2.2 ml/pound of body weight.

PHYSIOLOGIC DEAD SPACE

Another kind of wasted ventilation can occur in the lung—the ventilation of unperfused alveoli. Alveoli that are ventilated but not perfused are called *alveolar dead space;* they contribute nothing to gas exchange. Alveolar dead space may occur distal to portions of the pulmonary circulation that have become occluded by blood clots (pulmonary emboli) or if right ventricular output is unable to perfuse upper regions of the lungs. Young healthy adults usually do not have any alveolar dead space.

The *Bohr equation* is used to determine the alveolar dead space *plus* the anatomic dead space. This is called the *physiologic dead space* V_DCO_2:

Physiologic dead space = anatomic dead space + alveolar dead space

The Bohr equation is based on the concept that air expired from alveoli that are both ventilated and perfused with mixed venous blood contribute carbon dioxide to the mixed expired air, but air coming from anatomic or alveolar dead space contains only the tiny amount of carbon dioxide found in the inspired air.

$$\frac{V_D CO_2}{V_T} = \frac{Pa CO_2 - P\bar{E} CO_2}{Pa CO_2}$$

where $V_D CO_2$ is the physiologic dead space, V_T is the tidal volume, $Pa CO_2$ is the partial pressure of carbon dioxide in the arterial blood, and $P\bar{E} CO_2$ is the partial pressure of carbon dioxide in the mixed expired air.

Because alveolar dead space dilutes the CO_2 coming from alveoli that are both ventilated and perfused, it decreases the $P CO_2$ of end-tidal expired air (which is used to assess the alveolar $P CO_2$). Arterial $P CO_2$ is normally in equilibrium with the $P CO_2$ of alveoli that are ventilated *and* perfused. Thus the presence of *an arterial-alveolar $P CO_2$ gradient usually indicates the presence of alveolar dead space.*

EFFECTS OF ALVEOLAR VENTILATION ON OXYGEN AND CARBON DIOXIDE LEVELS

The levels of oxygen and carbon dioxide in the alveolar gas are determined by the alveolar ventilation, the fractional concentrations of oxygen and carbon dioxide breathed (the $F_I O_2$ and $F_I CO_2$), the oxygen consumption ($\dot{V}O_2$) of the body, the carbon dioxide production of the body ($\dot{V} CO_2$), and the flow of mixed venous blood to the lungs. Each tidal breath brings about 350 ml of fresh air, about 21 percent of which is oxygen, into the 3 liters of gas already in the lungs (the FRC) and removes about 350 ml of air, about 5 or 6 percent of which is carbon dioxide. Meanwhile, about 250 ml of carbon dioxide diffuses from the pulmonary capillary blood into the alveoli and about 300 ml of oxygen diffuses from the alveolar air into the pulmonary capillary blood each minute.

Partial Pressures of Respiratory Gases

According to Dalton's law, in a gas mixture, the pressure exerted by each individual gas in a space is independent of the pressures of other gases in the mixture. The *partial pressure* of a particular gas is therefore equal to its fractional concentration times the total pressure of all the gases in the mixture.

Oxygen constitutes 20.93 percent of dry atmospheric air. At a standard barometric pressure of 760 mmHg:

$$P O_2 = 0.2093 \times 760 \text{ torr} = 159 \text{ torr}$$

as shown in Table 13-1. (The units of pressure are expressed as mmHg, or torr, in honor of Torricelli, the inventor of the barometer.) Carbon dioxide constitutes

Table 13-1   Gas Partial Pressures at Standard Barometric Pressure Units torr, or mmHg

	P_{O_2}	P_{CO_2}	P_{H_2O}	P_{N_2}
Dry atmospheric air	159.0	0.3	0	600.6
Inspired air	149.0	0.3	47.0	564.0
Alveolar air	104.0	40.0	47.0	569.0
Mixed expired air	120.0	27.0	47.0	566.0

only about 0.04 percent of dry atmospheric air, so

$$P_{CO_2} = 0.0004 \times 760 \text{ torr} = 0.3 \text{ torr}$$

As air is inspired through the upper airways, it is heated and humidified. The partial pressure of water vapor is a relatively constant 47 torr at body temperature. Humidification (that is, saturating it with water vapor) of 1 liter of dry gas *in a container* at 760 torr would increase its total pressure to 807 torr (760 + 47 torr). In the body, the gas expands, according to Boyle's law, so that we can think of the 1 liter of gas at 760 torr as *diluted* by the added water vapor. The P_{O_2} of inspired air (saturated with water vapor at a standard barometric pressure) then is equal to 0.2093 (760 − 47) torr, or 149 torr. The P_{CO_2} of inspired air is 0.0004 (760 − 47) torr, or 0.29 torr, which is rounded off to 0.3 torr.

The partial pressures of oxygen and carbon dioxide in the alveolar air are determined by the alveolar ventilation, inspired P_{O_2} and P_{CO_2}, the oxygen uptake, and the carbon dioxide delivery to the lungs. Mixed venous blood, with a carbon dioxide partial pressure of 45 torr and an oxygen partial pressure of 40 torr, is continuously entering the pulmonary capillaries. As discussed later, alveolar ventilation is normally regulated by the respiratory control center in the brain to keep mean arterial and alveolar P_{CO_2} at about 40 torr. Mean alveolar P_{O_2} is about 104 torr.

Alveolar P_{O_2} increases by 2 to 4 torr with each normal tidal inspiration and falls slowly until the next inspiration. Similarly, the alveolar P_{CO_2} falls 2 to 4 torr with each inspiration and increases slowly until the next inspiration. Expired air is a mixture of about 350 ml of alveolar air and 150 ml of air from the dead space. Therefore, the P_{O_2} of mixed expired air is higher than alveolar P_{O_2} and less than the inspired P_{O_2}, or about 120 torr. Similarly, the P_{CO_2} of mixed expired air is much higher than the inspired P_{CO_2} but lower than the alveolar P_{CO_2}, or about 27 torr.

Alveolar Ventilation and Carbon Dioxide

The volume of carbon dioxide expired per unit of time $\dot{V}_E CO_2$ is equal to the alveolar ventilation $\dot{V}_A$ times the alveolar fractional concentration of carbon dioxide $F_A CO_2$. Remember that no carbon dioxide comes from the dead space.

$$\dot{V}_E CO_2 = \dot{V}_A \times F_A CO_2$$

Similarly, the fractional concentration of carbon dioxide in the alveoli is directly proportional to the carbon dioxide production by the body $\dot{V}CO_2$ and is inversely proportional to the alveolar ventilation:

$$F_ACO_2 \propto \frac{\dot{V}CO_2}{\dot{V}_A}$$

Because the alveolar fractional concentration of CO_2 times the total barometric pressure P_b minus water vapor pressure is equal to the alveolar partial pressure of CO_2:

$$F_ACO_2 \times (P_b - PH_2O) = P_ACO_2$$

then

$$P_ACO_2 \propto \frac{\dot{V}CO_2}{\dot{V}_A}$$

In healthy persons, alveolar PCO_2 is in equilibrium with arterial PCO_2 ($PaCO_2$). Thus, if alveolar ventilation is doubled (and carbon dioxide production is unchanged), the alveolar and arterial PCO_2 are reduced by one-half. If alveolar ventilation is cut in half, then alveolar and arterial PCO_2 double.

Alveolar Ventilation and Oxygen

As alveolar ventilation increases, the alveolar PO_2 should also increase. However, doubling alveolar ventilation cannot double P_AO_2 in a person whose alveolar PO_2 is already 104 torr because the highest P_AO_2 one can achieve (breathing air at sea level) is the inspired PO_2 (P_IO_2) of about 149 torr. The alveolar PO_2 can be calculated from the *alveolar air equation*.

$$P_AO_2 = P_IO_2 - \frac{P_ACO_2}{R} + F$$

where R is the respiratory exchange ratio ($R = \dot{V}CO_2/\dot{V}O_2$) and F is a correction factor.

As alveolar ventilation increases, the alveolar PCO_2 decreases, bringing the alveolar PO_2 closer to the inspired PO_2.

REGIONAL DISTRIBUTION OF ALVEOLAR VENTILATION

Although it is reasonable to assume that the alveolar ventilation is distributed evenly to alveoli throughout the lungs, such is not the case. Studies done on normal subjects seated upright and breathing from the FRC have shown that alveoli in the lower regions of the lung receive more ventilation per unit volume than those in the upper regions of the lung (see Fig. 15-2.)

If a similar study is done on a subject lying on his or her side, the regional differences in ventilation between the *anatomic* upper and lower regions of the lung disappear, although relative ventilation of the lower lung is greater than that of the upper lung. The regional differences in ventilation thus seem to be caused by gravity. Precise measurements have shown that intrapleural surface pressure is not uniform throughout the thorax but rather is *less negative* in the lower gravity-dependent regions of the thorax. There is a gradient of intrapleural surface pressure of $+0.2$ to $+0.3$ cmH$_2$O for every centimeter of vertical displacement down the lung.

The influence of this gradient of intrapleural surface pressure on regional alveolar ventilation can be explained by predicting its effect on the transpulmonary pressure in upper and lower regions of the lung. Because the alveolar pressure is zero throughout the lung at the FRC and intrapleural pressure is *more negative in upper regions* of the lung, the alveolar distending pressure (alveolar minus intrapleural) is greater in upper regions of the lung. Thus the alveoli in upper regions have greater *volumes* than the alveoli in more dependent regions.

We can see how this difference in alveolar volume results in a difference in ventilation between alveoli located in upper and lower regions of the lung by imagining a pressure-volume curve for each alveolus similar to the one in Fig. 12-2. Because an alveolus in the upper part of the lung is larger than an equivalent alveolus in the lower part of the lung, at the FRC, the upper alveolus is on a flatter portion of its pressure-volume curve (that is, it is less *compliant*) than the lower alveolus and therefore undergoes a smaller change in volume during the respiratory cycle. Lower alveoli are therefore better *ventilated* during eupneic breathing from the FRC.

The intrapleural pressure gradient in a person standing or seated upright also affects the regional static lung volume. At the FRC most of the alveolar air is in upper regions of the lung, because those alveoli have larger volumes. Most of the expiratory reserve volume is also in upper portions of the lung, as is most of the residual volume. On the other hand, most of the inspiratory reserve volume and inspiratory capacity is in lower regions of the lung.

In summary, most of the air inspired and expired during a tidal breath begun at the functional residual capacity ventilates the alveoli in lower regions of the lung. However, if a slow inspiration is begun at the *residual volume,* the initial part of the breath enters the upper alveoli, and alveoli in lower regions begin to fill later in the breath. During a forced expiration to the residual volume, alveoli in lower lung regions, which start at a lower volume than alveoli in upper lung regions, initially empty more rapidly. As positive intrapleural pressures are generated, small airways in lower regions of the lung are much more likely to be the first to collapse as a result of dynamic compression. This is because intrapleural pressure is slightly more positive in lower regions of the thorax and because smaller alveoli in lower lung regions have less elastic recoil, so they offer less alveolar septal traction to hold the small airways open.

Therefore, at the beginning of an inspiration from the residual volume, airways in the lowest regions of the lung may still be collapsed and require large transpulmonary pressure to open. At the same time, alveoli in upper lung regions, which are at lower volume than they would be at the functional residual capacity, are now on the steep portion of their pressure-volume curves. Thus they are more compliant at the residual volume than they are at the functional residual capacity, and they receive more of the air initially inspired in the breath.

The lung volume at which airways begin to close is called the *closing capacity* (or *closing volume*).

THE CLOSING VOLUME

To determine the closing capacity the subject, seated upright, starts from the *residual volume,* inspires a single breath of 100% oxygen to the total lung capacity, and then exhales back to the residual volume. The nitrogen concentration at the mouth and the volume of gas expired are monitored simultaneously throughout the second expiration.

During the first expiration to the residual volume the upper alveoli, which are larger, retain most of the residual volume and thus most of the nitrogen. At the bottom part of the lung, airways are closed, trapping whatever small volume of gas remains in these alveoli. Although the initial portion of the oxygen breath will likely enter the upper alveoli, as described previously, most of the oxygen enters the more dependent alveoli. If we could measure the nitrogen concentration of alveoli in different parts of the lung at this point, we would find the highest nitrogen concentration in upper regions of the lung. Figure 13-2 shows the nitrogen concentration trace as the subject exhales to the residual volume. The first gas exhaled (phase I) is from the anatomic dead space and is virtually 100% oxygen or 0% nitrogen. The second portion (phase II) is a mixture of dead-space gas and alveolar gas. The volume exhaled during the interval between the beginning of phase I and the midpoint of phase II represents the anatomic dead space. Quantification of the anatomic dead space in this manner is called *Fowler's test.* The third portion of gas expired by the subject is mixed alveolar gas from the upper and lower regions (phase III, or the "alveolar plateau").

Note that in a healthy person the slope of phase III is nearly horizontal. In patients with certain types of airways-resistance maldistribution, the phase III slope rises rapidly. This is because those alveoli that are supplied by high-resistance airways fill more slowly than those supplied by the normal airways during the 100% oxygen inspiration, and therefore retain relatively higher nitrogen concentrations. During expiration they empty more slowly, and when they do, the expired nitrogen concentration rises.

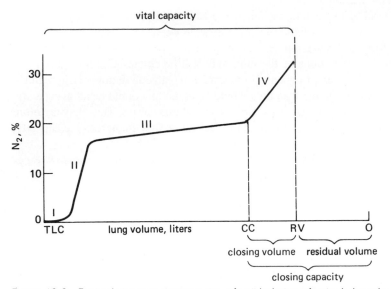

Figure 13-2 Expired nitrogen concentration after inhalation of a single breath of 100% O_2 from the residual volume to the total lung capacity. Subject exhales to the residual volume. Phase I: 0% nitrogen from anatomic dead space. Phase II: mixture of gas from anatomic dead space and alveoli. Phase III: "alveolar plateau" gas from alveoli. A steep slope of phase III indicates nonuniform distribution of alveolar gas. Phase IV: closing volume. Takeoff point of phase IV denotes beginning of airway closure in dependent portions of the lung. (*From Levitzky MG: Pulmonary Physiology, 4th ed., New York, McGraw-Hill, 1995, with permission.*)

As the expiration to the residual volume continues, the positive pleural surface pressure causes dynamic compression and ultimately airway closure. Because of the intrapleural pressure gradient from the upper parts of the lung to the lower parts of the lung, and because the smaller alveoli in lower parts of the lung have less elastic recoil, the airway closure first occurs in lower regions of the lung where the nitrogen concentration is the lowest. Thus, as airway closure begins, the expired nitrogen concentration rises abruptly because more and more of the expired gas is coming from alveoli in upper regions of the lung. The point at which the expired nitrogen concentration trace rises abruptly is the *closing capacity,* which is equal to the residual volume plus the volume expired between the beginning of airway closure and the residual volume. This volume is called the *closing volume.*

BIBLIOGRAPHY
Boggs DS, Kinasewitz GT: Review: Pathophysiology of the pleural space. *Am J Med Sci* 309:53–59, 1995.

Forster RE II, Dubois AB, Briscoe WA, Fisher AB: *The Lung: Physiologic Basis of Pulmonary Function Tests,* 3d ed. Chicago, Year Book Medical Publishers, 1986, pp 8–64.

Levitzky MG: *Pulmonary Physiology,* 4th ed. New York, McGraw-Hill, 1995, pp 55–86.

Levitzky MG, Cairo JM, Hall SM: *Introduction to Respiratory Care.* Philadelphia, Saunders, pp 111–116.

Nunn JF: *Nunn's Applied Respiratory Physiology,* 4th ed. Oxford, Butterworth-Heinemann, 1993, pp 156–163.

West JB: *Ventilation/Blood Flow and Gas Exchange,* 5th ed. Oxford, Blackwell, 1990, pp 25–30.

West JB: *Respiratory Physiology—The Essentials,* 5th ed. Baltimore, Williams & Wilkins, 1995, pp 11–20.

14

PULMONARY BLOOD FLOW

OBJECTIVES
The reader should be able to:

1   Compare and contrast the bronchial circulation and the pulmonary circulation.
2   Compare and contrast the pulmonary circulation and the systemic circulation.
3   Describe and explain the effects of lung volume, elevated intravascular pressure, and neural and humoral factors on pulmonary vascular resistance.
4   Describe the effects of gravity on pulmonary blood flow.
5   Describe the interrelationships of alveolar pressure, pulmonary arterial pressure, and pulmonary venous pressure and their effects on the regional distribution of pulmonary blood flow.

PERSPECTIVE
The lung receives blood flow via both the bronchial circulation and the pulmonary circulation. *Bronchial blood flow* constitutes a very small portion of the output of the left ventricle, and it supplies part of the tracheobronchial tree with systemic arterial blood. *Pulmonary blood flow* constitutes the entire output of the right ventricle, and it supplies the lung with the mixed venous blood draining all the tissues of the body. It is this blood that undergoes gas exchange with the alveolar air in the pulmonary capillaries. Because the right and left ventricles are arranged in series in normal adults, pulmonary blood flow is approximately equal to 100 percent of the output of the left ventricle.

BRONCHIAL CIRCULATION
The bronchial arteries arise variably, either directly from the aorta or by branching from the intercostal arteries. The bronchial blood flow constitutes about 2 percent of the output of the left ventricle. Blood pressure in the bronchial arteries is the same as that in the other systemic arteries.

Although some of the bronchial venous drainage is via the *azygous* and *hemiazygous veins,* a substantial portion of bronchial venous blood enters the *pulmonary veins,* and thus contributes to the normal anatomic right-to-left *shunt. Anastomoses,* or connections, between some bronchial and pulmonary capillaries and between bronchial arteries and branches of the pulmonary artery have also been demonstrated. These connections are probably not open in a normal healthy person but may open if either bronchial or pulmonary blood flow to a portion of lung is occluded, as by a pulmonary embolus.

PULMONARY CIRCULATION

In the normal adult the outputs of the two ventricles are approximately equal and are about 3.5 liters/min/m^2 body surface area. The pulmonary circulation contains about 250 to 300 ml of blood per m^2 of body surface area, about 60 to 70 ml/m^2 of which is in the pulmonary capillaries. It takes a red blood cell an average of 4 to 5 s to travel through the pulmonary circulation at resting cardiac outputs; about 0.75 to 1.2 s of that time is spent in pulmonary capillaries. In traveling through the lung, an erythrocyte passes through a number of successive pulmonary capillaries. Gas exchange starts to occur in smaller pulmonary arterial vessels, which are not truly capillaries by histologic standards. These arterial segments and successive capillaries may be thought of as *functional pulmonary capillaries.* Usually, when we refer to pulmonary capillaries, we mean functional pulmonary capillaries rather than anatomic capillaries.

Each alveolus is completely surrounded by pulmonary capillaries. The capillaries are so close to each other that some investigators have described pulmonary capillary blood flow as resembling blood flowing through two parallel sheets of endothelium held together by occasional connective tissue supports.

Determinants of Pulmonary Vascular Resistance

There is much less vascular smooth muscle in the vessel walls of the pulmonary arterial tree, and there are no highly muscular vessels that correspond to the systemic arterioles. Because of their thin walls and sparse smooth muscle the pulmonary vessels offer much less resistance to blood flow and are also much more *distensible* than systemic arterial vessels. They therefore have much lower intravascular pressures than those in the systemic arteries. As a result, the pulmonary arterial vessels are much more subject to *extravascular compression* than systemic arterial vessels. Because the pulmonary vessels are distensible and compressible and because they are located in the thorax and therefore subject to alveolar and intrapleural pressures (which can change greatly during inspiratory or forced expiratory efforts), factors other than the tone of the pulmonary vascular smooth muscle have profound effects on the pulmonary vascular resistance. These include gravity, body position, lung volume, alveolar and intrapleural pressure, right ventricular output, and pulmonary arterial, interstitial, and left atrial pressures.

Calculation of Pulmonary Vascular Resistance
According to Poiseuille's law:

$$R = \frac{P_1 - P_2}{\dot{Q}}$$

where P_1 is the pressure at the beginning of a tube, P_2 is the pressure at the end of the tube, $\dot{Q}$ equals the flow through the tube, and R is the resistance to flow through the tube.

For the pulmonary circulation, then,

$$PVR = \frac{MPAP - MLAP}{PBF}$$

That is, the pulmonary vascular resistance (PVR) is equal to the mean pulmonary artery pressure (MPAP) minus the mean left atrial pressure (MLAP), with the result divided by pulmonary blood flow (PBF) or cardiac output.

This formula is only an approximation even under the most optimal circumstances, because of these factors: Blood is not a Newtonian fluid, pulmonary blood flow is *pulsatile* (and may also be turbulent), the pulmonary circulation is distensible and *compressible,* and the pulmonary circulation is an extremely complex branching structure. Furthermore, as discussed later, the mean left atrial pressure may not always be the appropriate downstream pressure to use in the calculation of pulmonary vascular resistance.

If the outputs of the two ventricles are approximately equal and the measured pressure drops across the systemic circulation and the pulmonary circulation are about 98 and 10 mmHg, respectively, as shown in Fig. 14-1, then the pulmonary vascular resistance must be about one-tenth that of the systemic vascular resistance. This low resistance to blood flow offered by the pulmonary circulation is due to its structural aspects, as already discussed.

Pulmonary blood flow can be determined by several means. Clinically, the most commonly used method is the thermal dilution technique. Cold fluid, such as saline, is injected into a central vein and the change in temperature of the blood downstream is monitored continuously with a thermistor. With high cardiac outputs, the temperature returns to normal rapidly; with low cardiac outputs the temperature rises slowly. The advantages of this method are that the insertion of a single intravenous catheter is the only necessary surgical procedure and a fluoroscope is not usually necessary. A quadruple-lumen Swan-Ganz catheter is used. One lumen is connected to a tiny inflatable balloon at the end of the catheter. During the insertion of the catheter, the balloon is inflated so that the tip of the catheter "floats" in the direction of blood flow: through the right atrium and ventricle and into the pulmonary artery. The balloon is then deflated. A second lumen carries a thermistor wire to the end of the catheter. A third lumen travels only part of the way down the catheter so that it opens into a central vein. This

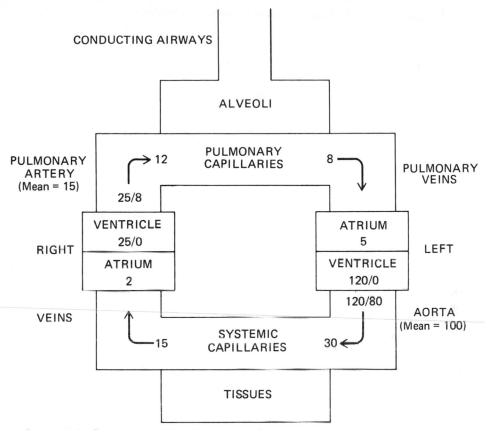

Figure 14-1 Comparison of the pulmonary and systemic circulations. *(From Levitzky MG, Pulmonary Physiology 4th ed. New York, McGraw-Hill, 1995, with permission.)*

lumen is used for the injection of the cold solution. The final lumen, at the end of the catheter, is open to the pulmonary artery, and it allows pulmonary artery pressure to be monitored. (It can also be used to sample mixed venous blood.) This monitoring is necessary because the only way the physician knows that the catheter is placed properly is by recognizing the characteristic pulmonary artery pressure trace (unless a fluoroscope is used). The temperature change after the injection is monitored by a cardiac output "computer" that automatically calculates the cardiac output from the temperature of the injected substance, the original blood temperature, and the temperature change of the blood with time.

Distribution of Pulmonary Vascular Resistance
As can be seen by looking at the pressure drops across the three major components of the pulmonary circulation, at the FRC the resistance to blood flow is fairly

evenly distributed among the pulmonary arteries, capillaries, and veins. This is in contrast to the systemic circulation, in which about 70 percent of the resistance to blood flow is located in the muscular systemic arterioles.

Effects of Lung Volume on Pulmonary Vascular Resistance

In considering the effects of lung volume on pulmonary vascular resistance, we must think in terms of two different groups of vessels: those exposed to alveolar pressure (*alveolar vessels,* mainly pulmonary capillaries) and those not exposed to alveolar pressure (*extraalveolar vessels*). As the alveoli expand during a normal negative-pressure inspiration, the vessels interposed between them, mainly pulmonary capillaries, are compressed and lengthened. At high lung volumes, the resistance to blood flow offered by the alveolar vessels increases; at low lung volumes, it decreases. These effects can be seen in the alveolar curve in Fig. 14-2.

Some of the extraalveolar vessels—the larger arteries and veins—are exposed to the intrapleural pressure. During inhalation the decrease in pleural pressure causes them to distend. Another factor tending to decrease the resistance to blood flow offered by the extraalveolar vessels at higher lung volumes is *radial traction* by the connective tissue and alveolar septa holding the larger vessels in place in the lung. Thus, at high lung volumes during normal negative-pressure breathing, the resistance to blood flow offered by the extraalveolar vessels decreases (Fig. 14-2). During a forced expiration to low lung volumes, however, intrapleural pressure becomes strongly positive and there is less traction. The resistance to blood flow offered by the extraalveolar vessels increases greatly, as seen at left in the figure.

Because the alveolar and extraalveolar vessels are in series, their resistances are additive at any lung volume. Thus the effect of changes in lung volume on the total pulmonary vascular resistance gives the V-shaped curve seen in Fig. 14-2. Pulmonary vascular resistance is lowest near the functional residual capacity and increases at both high and low lung volumes.

During *positive-pressure ventilation,* both the alveolar and extraalveolar vessels are compressed as lung volume increases (although radial traction may oppose this compression in the extraalveolar vessels), and the resistance to blood flow offered by both alveolar and extraalveolar vessels increases during lung inflation. Positive intrapleural pressures may also compress the vena cavae and other intrathoracic vessels and therefore decrease cardiac output.

Recruitment and Distention

During exercise, cardiac output can increase four- or fivefold. Mean pulmonary artery pressure increases by only a few mmHg, however, so some mechanism must be causing a decrease in pulmonary vascular resistance. This fall in pul-

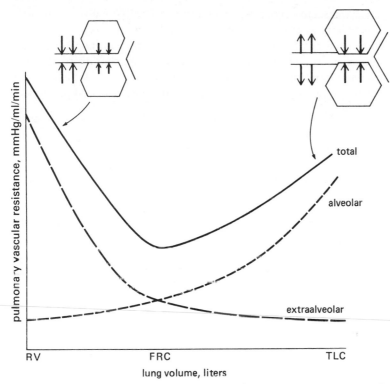

Figure 14-2   The effects of lung volume on pulmonary vascular resistance. PVR is lowest near the FRC and increases at both high and low lung volumes because of the combined effects on the alveolar and extraalveolar vessels. To achieve low lung volumes, positive intrapleural pressures must be generated, which compress the extraalveolar vessels, as seen at left in the figure. (From Murray JF: The Normal Lung, 2d ed. Philadelphia, Saunders, 1986, with permission.)

monary vascular resistance is *passive*—that is, it does not result from changes in the tone of pulmonary vascular smooth muscle caused by neural mechanisms or humoral agents. This can be demonstrated in an isolated perfused lung. Two mechanisms are involved: *recruitment* and *distention.*

Not all the pulmonary capillaries are perfused at resting cardiac outputs. Some are not perfused as a result of hydrostatic effects; others may be unperfused because they have a relatively high *critical opening pressure,* either because of their high vascular smooth muscle tone or because of elevated alveolar pressure. As blood flow increases, the increase in mean pulmonary artery pressure tends to overcome hydrostatic forces and exceeds the critical opening pressure of some previously closed vessels. These changes cause new parallel pathways for blood flow to open, thus decreasing the pulmonary vascular resistance. The opening of these new pathways is called *recruitment,* and it increases the surface area available for gas diffusion. It is important to understand that as the cardiac output or pulmonary artery pressure decreases, a *derecruitment* of pulmonary capillaries can result, which decreases the gas exchange capability of the lung.

Because pulmonary vessels are relatively distensible, an increase in perfusion pressure increases the lateral pressure component, thus increasing the transmural pressure gradient and causing them to distend. This decreases their resistance to blood flow. Increased left atrial pressure and increased pulmonary blood volume also decrease pulmonary vascular resistance by recruitment and distention.

Regional Distribution of Pulmonary Blood Flow

Gravity is one of the most important passive factors affecting local pulmonary vascular resistance and regional pulmonary blood flow within the lung. The interaction of gravity and extravascular pressures may profoundly influence the relative perfusion of different areas of the lung.

If the vertical distribution of pulmonary blood flow is determined, a pattern like that shown for the *perfusion* line in Fig. 15-2 is seen. There is more blood flow per unit volume to lower regions of the lung than to upper regions of the lung. If a person lies down, this pattern changes so that blood flow per unit volume is greater in the more gravity-dependent regions of the lung; thus if a person lies on the left side, blood flow per unit volume is greater in the left lung than in the right.

Gravity creates this gradient of perfusion because the pressure at the bottom of a column of liquid is equal to the product of the column's height, the liquid's density, and the force of gravity (Pascal's law). The blood toward the bottom is thus under greater pressure and therefore causes recruitment and distention of vessels, reducing the vascular resistance and increasing flow. Thus both gravity and the peculiar characteristics of the pulmonary circulation cause the flow gradient. The same hydrostatic effects occur to an even greater extent in the left side of the circulation, but the thick walls of the systemic arterioles are not affected by the higher intravascular pressures.

Experiments done on excised, perfused animal lungs have shown the same gradient of increased perfusion per unit volume from the top to the bottom of the lung. When the pump outputs were low, so that the pulmonary artery pressure was low, the uppermost regions of the lung received no blood flow. Perfusion of the lung ceased at the point at which alveolar pressure P_A was just equal to pulmonary arterial pressure Pa.

Thus, under circumstances in which alveolar pressure is higher than pulmonary artery pressure in the upper parts of the lung, no blood flow occurs in that region. This is referred to as *zone 1* (Fig. 14-3). If it is ventilated, it is *alveolar dead space,* because it is ventilated but not perfused. During negative-pressure breathing a normal person has no zone 1.

The lowest portion of the lung, in which pulmonary artery pressure and pulmonary vein pressure Pv both exceed alveolar pressure, is called *zone 3*. The

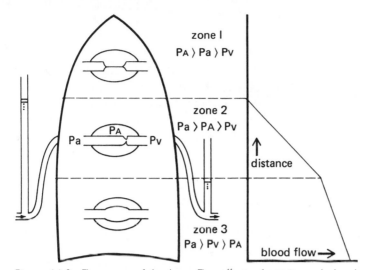

Figure 14-3   The zones of the lung: The effects of gravity and alveolar pressure on the perfusion of the lung. (From West JB, Dollery CT, Naimark A: Distribution of blood flow in isolated lung: Related to vascular and alveolar pressure. J Appl Physiol 19:713–724, 1964, with permission.)

driving pressure for blood flow through the lung in that region is simply pulmonary artery pressure minus pulmonary vein pressure. Note that this driving pressure remains constant as one moves farther down the lung in zone 3 because the hydrostatic pressure effects are the same for both the arteries and the veins.

The middle portion of the lung in Fig. 14-3 is *zone 2*. Pulmonary artery pressure exceeds alveolar pressure, so blood flows. Nevertheless, because alveolar pressure is greater than pulmonary vein pressure, the *effective* driving pressure for blood flow is pulmonary artery pressure minus *alveolar pressure*. Notice that, in zone 2, the increase in blood flow per unit of distance down the lung is greater than in zone 3. This difference occurs because the upstream driving pressure, the pulmonary artery pressure, increases according to the hydrostatic pressure increase, but the effective downstream pressure, alveolar pressure, is constant throughout the lung at any instant.

To summarize then, in zone 1:

$$P_A > Pa > Pv$$

and blood does not flow.

In zone 2:

$$Pa > P_A > Pv$$

and the effective driving pressure for blood flow is $Pa - P_A$.

In zone 3:

$$Pa > Pv > P_A$$

and the driving pressure for blood flow is Pa − Pv.

It is important to realize that the boundaries between the zones are physiologic, not anatomic. During the course of each breath, alveolar pressure changes. During eupneic breathing, these changes amount to only a few cmH_2O, but they may be much greater during speech, exercise, or positive-pressure ventilation. Similarly, after a hemorrhage or during general anesthesia, pulmonary blood flow and pulmonary artery pressure are low and zone 1 conditions are also likely. On the other hand, increases in cardiac output and/or pulmonary artery pressure move the boundaries between the zones upward, converting some zone 2 to zone 3 and possibly eliminating any zone 1 present. Changes in body position alter the orientation of the zones with regard to the anatomic locations in the lung, but the same relationships exist with regard to gravity and alveolar pressure. Passive influences on pulmonary vascular resistance are summarized in Table 14-1.

Active Control of Pulmonary Vascular Smooth Muscle

Pulmonary vascular smooth muscle responds to both *neural* and *humoral* influences. Both can produce active changes in pulmonary vascular resistance, in contrast to the passive factors discussed previously.

The pulmonary vasculature is innervated by sympathetic and parasympathetic fibers. This innervation is relatively sparse compared with the innervation of systemic vessels. The larger elastic vessels receive relatively more innervation than the smaller muscular vessels.

The effects of sympathetic stimulation of the pulmonary vessels are somewhat controversial. Some investigators have shown that the pulmonary vascular resistance increases when the sympathetic innervation of the pulmonary vasculature is stimulated, whereas others have found that large-vessel *distensibility* decreases but that the calculated pulmonary vascular resistance remains unchanged. Stimulation of parasympathetic innervation of the pulmonary vessels may cause vasodilation, particularly if the vessels are already constricted. The physiologic importance of this response is not known.

When injected into the pulmonary circulation, the catecholamines epinephrine and norepinephrine increase pulmonary vascular resistance, probably by stimulating α-adrenergic receptors. Pulmonary vascular constrictors include angiotensin, histamine (which is found in the lung mast cells and appears to be mainly a venoconstrictor), some prostaglandins (such as PGE_2, $PGF_{2\alpha}$, and thromboxane), and some prostaglandin precursors and breakdown products. Alveolar hypoxia and hypercapnia can also cause pulmonary vascular constriction. Pulmonary vasodilators include acetylcholine, the β-adrenergic agonist isoproterenol, and certain prostaglandins, such as PGE_1, prostacyclin, and nitric oxide (NO).

Table 14-1   Passive Influences on Pulmonary Vascular Resistance

Causes	Effect on pulmonary vascular resistance	Mechanism
Increased lung volume (above FRC)	Increases	Compression and lengthening of alveolar vessels
Decreased lung volume (below FRC)	Increases	Compression of and less traction on extraalveolar vessels
Increased pulmonary artery pressure; Increased left atrial pressure; Increased pulmonary blood volume; Increased cardiac output	Decreases	Recruitment and distention
Gravity; body position	Decreases in gravity-dependent regions of the lungs	Hydrostatic effects lead to recruitment and distention
Increased (more positive) interstitial pressure	Increases	Compression of vessels
Increased blood viscosity	Increases	Viscosity (the internal friction between layers of a fluid) directly increases resistance. See discussion of Poiseuille's law
Positive-pressure ventilation; Increased alveolar pressure	Increases	Compression and derecruitment of alveolar vessels
Positive intrapleural pressure	Increases	Compression of extraalveolar vessels; compression of vena cavae decreases pulmonary blood flow and leads to derecruitment and less distention

(From Levitzky MG, Pulmonary Physiology, 4th ed. New York, McGraw-Hill, 1995, with permission.)

Alveolar hypoxia or atelectasis causes an active vasoconstriction in the pulmonary circulation. The site of vascular smooth muscle constriction appears to be in the arterial (precapillary) vessels close to the alveoli. The mechanism of this *hypoxic pulmonary vasoconstriction* is not completely understood. The response is local, that is, it occurs only in the area of the alveolar hypoxia. Connections to the central nervous system are not necessary; the response occurs in isolated perfused lungs. Hypoxia may act directly on the vascular smooth muscle or may cause the release of a vasoactive substance from the pulmonary parenchyma or mast cells in the area.

Table 14-2   Active Influences on Pulmonary Vascular Resistance

Increase	Decrease
Stimulation of sympathetic innervation (may have greater effect by decreasing large-vessel distensibility)	Stimulation of parasympathetic innervation (if vascular tone is already elevated)
Norepinephrine, epinephrine	Acetylcholine
α-adrenergic agonists	β-adrenergic agonists
$PGF_{2\alpha}$, PGE_2	Bradykinin
Thromboxane	PGE_1
Angiotensin	Prostacyclin (PGI_2)
Histamine (primarily a pulmonary venoconstrictor)	Nitric Oxide (NO)
Alveolar hypoxia	
Alveolar hypercapnia	
Low pH of mixed venous blood	

(From Levitzky MG, Pulmonary Physiology, 4th ed. New York, McGraw Hill, 1995, with permission.)

The function of the hypoxic pulmonary vasoconstriction response is to help match perfusion to ventilation within the lung. The mixing of venous blood from a hypoxic area with blood draining well-ventilated areas of the lung is called an *intrapulmonary shunt*. Intrapulmonary shunts lower the overall arterial PO_2 and may even increase the arterial PCO_2. The hypoxic pulmonary vasoconstriction diverts mixed venous blood flow away from poorly ventilated areas of the lung, shifting blood flow to better-ventilated areas. The hypoxic pulmonary vasoconstriction, however, is not a very strong response, which is not surprising because pulmonary arteries have so little smooth muscle. Very high pulmonary artery pressures can interfere with hypoxic pulmonary vasoconstriction, as can other physiologic disturbances, such as alkalosis.

Alveolar hypercapnia (high carbon dioxide) also causes pulmonary vasoconstriction. Whether this occurs by the same mechanism as the hypoxic pulmonary vasoconstriction is not clear. Low pulmonary blood pH may also cause pulmonary vasoconstriction. Active influences on pulmonary vascular resistance are summarized in Table 14-2.

Pulmonary Edema

Pulmonary edema, the extravascular accumulation of fluid in the lung, may be caused by one or more physiologic abnormalities. The result is inevitably impaired gas transfer. As the fluid accumulates, first in the interstitium and later in alveoli, diffusion of gases, particularly oxygen, decreases.

We have already discussed the Starling equation in Chap. 7:

$$\dot{Q}_f = K_f[(P_c - P_{is}) - \sigma(\pi_{pl} - \pi_{is})]$$

Factors that may predispose to pulmonary edema are summarized in Table 14-3.

Pulmonary capillary hydrostatic pressure is estimated to be about 7 to 12 mmHg under normal conditions. Although some investigators believe that the

Table 14-3   Factors Predisposing to Pulmonary Edema

Factor in Starling equation	Clinical problems
Increased capillary permeability ($K_{f;\sigma}$)	Adult respiratory distress syndrome
	Oxygen toxicity
	Inhaled or circulating toxins
Increased capillary hydrostatic pressure (P_c)	Increased left atrial pressure resulting from left ventricular infarction, or mitral stenosis
	Overadministration of intravenous fluids
Decreased interstitial hydrostatic pressure (P_{is})	Too rapid evacuation of pneumothorax or hemothorax
Decreased colloid osmotic pressure (π_{pl})	Protein starvation
	Dilution of blood proteins by intravenous solutions
	Renal problems resulting in urinary protein loss (proteinuria)

Other Etiologies	Clinical problems
Insufficient pulmonary lymphatic drainage	Tumors
	Interstitial fibrosing diseases
Unknown etiology	High-altitude pulmonary edema
	Pulmonary edema after head injury (neurogenic pulmonary edema)
	Drug overdose

From Levitzky MG, Cairo JM, Hall SM: *Introduction to Respiratory Care.* Philadelphia, Saunders, 1990, with permission.

pulmonary interstitial hydrostatic pressure is slightly positive, many recent studies have determined it to be negative, in the range of -5 to -7 mmHg. This seems reasonable in light of the normally negative intrapleural pressure, which may be transmitted through much of the pulmonary interstitium.

BIBLIOGRAPHY

Barnes PJ, Liu SF: Regulation of pulmonary vascular tone. *Pharm Rev* 47:87–131, 1995.

Deffebach ME, Charan NB, Lakshminarayan S, Butler J: The bronchial circulation: Small, but a vital attribute of the lung. *Am Rev Resp Dis* 135:463–481, 1987.

Fishman AP (ed): *The Pulmonary Circulation: Normal and Abnormal.* Philadelphia, University of Pennsylvania Press, 1990.

Fishman AP, Fisher AB (eds): *Handbook of Physiology,* sec 3, *The Respiratory System,* vol I, *Circulation and Nonrespiratory Functions.* Bethesda, MD, American Physiological Society, 1985, pp 93–230.

Harris P, Heath D: *The Human Pulmonary Circulation,* 3d ed. Edinburgh, Churchill Livingstone, 1986.

Levitzky MG: *Pulmonary Physiology,* 4th ed. New York, McGraw-Hill, 1995, pp 87–113.

Levitzky MG, Cairo JM, Hall SM: *Introduction to Respiratory Care.* Philadelphia, Saunders, pp 116–123.

Malik AB, Feustel PJ: Pulmonary circulation and lung fluid and solute exchange, in Murray JF and Nadel JA (eds): *Textbook of Respiratory Medicine,* 2nd ed. Philadelphia, Saunders, 1994, pp 139–174.

Murray JF: *The Normal Lung,* 2d ed. Philadelphia, Saunders, 1986, pp 139–162.

Nunn JF: *Nunn's Applied Respiratory Physiology,* 4th ed. Oxford, Butterworth-Heinemann, 1993, pp 135–155.

Weibel ER: *The Pathway for Oxygen: Structure and Function in the Mammalian Respiratory System.* Cambridge, MA, Harvard University Press, 1984, pp 272–301, 339–343.

West JB: *Ventilation/Blood Flow and Gas Exchange,* 5th ed. Oxford, Blackwell, 1990, pp 27–30.

West JB: *Respiratory Physiology—The Essentials,* 5th ed. Baltimore, Williams & Wilkins, 1995, pp 31–50.

West JB, Dollery CT, Naimark A: Distribution of blood flow in isolated lung: Relation to vascular and alveolar pressure. *J Appl Physiol* 19:713–724, 1964.

15

VENTILATION-PERFUSION RELATIONSHIPS

OBJECTIVES

The reader should be able to:

1 Predict the consequences of mismatched ventilation and perfusion.
2 Explain the regional differences in the matching of ventilation and perfusion of the normal upright lung.
3 Predict the consequences of the regional differences in the ventilation and perfusion of the normal upright lung.
4 Classify and explain the causes of tissue hypoxia.

PERSPECTIVE

Alveolar ventilation brings inspired gas with a PO_2 of about 150 mmHg and a PCO_2 of about 0.3 mmHg into the alveoli. At the same time, the right ventricle pumps mixed venous blood with a PO_2 of about 40 mmHg and a PCO_2 of about 45 mmHg into the pulmonary capillaries. Oxygen diffuses from the alveoli into the pulmonary capillaries at the same time that carbon dioxide diffuses from the pulmonary capillaries. The PO_2 and PCO_2 of an alveolar-capillary unit are *determined* by the relative ventilation and perfusion of the unit. Increasing the ventilation relative to the perfusion increases the PO_2 and decreases the PCO_2 of the alveolus. Increasing the perfusion relative to the ventilation decreases the PO_2 and increases the PCO_2 of that alveolus.

IMPORTANCE OF MATCHING VENTILATION AND PERFUSION

Alveolar ventilation $\dot{V}_A$ is normally about 4 to 6 liters of air per minute, and pulmonary capillary blood flow $\dot{Q}c$ has a similar range, so the ratio of ventilation to perfusion for the whole lung is about 0.8 to 1.2. However, ventilation and perfusion must be matched on the *alveolar-capillary level*. The $\dot{V}_A/\dot{Q}c$ for the whole lung is really of interest only as an approximation of the situation in all the alveolar-capillary units of the lung.

Clearly, alveoli that are ventilated but not perfused constitute alveolar dead space and contribute nothing to gas exchange in the lung (Fig. 15-1). Similarly, alveoli that are perfused but not ventilated constitute an *intrapulmonary shunt* and return mixed venous blood to the systemic circulation.

CONSEQUENCES OF $\dot{V}_A/\dot{Q}c$ MISMATCH

Alveolar-capillary unit A in Fig. 15-1 has a normal ventilation-perfusion ratio. Inspired air entering the alveolus has a PO_2 of about 150 torr and a PCO_2 of nearly 0 torr. Mixed venous blood entering the pulmonary capillary has a PO_2 of about 40 torr and a PCO_2 of about 45 torr. This results in an alveolar PO_2 of about 100 torr and an alveolar PCO_2 of 40 torr. The partial pressure gradient for oxygen diffusion is thus about $100 - 40$, or 60 torr; the partial pressure gradient for carbon dioxide is about $45 - 40$, or 5 torr.

The airway supplying unit B has become completely occluded. Its $\dot{V}_A/\dot{Q}c$ is zero. In time, the air trapped in the alveolus equilibrates by diffusion with the gas dissolved in the mixed venous blood entering the alveolar-capillary unit. (If the blockage persists, the alveolus will likely collapse.) No gas can be exchanged, and any blood perfusing this alveolus is the same at exit as at entry. Unit B, therefore, acts as a right-to-left shunt.

A pulmonary embolus blocks the blood flow to unit C, which is therefore completely unperfused. The unit has an infinite $\dot{V}_A/\dot{Q}c$. Because no oxygen can diffuse from the alveolus into pulmonary capillary blood, and no carbon dioxide can enter the alveolus from the blood, the PO_2 of the alveolus is about 150 torr, and its PCO_2 is about zero. Thus the gas composition of this unperfused alveolus is the same as that of inspired air. Unit C is alveolar dead space. If unit C were unperfused because its alveolar pressure exceeded its precapillary pressure (instead of as the result of an embolus), it would also correspond to part of zone 1.

Units B and C represent the two extremes of a *continuum* of ventilation-perfusion ratios. The ventilation-perfusion ratio of a particular alveolar-capillary unit can fall anywhere along this continuum, as the line along the bottom of Fig. 15-1 shows. The alveolar PO_2 and PCO_2 of such units fall between the two extremes shown in the figure.

REGIONAL $\dot{V}/\dot{Q}$ IN THE LUNG

We have already discussed the regional differences in ventilation and pulmonary blood flow in Chaps 13 and 14. During normal ventilation from the functional residual capacity in a person in an upright posture, the lower regions of the lung are both better ventilated and better perfused. Figure 15-2 shows that the perfusion

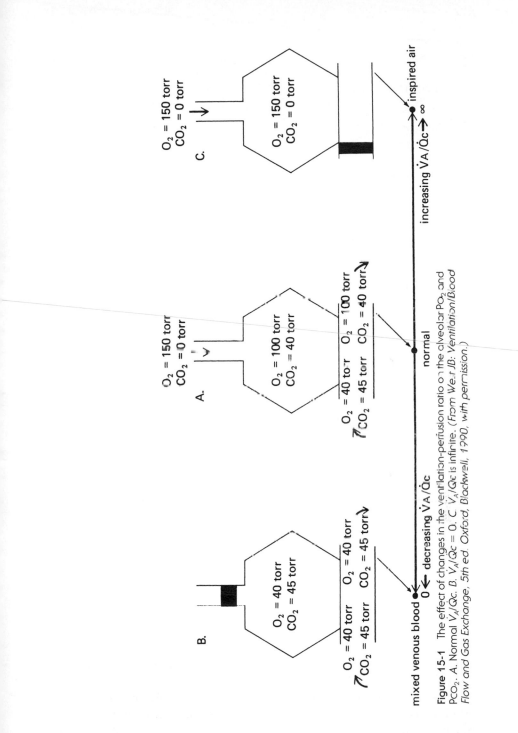

Figure 15-1 The effect of changes in the ventilation-perfusion ratio on the alveolar P_{O_2} and P_{CO_2}. A. Normal $\dot{V}_A/\dot{Q}c$. B. $\dot{V}_A/\dot{Q}c = 0$. C. $\dot{V}_A/\dot{Q}c$ is infinite. (From West JB: *Ventilation/Blood Flow and Gas Exchange,* 5th ed. Oxford, Blackwell, 1990, with permission.)

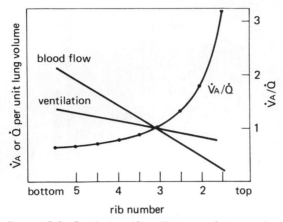

Figure 15-2 Distribution of ventilation, perfusion, and ventilation-perfusion ratio down the upright dog lung. (*From West JB: Ventilation/Blood Flow and Gas Exchange, 5th ed. Oxford, Blackwell, 1990, with permission.*)

gradient exceeds the ventilation gradient so that the ventilation-perfusion ratio is lower in the lower regions and higher in the upper regions of the lung. In fact, if pulmonary perfusion pressure is low (for example, from hemorrhage), and/or if alveolar pressure is high (from positive pressure ventilation with positive end-expiratory pressure), there may be areas of zone 1 in the upper parts of the lung.

The effects of regional differences in $\dot{V}_A/\dot{Q}c$ on the alveolar PO_2 and PCO_2 can be estimated by looking at Fig. 15-1 and 15-2. Under normal circumstances, the blood in the pulmonary capillaries equilibrates with the alveolar PO_2 (P_AO_2) and PCO_2 (P_ACO_2), so blood in the pulmonary venule draining an alveolar-capillary unit has the same PO_2 and PCO_2 as the alveolus.

Because the ventilation-perfusion ratio is much higher in upper regions of the lung, the alveolar PO_2 is higher and the alveolar PCO_2 is lower in upper than in lower regions. This means that the blood draining the upper regions has a higher oxygen *content* and lower carbon dioxide content than the blood draining the lower regions. However, because there is much less blood flow to upper than to lower regions, more total *gas exchange* occurs in the lower sections.

CLINICAL ASSESSMENT OF $\dot{V}/\dot{Q}$

Several methods can demonstrate the presence or location of areas of the lung with mismatched ventilation and perfusion. These methods include calculations of the physiologic shunt, the physiologic dead space, differences between the alveolar and arterial PO_2's and PCO_2's, and lung scans after inhaled and intra-venously administered ^{133}Xe or ^{99m}Tc labeled diethylene triamine pentaacetic acid (^{99m}Tc DTPA).

A *right-to-left shunt* is the mixing of venous blood that has not been oxygenated (or not fully oxygenated) into the arterial blood. The *physiologic shunt*, which corresponds to the physiologic dead space, consists of the anatomic shunts plus the intrapulmonary shunts. The intrapulmonary shunts can be *absolute shunts* (true shunts) or they can be *"shuntlike states,"* i.e., areas of low ventilation-perfusion ratios in which alveoli are underventilated and/or overperfused. Anatomic shunts consist of systemic venous blood entering the left ventricle without having entered the pulmonary vasculature. In a normal healthy adult about 2 to 5 percent of the cardiac output, including venous blood from the bronchial veins, the thebesian veins, the anterior cardiac veins, and the pleural veins, enters the left side of the circulation directly without passing through the pulmonary capillaries. Pathological anatomical shunts such as right-to-left intracardiac shunts can also occur, as in tetralogy of Fallot.

The Shunt Equation   The shunt equation conceptually divides all alveolar-capillary units into two groups: those with well-matched ventilation and perfusion and those with ventilation-perfusion ratios of zero. Thus the shunt equation combines the areas of absolute shunt (including the anatomic shunts) and the shuntlike areas into a single conceptual group. The resulting ratio of shunt flow to the cardiac output, often referred to as the *venous admixture*, is the part of the cardiac output that would have to be perfusing *absolutely unventilated alveoli* to cause a systemic arterial oxygen content equivalent to that from a particular patient. A much larger portion of the cardiac output could be *overperfusing* poorly ventilated alveoli and yield the same ratio.

The shunt equation is derived by assuming that the total amount of oxygen entering the systemic arteries must equal the sum of that coming from alveolar-capillary units with well-matched ventilation and perfusion plus that coming from the shunt flow ($\dot{Q}s$).

The total volume of oxygen per time entering the systemic arteries is

$$\dot{Q}t \times CaO_2$$

where CaO_2 equals the oxygen content of arterial blood in milliliters of oxygen per 100 ml of blood and $\dot{Q}t$ is the cardiac output. This total amount of oxygen per time entering the systemic arteries is composed of the oxygen coming from the well-ventilated and well-perfused alveolar-capillary units:

$$(\dot{Q}t - \dot{Q}s) \times Cc'O_2$$

where $\dot{Q}t - \dot{Q}s$ equals the cardiac output minus the shunt flow and $Cc'O_2$ equals the oxygen content of the blood at the end of the ventilated and perfused pulmonary capillaries, plus the oxygen in the unaltered mixed venous blood coming from the shunt, $\dot{Q}s \times C\bar{v}O_2$ (where $C\bar{v}O_2$ is equal to the oxygen content of the mixed venous blood). That is,

$$\underbrace{\dot{Q}t \times CaO_2}_{\substack{\text{Oxygen delivery} \\ \text{to systemic arteries}}} = \underbrace{(\dot{Q}t - \dot{Q}s) \times Cc'O_2}_{\substack{\text{Oxygen coming} \\ \text{from normal} \\ \dot{V}_A/\dot{Q}c \text{ units}}} + \underbrace{\dot{Q}s \times C\overline{v}O_2}_{\substack{\text{Oxygen from} \\ \text{shunted blood} \\ \text{flow}}}$$

This can be rearranged to

$$\frac{\dot{Q}s}{\dot{Q}t} = \frac{Cc'O_2 - CaO_2}{Cc'O_2 - C\overline{v}O_2}$$

The shunt fraction $\dot{Q}s/\dot{Q}t$ is usually multiplied by 100 percent so that the shunt flow is expressed as a percent of the cardiac output.

The arterial and mixed venous oxygen content can be determined if blood samples are obtained from a systemic artery and from the pulmonary artery (for mixed venous blood), but the oxygen content of the blood at the end of the pulmonary capillaries with well-matched ventilation and perfusion is impossible to measure directly. This must be calculated from the *alveolar air equation* and the patient's hemoglobin concentration, which will be discussed shortly.

The relative contributions of the true intrapulmonary shunts and the shuntlike states to the calculated shunt flow can be estimated by repeating the measurements and calculations with the patient breathing first air with a normal or slightly elevated oxygen concentration and then nearly pure oxygen (F_IO_2's of 0.95 to 1.00). At the lower inspired oxygen concentrations, the calculated $\dot{Q}s/\dot{Q}t$ will include both the true shunts and the alveolar-capillary units with low ventilation-perfusion ratios. After a patient has inspired nearly 100% oxygen for 20 to 30 min, even alveoli with very low $\dot{V}_A/\dot{Q}c$'s will have high enough alveolar PO_2's to completely saturate the hemoglobin in the blood perfusing them. These units will therefore no longer contribute to the calculated $\dot{Q}s/\dot{Q}t$, and the new calculated shunt should include only areas of absolute shunt. Unfortunately, very high inspired oxygen concentrations may lead to absorption atelectasis of very poorly ventilated alveoli that remain perfused, and so this test may alter what it is trying to measure when the high F_IO_2's are used.

Physiologic Dead Space   The use of the Bohr equation to determine the physiologic dead space has already been discussed. If the anatomic dead space is subtracted from the physiologic dead space, the difference (if any) is *alveolar dead space,* or areas of infinite ventilation-perfusion ratios. Alveolar dead space also results in an *arterial-alveolar* CO_2 difference, as discussed in Chap. 13.

Alveolar-Arterial Oxygen Difference   Larger-than-normal differences between the alveolar and arterial PO_2 may indicate a degree of ventilation-perfusion mismatch or the presence of intrapulmonary shunts; however, the alveolar-arterial oxygen difference, normally 5 to 15 torr, is not caused only by ventilation-perfusion mismatch. It may also be caused by anatomic shunts, diffusion block, low mixed venous P_{O_2}'s, high inspired oxygen concentrations, and shifts in the oxyhemoglobin dissociation curve.

Lung Scans   Lung scans after both inhaled and injected radioactive markers can be used to inspect the location and amount of ventilation and perfusion to the various regions of the lung, as already described.

THE CAUSES OF HYPOXIA

At this point the various causes of tissue hypoxia can be considered. These causes can be classified (in some cases rather arbitrarily) into four or five major groups, as shown in Table 15-1. The underlying physiology of some of these types of hypoxia has already been discussed; others will be discussed in greater detail in subsequent chapters.

Hypoxic Hypoxia

Hypoxic hypoxia refers to conditions in which the arterial P_{O_2} is abnormally low. Because the amount of oxygen that will combine with hemoglobin is mainly determined by the P_{O_2}, these conditions may lead to decreased oxygen delivery to the tissues. Conditions causing *low alveolar* P_{O_2}'s inevitably lead to low arterial P_{O_2}'s and oxygen contents because the alveolar P_{O_2} determines the upper limit of arterial P_{O_2}. *Hypoventilation* leads to both alveolar hypoxia and hypercapnia (high CO_2). *Ascent to high altitudes* causes alveolar hypoxia because of the reduced total barometric pressure encountered above sea level. Reduced $F_{I_O_2}$'s have similar effects. Under these conditions, alveolar CO_2 is decreased because of the reflex increase in ventilation caused by hypoxic stimulation, as will be discussed in Chapter 18. Hypoventilation and ascent to high altitude lead to decreased venous P_{O_2} and oxygen content as oxygen is extracted from the already hypoxic

Table 15-1   A Classification of the Causes of Hypoxia

Classification	$P_{A_O_2}$	$P_{a_O_2}$	$C_{a_O_2}$	$P\bar{v}_{O_2}$	$C\bar{v}_{O_2}$	Increased $F_{I_O_2}$ helpful?
Hypoxic hypoxia:						
Low alveolar P_{O_2}	Low	Low	Low	Low	Low	Yes
Diffusion impairment	Normal	Low	Low	Low	Low	Yes
Right-to-left shunts	Normal	Low	Low	Low	Low	No
$\dot{V}/\dot{Q}$ mismatch	Normal	Low	Low	Low	Low	Yes
Anemic hypoxia	Normal	Normal	Low	Low	Low	No
CO poisoning	Normal	Normal	Low	Low	Low	Possibly
Hypoperfusion hypoxia	Normal	Normal	Normal	Low	Low	No
Histotoxic hypoxia	Normal	Normal	Normal	High	High	No

From Levitzky MG: *Pulmonary Physiology*, 4th ed. New York, McGraw-Hill, 1995, with permission.

arterial blood. Administration of elevated oxygen concentrations in the inspired gas (F_IO_2's) can alleviate the alveolar and arterial hypoxia in hypoventilation and in ascent to high altitude, but it cannot reverse the hypercapnia of hypoventilation. In fact, administration of elevated F_IO_2's to spontaneously breathing patients hypoventilating because of a depressed central response to CO_2 can further depress ventilation.

Impairment of alveolar-capillary diffusion, which will be discussed in greater detail in the next chapter, can cause hypoxia. Conditions such as interstitial fibrosis and interstitial or alveolar edema can lead to low arterial PO_2's and contents with normal or elevated alveolar PO_2's. High F_IO_2's that increase the alveolar PO_2 to very high levels may raise the arterial PO_2 by increasing the partial pressure gradient for oxygen diffusion. True *right-to-left shunts,* such as anatomic shunts and absolute intrapulmonary shunts, can cause decreased arterial PO_2's with normal or even elevated alveolar PO_2's. Arterial hypoxia caused by true shunts is not relieved by high F_IO_2's because the shunted blood does not come into contact with the high levels of oxygen. The hemoglobin of the unshunted blood is nearly completely saturated with oxygen at a normal F_IO_2 of 0.21, and the small additional volume of oxygen dissolved in the blood at high F_IO_2's cannot make up for the low hemoglobin saturation of the shunted blood. $\dot{V}_A/\dot{Q}c$ *mismatch* can cause hypoxia. Alveolar-capillary units with low ventilation-perfusion ratios contribute to arterial hypoxia, as already discussed. Units with high $\dot{V}_A/\dot{Q}c$'s do not by themselves lead to arterial hypoxia, of course, but large lung areas that are underperfused are usually associated with either overperfusion of other units or low cardiac output. Hypoxic pulmonary vasoconstriction and local airway responses normally help to minimize ventilation-perfusion mismatch.

Anemic Hypoxia

Anemic hypoxia is caused by a decrease in the amount of functioning hemoglobin, which can be a result of decreased hemoglobin or erythrocyte production, the production of abnormal hemoglobin or red blood cells, pathological destruction of erythrocytes, or interference with the chemical combination of oxygen and hemoglobin. Carbon monoxide poisoning, for example, results from the greater affinity of hemoglobin for carbon monoxide than for oxygen. Methemoglobinemia is a condition in which the iron in hemoglobin has been altered from the Fe^{2+} to the Fe^{3+} form, which does not combine with oxygen.

Anemic hypoxia results in a decreased oxygen content even when both alveolar and arterial PO_2 are normal. Venous PO_2 and oxygen content are both decreased. Administration of high F_IO_2's is not effective in greatly increasing the arterial oxygen content (except possibly in carbon monoxide poisoning).

Hypoperfusion Hypoxia

Hypoperfusion hypoxia (sometimes called *stagnant hypoxia*) results from low blood flow. This can occur either locally, in a particular vascular bed, or systemically, in the case of a low cardiac output. The alveolar P_{O_2} and the arterial P_{O_2} and oxygen content may be normal, but the reduced oxygen delivery to the tissues may result in tissue hypoxia. Venous P_{O_2} and oxygen content are low. Raising the F_IO_2 is of little value in hypoperfusion hypoxia (unless it directly increases the perfusion) because the blood flowing to the tissues is already oxygenated normally.

Histotoxic Hypoxia

Histotoxic hypoxia refers to a poisoning of the cellular machinery that uses oxygen to produce energy. Cyanide, for example, binds to cytochrome oxidase in the respiratory chain and effectively blocks oxidative phosphorylation. Alveolar P_{O_2} and arterial P_{O_2} and oxygen content may be normal (or even *elevated,* because low doses of cyanide increase ventilation by stimulating the arterial chemoreceptors). Venous P_{O_2} and oxygen content are elevated because oxygen is not utilized.

Other Causes of Hypoxia

Tissue edema or fibrosis may result in impaired diffusion of oxygen from the blood to the tissues. It is also conceivable that the delivery of oxygen to a tissue is completely normal, but the tissue's metabolic demands still exceed the supply and tissue hypoxia could result. This is known as *overutilization hypoxia.* Conditions such as malignant hyperthermia or thyroid storm could produce this.

BIBLIOGRAPHY
Forster RE II, Dubois AB, Briscoe WA, Fisher AB: *The Lung: Physiologic Basis of Pulmonary Function Tests,* 3d ed. Chicago, Year Book Medical Publishers, 1986, pp 163–189.

Levitzky MG: *Pulmonary Physiology,* 4th ed. New York, McGraw-Hill, 1995, pp 114–129; 182–186.

Nunn JF: *Nunn's Applied Respiratory Physiology,* 4th ed. Oxford, Butterworth-Heinemann, 1993, pp 156–197.

Siggaard-Andersen O, Ulrich A, Gothgen IH: Classes of tissue hypoxia. *Acta Anaesthesiol Scand* 39 (Suppl 107): 137–142, 1995.

West JB: *Ventilation/Blood Flow and Gas Exchange,* 5th ed. Oxford, Blackwell, 1990.

West JB: *Respiratory Physiology—The Essentials,* 5th ed. Baltimore, Williams & Wilkins, 1995, pp 51–69.

West JB: *Pulmonary Pathophysiology—The Essentials,* 4th ed. Baltimore, Williams & Wilkins, 1992, pp 18–40.

16

DIFFUSION OF GASES

OBJECTIVES

The reader should be able to:

1 Define diffusion and distinguish it from "bulk flow."
2 State Fick's law for diffusion.
3 Distinguish between perfusion limitation and diffusion limitation of gas transfer in the lung.
4 Describe the diffusion of oxygen from the alveoli into the blood and the diffusion of carbon dioxide from the blood to the alveoli.

PERSPECTIVE

Diffusion of a gas occurs when there is a net movement of molecules from a region in which that particular gas exerts a high partial pressure to a region in which it exerts a lower partial pressure. Movement by diffusion therefore differs from the movement of gases through the conducting airways, which occurs by bulk flow (mass movement or convection). During bulk flow, gas movement results from differences in *total* pressure, and molecules of different gases move together along the total pressure gradient. During diffusion, gas movement occurs in both directions, but because of its greater number of molecules per unit volume, the area of higher partial pressure has proportionately more random departures. The *net* movement of gas therefore depends on the partial pressure difference between the two areas. The rate of diffusion is temperature-dependent because random molecular movement increases at higher temperatures. In a static situation, diffusion continues until no partial pressure differences exist. In the lungs, oxygen and carbon dioxide continuously enter and leave the alveoli, so such an equilibrium is never reached.

FICK'S LAW FOR DIFFUSION

By the time inspired air reaches the alveoli, the linear velocity of bulk flow decreases to zero. This decrease results mainly from the tremendous increase in

178

the total cross-sectional area of the branching conducting airways, respiratory bronchioles, and alveolar ducts. As the total cross-sectional area increases, the linear velocity decreases:

Flow (cm³/s) = cross-sectional area (cm²) × linear velocity (cm/s)

In the alveoli, oxygen then moves through the gas phase according to its own partial pressure gradient. The distance from the alveolar duct to the alveolar-capillary interface is usually less than 1 mm. In the alveolar gas phase, diffusion occurs very rapidly and is believed to be assisted by the pulsations of the heart.

Oxygen then diffuses through the alveolar-capillary interface. First, it must move from the gas phase to the liquid phase, according to *Henry's law,* which states that the amount of a gas absorbed by a liquid with which it does not combine chemically is directly proportional to the partial pressure of the gas and the solubility of the gas in the liquid. Oxygen must dissolve in and diffuse through the thin layer of pulmonary surfactant, the alveolar epithelium, the interstitium, and the capillary endothelium. It must then diffuse through the plasma, where some remains dissolved but most diffuses through the erythrocyte cell membrane and combines with hemoglobin. The thickness of this alveolar-capillary diffusion barrier is normally only about 0.5 μm, but this barrier thickness can increase in interstitial fibrosis or interstitial edema.

The blood then carries the oxygen out of the lung and distributes it to the other tissues of the body. At the tissues, oxygen diffuses from the red blood cell through the cell membrane, plasma, capillary endothelium, interstitium, tissue cell membrane, and cell interior into the mitochondrion. For carbon dioxide, the process is reversed.

Factors that determine the rate of diffusion of a gas through the alveolar-capillary barrier are described by Fick's law for diffusion:

$$\dot{V}_{gas} = \frac{A \times D \times (P_1 - P_2)}{T}$$

where $\dot{V}_{gas}$ is the volume of gas diffusing through the tissue barrier per unit of time (ml/min); A is the surface area of the barrier available for diffusion; D is the diffusion coefficient, or diffusivity, for the particular gas in the barrier; T is the thickness of the barrier, or the diffusion distance; and $P_1 - P_2$ is the partial pressure difference of the gas across the barrier.

Thus the volume of gas moving across the alveolar-capillary barrier per unit of time is directly proportional to the surface area of the barrier, the diffusivity, and the difference in concentration between the two sides, but it is inversely proportional to the barrier thickness.

The surface area of the blood-gas barrier is believed to be at least 70 m² in a healthy average-sized adult at rest. That is, about 70 m² of the *potential* surface area is both ventilated and perfused at rest. If more capillaries are recruited, the surface area available for diffusion increases; if venous return falls, capillaries may be derecruited, and the surface area available for diffusion may decrease.

The diffusivity, or diffusion constant, for a gas is directly proportional to the solubility of the gas in the diffusion barrier and inversely proportional to the square root of the molecular weight of the gas:

$$D \propto \frac{\text{solubility}}{\sqrt{\text{M.W.}}}$$

The diffusivity is inversely proportional to the square root of the molecular weight of the gas because, at the same temperature, different gases with equal numbers of molecules in equal volumes have the same molecular energy. Therefore, light molecules travel faster, have more frequent collisions, and diffuse more rapidly. Because carbon dioxide is more dense than oxygen, it diffuses only 0.85 times as fast as it moves through the gas phase in the alveoli. However, in the liquid phase, the solubility of carbon dioxide is about 24 times that of oxygen, so carbon dioxide diffuses about 0.85×24, or about *20 times* more rapidly than does oxygen through the alveolar-capillary barrier. Thus, in situations of diffusion impairment, patients usually develop problems in oxygen diffusion through the alveolar-capillary barrier before they develop carbon dioxide retention.

PERFUSION LIMITATION OF GAS TRANSFER

At resting cardiac outputs, a red blood cell, along with the plasma surrounding it, spends an average of about 0.75 to 1.20 s inside a functional pulmonary capillary. If the partial pressure of a gas in the blood traveling through a pulmonary capillary equilibrates with the alveolar partial pressure before the blood has finished moving through the capillary, no further gas exchange takes place for that blood because there is no longer a pressure gradient for diffusion. Of course, new mixed venous blood just entering the capillary at the arterial end is not equilibrated with the alveolar partial pressure, so gas exchange occurs at the arterial end. To increase the gas exchange in that alveolar-capillary unit, the rate of blood flow through the capillary must be increased to expose unequilibrated blood to the alveolar air. This is called *perfusion* limitation of diffusion.

Nitrous oxide normally shows perfusion limitation of diffusion (as shown in Fig. 16-1) because it is so soluble in the alveolar-capillary barrier that its pulmonary capillary partial pressure equilibrates with the alveolar partial pressure within about 0.10 s. The remaining time that the equilibrated blood spends in the pulmonary capillary results in no further gas exchange. Nitrous oxide uptake is therefore perfusion-limited. Volatile anesthetic agents such as halothane are much more soluble than nitrous oxide and so they are also perfusion-limited.

It is important to realize that increasing the cardiac output normally increases gas diffusion in the lung not only by increasing the velocity of blood flow through the pulmonary capillaries but also by recruiting more pulmonary capillaries, thus increasing the surface area for diffusion.

DIFFUSION LIMITATION OF GAS TRANSFER

Carbon monoxide is an example of a gas whose diffusion into the blood is not perfusion-limited but *diffusion-limited*. The partial pressure of carbon monoxide breathed into the alveoli does not equilibrate with that of the plasma in the amount of time the blood spends in the pulmonary capillary (as shown in Fig. 16-1). This is because carbon monoxide binds chemically to hemoglobin (and thus is removed from solution). In fact, the affinity of carbon monoxide for hemoglobin is more than 200 times that of oxygen. The carbon monoxide that chemically combines with hemoglobin does not contribute to the partial pressure of carbon monoxide in the blood. Therefore, the partial pressure of carbon monoxide in the pulmonary capillary blood does not approach the partial pressure of carbon monoxide in the alveoli. The partial pressure gradient across the alveolar-capillary barrier for carbon monoxide is thus well maintained, and the diffusion of carbon monoxide is limited only by its diffusivity in the barrier, by the surface area, and by the thickness of the barrier. For this reason, carbon monoxide is used (in very low, nonlethal concentrations, of course) to test the diffusion characteristics of the alveolar-capillary barrier.

DIFFUSION OF OXYGEN

The time course for oxygen transfer is shown in Fig. 16-1A. The PO_2 of mixed venous blood entering the functional pulmonary capillary is 40 torr, and the PO_2 in the alveolus is 100 torr. The PO_2 of the blood equilibrates with the alveolar PO_2 within about 0.25 s, or about one-third of the time the blood spends in the pulmonary capillary at normal resting cardiac outputs. As oxygen enters the blood it is rapidly taken up by hemoglobin, which removes it from solution and thus maintains the partial pressure gradient across the alveolar-capillary barrier. The chemical combination of oxygen and hemoglobin, however, occurs rapidly (within hundredths of a second), and at the normal alveolar PO_2, the hemoglobin very quickly becomes nearly saturated with oxygen. The partial pressure of oxygen in the plasma then rises rapidly to equilibrium with the alveolar PO_2, and diffusion ceases. Therefore, oxygen transfer from alveolus to pulmonary capillary is perfusion-limited at a normal resting cardiac output.

During exercise, the movement of blood through the pulmonary capillary is much more rapid than at resting cardiac outputs. In fact, during severe

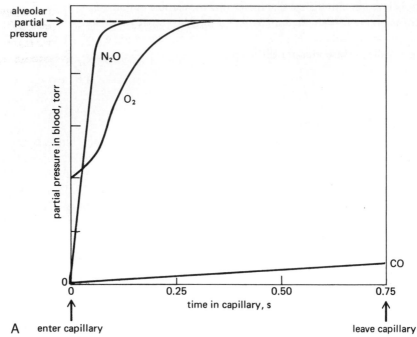

Figure 16-1 *A,* Calculated changes in the partial pressure of oxygen nitrous oxide, and carbon monoxide as blood passes through a pulmonary capillary. The alveolar P_{O_2} of about 100 torr is denoted by the dotted line. Note that the partial pressure of oxygen normally equilibrates rapidly with the alveolar P_{O_2}. (Forster RE II, Dubois AB, Briscoe WA Fisher AB: *The Lung: Physiologic Basis of Pulmonary Function Tests,* 3d ed. Chicago. Year Book Medical Publishers, 1986, pp. 190–222.) *B.* Calculated changes in the partial pressure of carbon dioxide as blood passes through a pulmonary capillary. The mixed venous P_{CO_2} is about 45 torr. The alveolar P_{CO_2} is indicated by the dotted line. Note that the partial pressure of CO_2 in the pulmonary capillary blood normally equilibrates rapidly with the alveolar P_{CO_2}. *(From Wagner PD, West JB: Effects of diffusion impairment on O_2 and CO_2 time courses in pulmonary capillaries. J Appl Physiol 33:62–71, 1972, with permission.)*

exercise blood may stay in the functional pulmonary capillary an average of only about 0.25 s. The rate of oxygen transfer into the blood per unit of time increases greatly because little or no perfusion limitation occurs. (Indeed, the blood that stays in the capillary *less* than the average time may be subjected to diffusion limitation of oxygen transfer.) Note that *total* oxygen transfer also increases during exercise because of recruitment of previously unperfused capillaries, and because of better matching of ventilation and perfusion. A person with an abnormal alveolar-capillary barrier due to a fibrotic thickening or interstitial edema may approach diffusion limitation of oxygen transfer at rest and may have a serious diffusion limitation of oxygen transfer during strenuous exercise. A person with an extremely abnormal alveolar-capillary barrier might have diffusion limitation of oxygen transfer even at rest. Emphysema can also cause diffusion limitation of oxygen transfer during exercise, because the destruction of alveolar septa decreases the surface area for diffusion.

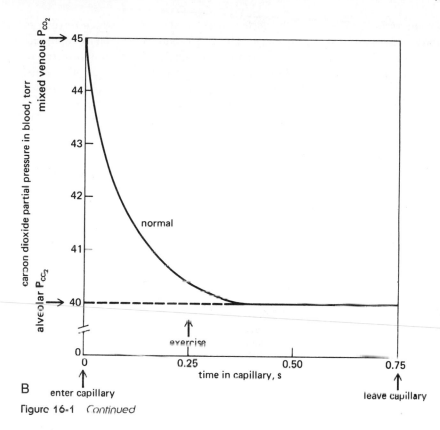

B   enter capillary   leave capillary

Figure 16-1   Continued

DIFFUSION OF CARBON DIOXIDE

Figure 16-1B shows the time course of carbon dioxide transfer from the pulmonary capillary blood to the alveolus. In a normal person having a mixed venous partial pressure of carbon dioxide of 45 torr and an alveolar partial pressure of carbon dioxide of 40 torr, an equilibrium is reached in about 0.25 s, or about the same time as that for oxygen. This may seem surprising, since the diffusivity of carbon dioxide is about 20 times that of oxygen, but the partial pressure gradient is normally only about 5 torr for carbon dioxide, whereas it is about 60 torr for oxygen. Carbon dioxide transfer is also normally *perfusion-limited,* as shown in the figure; it may be diffusion-limited in a person with an abnormal alveolar-capillary barrier.

MEASUREMENT OF DIFFUSING CAPACITY

It is often useful to assess the diffusion characteristics of a patient's lungs, particularly whether an apparent impairment in diffusion is a result of *perfusion limitation* or *diffusion limitation.*

The *diffusing capacity* (or transfer factor) is the rate at which oxygen or carbon monoxide is absorbed from the alveolar gas into the pulmonary capillaries (in milliliters per minute) per unit of partial pressure gradient (in millimeters of mercury). The diffusing capacity of the lung (for gas x), DL_x, is therefore equal to the uptake of gas x, $\dot{V}_x$, divided by the difference between the alveolar partial pressure of gas x, P_{A_x}, and the mean capillary partial pressure of gas x, $P\bar{c}_x$:

$$DL_x = \frac{\dot{V}_x}{P_{A_x} - P\bar{c}_x} \quad \text{ml/min/mmHg}$$

This is really just a rearrangement of the Fick equation. The terms for area, diffusivity, and thickness have been combined into DL_x and the equation has been rearranged:

$$\dot{V}_x = \frac{A \times D \times (P_1 - P_2)}{T}$$

$$\frac{\dot{V}_x}{P_1 - P_2} = \frac{A \times D}{T}$$

$$DL_x = \frac{\dot{V}_x}{P_1 - P_2}$$

The mean partial pressures of oxygen or carbon monoxide are, as already discussed, affected by their chemical reactions with hemoglobin, as well as by their transfer through the alveolar-capillary barrier. For this reason, the diffusing capacity of the lung is determined by both the diffusing capacity of the membrane D_M and the reaction with hemoglobin, expressed as $\theta \times Vc$, where θ is the volume of gas in milliliters per minute taken up by the erythrocytes in 1 ml of blood per millimeter of mercury partial pressure gradient between the plasma and the erythrocyte and Vc is the capillary blood volume in milliliters. (The units of $\theta \times Vc$ are therefore ml/min/mmHg.) The diffusing capacity of the lung D_L can be shown to be related to D_M and $\theta \times Vc$ as follows:

$$\frac{1}{DL} = \frac{1}{DM} + \frac{1}{\theta \times VC}\left(+\frac{1}{DA}\right)$$

DA, or diffusion through the alveolus, is normally very rapid and may be disregarded.

Carbon monoxide is most frequently used in determinations of the diffusing capacity because the mean pulmonary capillary partial pressure of carbon monoxide is virtually zero when nonlethal alveolar partial pressures of carbon monoxide are used:

$$DL_{CO} = \frac{\dot{V}_{CO}}{PA_{CO} - P\bar{c}_{CO}}$$

but

$$P\bar{c}_{CO} \simeq 0$$

and so

$$DL_{CO} = \frac{\dot{V}_{CO}}{PA_{CO}}$$

Several different methods are used clinically to measure the carbon monoxide diffusing capacity and involve both single-breath and steady-state techniques, sometimes during exercise. The DL_{CO} is decreased in diseases associated with thickening of the barrier, such as interstitial or alveolar fibrosis, sarcoidosis, scleroderma, and asbestosis, or conditions causing interstitial or alveolar pulmonary edema as shown in Table 16-1. It is also decreased in conditions causing a decrease in the surface area available for diffusion, such as emphysema, tumors, low cardiac output, or a low pulmonary capillary blood volume; conditions causing decreased uptake by red blood cells; as well as in conditions leading to ventilation-perfusion mismatch, which effectively decrease the surface area for diffusion.

Table 16-1   Conditions That Decrease the Diffusing Capacity

Thickening of the barrier
  Interstitial or alveolar edema
  Interstitial or alveolar fibrosis
    Sarcoidosis
    Scleroderma
Decreased surface area
  Emphysema
  Tumors
  Low cardiac output
  Low pulmonary capillary blood volume
Ventilation-perfusion mismatch
Decreased uptake by erythrocytes
  Anemia
  Low pulmonary capillary blood volume

From Levitzky MG: *Pulmonary Physiology,* 4th ed. New York, McGraw-Hill, 1995, with permission.

BIBLIOGRAPHY

Forster RE II, Dubois AB, Briscoe WA, Fisher AB: *The Lung: Physiologic Basis of Pulmonary Function Tests,* 3d ed. Chicago, Year Book Medical Publishers, 1986, pp 190–222.

Levitzky MG: *Pulmonary Physiology,* 4th ed. New York, McGraw-Hill, 1995, pp 130–141.

Nunn JF: *Nunn's Applied Respiratory Physiology,* 4th ed. Oxford, Butterworth-Heinemann, 1993, pp 198–218.

Wagner PD, West JB: Effects of diffusion impairment on O_2 and CO_2 time courses in pulmonary capillaries. *J Appl Physiol* 33:62–71, 1972.

West JB: *Respiratory Physiology—The Essentials,* 5th ed. Baltimore, Williams & Wilkins, 1995, pp 21–30.

17

OXYGEN AND CARBON DIOXIDE TRANSPORT

OBJECTIVES
The reader should be able to:

1 State the relationship between the partial pressure of oxygen in the blood and the amount of oxygen physically dissolved in the blood.
2 Describe the chemical combination of oxygen with hemoglobin and the "oxygen dissociation curve."
3 Define hemoglobin *saturation,* the oxygen-carrying *capacity,* and the oxygen *content* of blood.
4 State the physiologic consequences of the shape of the oxygen dissociation curve and discuss the physiologic factors that can influence the oxygen dissociation curve.
5 State the relationship between the partial pressure of carbon dioxide in the blood and the amount of carbon dioxide physically dissolved in the blood.
6 Describe the transport of carbon dioxide as carbamino compounds with blood proteins
7 Explain how most of the carbon dioxide in the blood is transported as bicarbonate.
8 Describe the carbon dioxide dissociation curve for whole blood.

PERSPECTIVE
The blood carries oxygen both physically dissolved in the blood and chemically bound to the hemoglobin in red blood cells. Normally, much more oxygen is transported in combination with hemoglobin than physically dissolved in the blood. Without hemoglobin, the cardiovascular system could not transport sufficient oxygen to meet tissue demands. The blood carries carbon dioxide in physical solution, chemically combined to amino acids in blood proteins, and as bicarbonate ions.

TRANSPORT OF OXYGEN IN THE BLOOD

Transport of Physically Dissolved Oxygen

The solubility of oxygen in plasma is such that at a temperature of 37°C, 1 ml of plasma contains 0.00003 ml of oxygen per torr P_{O_2}. This corresponds to Henry's law. Oxygen dissolves in the fluid inside the red blood cells in about the same amount, so *whole blood* contains a similar amount of dissolved oxygen per milliliter.

Blood oxygen content is conventionally expressed in milliliters of oxygen per 100 ml of blood, which is called *volume percent,* so there is 0.003 ml of oxygen per torr P_{O_2} physically dissolved in 100 ml of whole blood. Thus, at an arterial P_{O_2} of 100 torr, there is only 0.3 ml of oxygen transported physically dissolved in the 100 ml of blood.

Chemically Combined with Hemoglobin

Hemoglobin has a molecular weight of about 65,000 daltons. The protein portion (globin) consists of four linked polypeptide chains, each of which is attached to a protoporphyrin (heme) group. Each heme group consists of four symmetrically arranged pyrrol groups with a ferrous (Fe^{++}) iron atom at its center. The iron atom is bound to each of the pyrrol groups and to one of the four polypeptide chains. A sixth binding site on the ferrous iron atom can bind with oxygen (or carbon monoxide). Therefore, *each* of the four polypeptide chains is able to bind an oxygen (or carbon monoxide) molecule to the iron atom in its own heme group. Thus, the tetrameric hemoglobin molecule can combine chemically with four oxygen molecules.

Hemoglobin rapidly combines *reversibly* with oxygen. The reversibility of the reaction allows oxygen to be released to the tissues. The reaction is extremely fast, with a half time of 0.01 s or less. Each gram of hemoglobin can theoretically combine with about 1.39 ml of oxygen under optimal conditions, but normally some hemoglobin may be in forms that cannot bind oxygen, such as methemoglobin (the iron atom is in the ferric [Fe^{+++}] state) or combined with carbon monoxide. For this reason, the oxygen-carrying *capacity* of hemoglobin is conventionally considered to be 1.34 ml of oxygen per gram of hemoglobin. That is, each gram of hemoglobin, when *fully saturated* with oxygen, binds 1.34 ml of oxygen.

The reaction of hemoglobin and oxygen is conventionally written:

$$Hb + O_2 \rightleftharpoons HbO_2$$

Deoxyhemoglobin   Oxyhemoglobin

The equilibrium point of the reversible reaction of hemoglobin and oxygen depends on how much oxygen the hemoglobin in blood is exposed to. This exposure corresponds directly to the P_{O_2} in the plasma under the conditions in the body. Thus the P_{O_2} of the plasma *determines* the amount of oxygen that binds to the hemoglobin in the red blood cells.

One way to express the proportion of hemoglobin that is bound to oxygen is as *percent saturation* (Sa_{O_2}). This is equal to the amount of oxygen in the blood (minus that part physically dissolved), divided by the oxygen-carrying capacity of the hemoglobin in the blood times 100 percent.

$$\%\text{Hb saturation} = \frac{O_2 \text{ content of hemoglobin}}{O_2 \text{ capacity of hemoglobin}} \times 100\%$$

Note that a person's oxygen-carrying *capacity* depends on the amount of hemoglobin in that person's blood. The blood oxygen *content* also depends on the amount of hemoglobin present (as well as the P_{O_2}). Both content and capacity are expressed as milliliters of oxygen per 100 ml of blood. The percent hemoglobin saturation, on the other hand, expresses only a percentage and not an amount or volume of oxygen. Therefore, percent saturation is not interchangeable with oxygen content. For example, two patients may have the same arterial P_{O_2} and the same percent hemoglobin saturation, but if one has a lower blood hemoglobin concentration because of anemia, he or she also has a lower blood oxygen content and capacity.

OXYHEMOGLOBIN DISSOCIATION CURVE

The relationship between the P_{O_2} of the plasma and the percent of hemoglobin saturation is demonstrated by the *oxyhemoglobin dissociation curve* shown in Fig. 17-1. The curve shown is for blood at 37°C with a pH of 7.40 and a P_{CO_2} of 40 torr.

The oxyhemoglobin dissociation curve is a way of expressing how the availability of one reactant, oxygen (expressed as the P_{O_2} of the plasma), affects the reversible chemical reaction of oxygen and hemoglobin. The product, oxyhemoglobin, is expressed as percent saturation—really a percent of the maximum for any given amount of hemoglobin.

Figure 17-1 shows that the relationship between P_{O_2} and HbO_2 is not linear; it is an S-shaped curve, steep at lower P_{O_2}'s and nearly flat when the P_{O_2} is above 70 torr. The reason that the curve is not linear is that it is actually a plot of four successive reactions, as each of the four hemoglobin subunits combines with a molecule of oxygen.

OXYGEN LOADING IN THE LUNG

Mixed venous blood entering the pulmonary capillaries normally has a P_{O_2} of about 40 torr, at which hemoglobin is about 75 percent saturated with oxygen. If

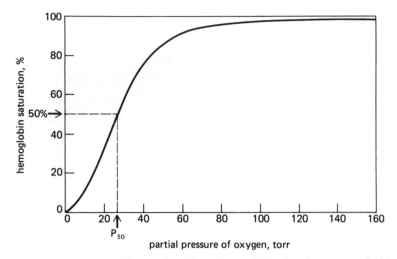

Figure 17-1 A typical "normal" adult oxyhemoglobin dissociation curve for blood at a pH of 7.40, a P_{CO_2} of 40 torr, and at 37°C. The P_{50} is the partial pressure of oxygen at which hemoglobin is 50 percent saturated with oxygen. *(From Levitzky MG, Pulmonary Physiology, 4th ed., New York, McGraw-Hill, 1995, with permission.)*

we assume the blood hemoglobin concentration to be 15 g of hemoglobin per 100 ml of blood, this corresponds to 15.08 ml of oxygen per 100 ml of blood *bound to hemoglobin* plus an additional 0.12 ml of oxygen per 100 ml of blood *physically dissolved,* so the *total oxygen content* is about 15.20 ml of oxygen per 100 ml of blood.

As the blood passes through the pulmonary capillaries, it equilibrates with the alveolar P_{O_2} of about 100 torr. At a P_{O_2} of 100 torr, hemoglobin is about 97.4 percent saturated with oxygen (see Fig. 17-1). This corresponds to 19.58 ml of oxygen per 100 ml of blood bound to hemoglobin plus 0.3 ml of oxygen per 100 ml of blood physically dissolved, or a *total oxygen content* of 19.88 ml of oxygen per 100 ml of blood.

Note that the oxyhemoglobin dissociation curve is relatively flat at P_{O_2}'s greater than about 70 torr. This is important physiologically, because it means that the oxygen content of blood decreases only slightly if it is equilibrated with a P_{O_2} of 70 torr instead of 100 torr. Similarly, because hemoglobin is about 97.4 percent saturated at a P_{O_2} of 100 torr, raising the alveolar P_{O_2} above 100 torr can load little additional oxygen onto hemoglobin. Hemoglobin is fully saturated with oxygen at a P_{O_2} of about 250 torr.

OXYGEN UNLOADING AT THE TISSUES

As blood passes from the arteries into the systemic capillaries, it is exposed to lower P_{O_2}'s, and oxygen is released by the hemoglobin. The P_{O_2} in the capillaries varies from tissue to tissue, being very low in some (e.g., the myocardium) and relatively higher in others (e.g., the kidney). As Fig. 17-1 shows, the oxyhemoglobin dissociation curve is rather steep in the range of 10 to 40 torr. This means that small decreases in PO_2 can result in a substantial further dissociation of oxygen and hemoglobin, unloading more oxygen for use by the tissues.

INFLUENCES ON THE OXYHEMOGLOBIN DISSOCIATION CURVE

The unloading of oxygen at the tissues is facilitated by other physiologic factors that can influence the chemical reaction of oxygen and hemoglobin and therefore *alter the shape and position* of the oxyhemoglobin dissociation curve. These factors include the pH, PCO_2, and temperature of the blood, and the concentration of 2,3-diphosphoglycerate (2,3-DPG; also called 2,3-BPG) in the red blood cells.

Figure 17-2 shows the influence of temperature, pH, PCO_2, and the concentration of 2,3-DPG on the oxyhemoglobin dissociation curve. Elevated temperature, low pH, high PCO_2, and elevated levels of 2,3-DPG all shift the oxyhemoglobin dissociation curve to the right, so that less oxygen combines with hemoglobin at a given PO_2. The influence of pH (and PCO_2) on the oxyhemoglobin dissociation curve, referred to as the *Bohr effect,* is discussed later.

Low temperatures shift the curve to the left; high temperatures shift the curve to the right. At extremely low blood temperatures, hemoglobin has such high affinity for oxygen that it does not release it even at very low PO_2's. Note that oxygen is *more* soluble in water or plasma at lower temperatures than at normal body temperature. At 20°C, about 50 percent more oxygen dissolves in plasma.

The metabolite 2,3-DPG is produced by red blood cells during anaerobic glycolysis, and normally is present in fairly high concentrations in red cells. High concentrations of 2,3-DPG shift the oxyhemoglobin dissociation curve to the right (see Fig. 17-2). More 2,3-DPG is produced during chronic hypoxia, thereby shifting the dissociation curve farther to the right and allowing more oxygen to be released from hemoglobin at a particular PO_2. Very low levels of 2,3-DPG shift the curve far to the left. Blood deficient in 2,3-DPG therefore does not unload much oxygen except at very low PO_2's.

The physiologic consequences of the effects on the oxyhemoglobin dissociation curve shown in Fig. 17-2 make sense if we think of the situation in a metabolically active tissue like skeletal muscle during exercise. The muscle releases carbon dioxide as the end product of aerobic metabolism and hydrogen ions (lactic acid) as an end product of anaerobic metabolism. The temperature increases because heat is released. These changes all shift the oxyhemoglobin dissociation curve to the right, facilitating release of oxygen. Mixed venous blood has a lower pH and higher PCO_2 and may even have a higher temperature and 2,3-DPG concentration than the normal arterial blood shown in Fig. 17-1. Thus the oxyhemoglobin dissociation curve is shifted to the right for venous blood.

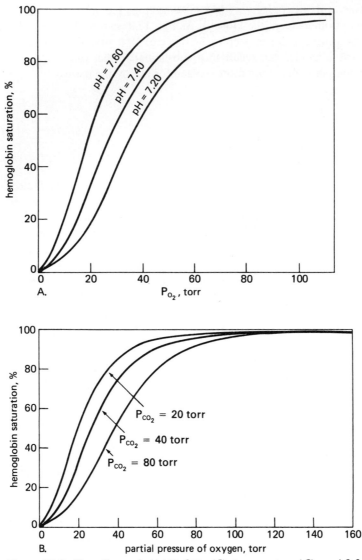

Figure 17-2 The effects of pH (*A*), P_{CO_2} (*B*), temperature (*C*), and 2,3-DPG (*D*) on the oxyhemoglobin dissociation curve. (*From Levitzky MG, Pulmonary Physiology, 4th ed., New York, McGraw-Hill, 1995, with permission.*)

Note that the effects of pH, P_{CO_2}, and temperature shown in Fig. 17-2 are all more pronounced at lower P_{O_2}'s. That is, they enhance oxygen unloading at the tissues more profoundly than they interfere with oxygen loading in the lungs.

The P_{50} shown in Fig. 17-1 is a convenient term for discussing shifts in the oxyhemoglobin dissociation curve. The P_{50} is the P_{O_2} at which 50 percent of the

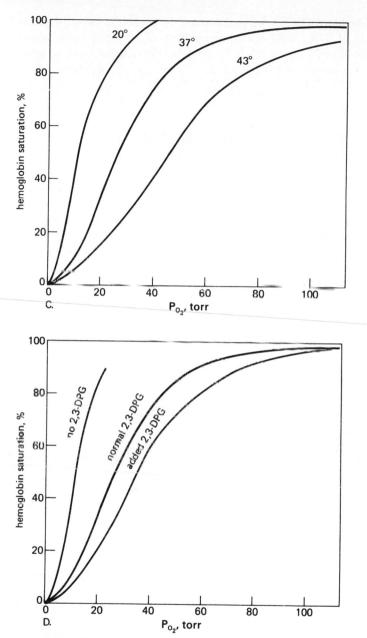

Figure 17-2   *Continued*

hemoglobin in the blood is deoxyhemoglobin and 50 percent is oxyhemoglobin. At a temperature of 37°C, a pH of 7.4, and a PCO_2 of 40 torr, normal human blood has a P_{50} of 26 or 27 torr. If the oxyhemoglobin dissociation curve is shifted to the right, the P_{50} increases; if it is shifted to the left, the P_{50} decreases.

OTHER FACTORS AFFECTING OXYGEN TRANSPORT

Anemia, carbon monoxide poisoning, methemoglobinemia, and abnormal kinds of hemoglobin can all affect oxygen transport adversely. Most forms of anemia do not affect the oxyhemoglobin dissociation curve if the association of oxygen and hemoglobin is expressed as *percent saturation*. For example, anemia secondary to blood loss does not affect the combination of oxygen and hemoglobin for the remaining erythrocytes. It is the *amount* of functional hemoglobin, and, therefore, the oxygen-carrying capacity and the arterial *content* of oxygen that decrease.

Carbon monoxide not only decreases oxygen transport by combining with hemoglobin, it also shifts the oxyhemoglobin dissociation curve to the left. Thus carbon monoxide can both prevent the loading of oxygen into the blood in the lungs and interfere with the unloading of oxygen at the tissues. Methemoglobin—hemoglobin with its iron in the ferric (Fe^{3+}) state—can be caused by nitrite poisoning or toxic reactions to oxidant drugs. It is also a congenital aberration in patients with hemoglobin M. In the Fe^{3+} state, iron atoms do not combine with oxygen.

Abnormal hemoglobins may have affinities for oxygen different from that of normal adult hemoglobin A (HbA). The best known of the abnormal hemoglobins, hemoglobin S, is responsible for *sickle cell anemia*. Deoxygenated hemoglobin S is not very soluble in the intracellular fluid of erythrocytes. At low PO_2's, therefore, it may crystallize within the red blood cells. This crystallization changes the shape of the erythrocyte from the normal biconcave disk to a crescent or sickle shape. Sickle cells are more fragile than normal red blood cells, and they also have a greater tendency to adhere to each other. This adherence increases blood viscosity and may also cause thrombosis and blood vessel blockage. Other abnormal hemoglobins, which, like hemoglobin S, are usually of genetic origin, may have either increased or decreased affinities for oxygen. Fetal hemoglobin (HbF) has a greater affinity for oxygen than HbA does.

TRANSPORT OF CARBON DIOXIDE IN THE BLOOD

Transport of Physically Dissolved Carbon Dioxide

Carbon dioxide is about 20 times more soluble in plasma (and inside the erythrocytes) than oxygen. About 5 to 10 percent of the total carbon dioxide transported by the blood is carried in physical solution.

Transport of Carbon Dioxide as Carbamino Compounds

Carbon dioxide can combine chemically with the terminal amine groups in blood proteins to form *carbamino compounds:*

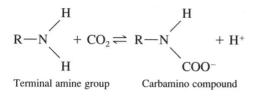

Terminal amine group   Carbamino compound

The reaction occurs rapidly; no enzymes are necessary.

Because hemoglobin is the most abundant blood protein, most of the carbon dioxide carried as carbamino compounds is bound to the amino acids of hemoglobin. Deoxyhemoglobin can bind more carbon dioxide as carbamino groups than can oxyhemoglobin. Therefore, as the venous blood enters the lung and the hemoglobin combines with oxygen, carbon dioxide is released from its terminal amine groups. About 5 to 10 percent of the blood's total carbon dioxide content is in the form of carbamino compounds.

Transport of Carbon Dioxide as Bicarbonate

The remaining 80 to 90 percent of the carbon dioxide in the blood is carried as bicarbonate ions. The following reaction shows how this occurs:

$$CO_2 + H_2O \underset{\text{anhydrase}}{\overset{\text{carbonic}}{\rightleftharpoons}} H_2CO_3 \rightleftharpoons H^+ + HCO_3$$

Carbon dioxide forms carbonic acid by combining with water. It can then dissociate into a hydrogen ion and a bicarbonate ion. Except in the presence of carbonic anhydrase, an enzyme found in the erythrocytes, this reaction is too slow to be physiologically significant. Hemoglobin also plays a critical role in the transport of carbon dioxide as bicarbonate because it can accept the hydrogen ion liberated by the dissociation of carbonic acid and it thereby allows the reaction to continue. This is discussed in greater detail later.

CARBON DIOXIDE DISSOCIATION CURVE

The carbon dioxide dissociation curve for whole blood is depicted in Fig. 17-3 (note that the Y axis is CO_2 *content*). It shows that, within the normal physiologic range of P_{CO_2}'s, the curve is nearly a straight line. If plotted on axes similar to those for oxygen content, the carbon dioxide dissociation curve for whole blood is steeper than the oxygen dissociation curve for whole blood. That is, the change in carbon dioxide content per torr change in P_{CO_2} is greater than the change in oxygen content per torr change in P_{O_2}.

The carbon dioxide dissociation curve for whole blood shifts to the right when blood contains mainly oxyhemoglobin; it shifts to the left when blood contains mainly deoxyhemoglobin. This is known as the *Haldane effect*. The Haldane effect allows the blood to load more carbon dioxide at the tissues, where more deoxyhemoglobin is present, and unload more carbon dioxide in the lungs, where more oxyhemoglobin is present.

The Bohr and Haldane effects are both mainly explained by the fact that *deoxyhemoglobin is a weaker acid than oxyhemoglobin.* That is, deoxyhemoglobin more readily accepts the hydrogen ion liberated by the dissociation of carbonic acid, thus permitting more carbon dioxide to be carried in the form of bicarbonate ions. Conversely, the association of hydrogen ions with the amino acids of hemoglobin lowers the affinity of hemoglobin for oxygen, thereby shifting the oxyhemoglobin dissociation curve to the right at low pH's or high PCO_2's. The following equation shows these actions:

$$H^+Hb + O_2 \rightleftharpoons H^+ + HbO_2$$

These effects of oxygen and carbon dioxide transport can be seen in Fig. 17-4. At the tissues, the PO_2 is low and the PCO_2 is high. Carbon dioxide dissolves

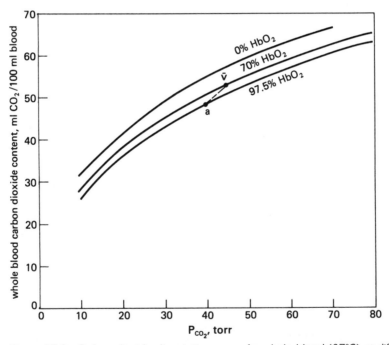

Figure 17-3 Carbon dioxide dissociation curves for whole blood (37°C) at different oxyhemoglobin saturations. Note that the ordinate is whole blood CO_2 content in milliliters of CO_2 per 100 ml of blood. *(From Levitzky MG, Pulmonary Physiology, 4th ed., New York, McGraw-Hill, 1995, with permission.)*

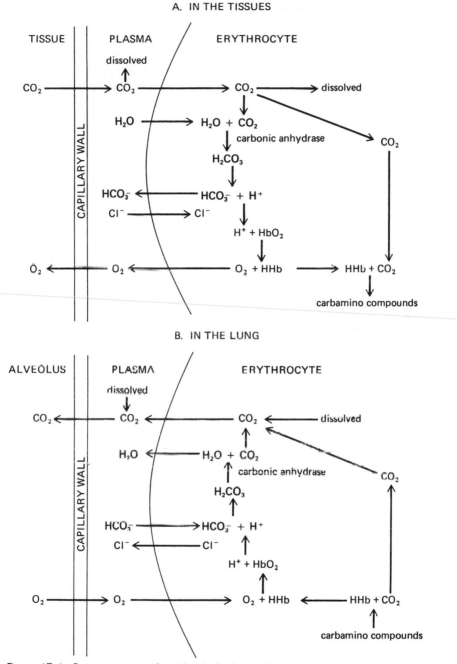

Figure 17-4 Representation of uptake and release of carbon dioxide and oxygen at the tissues (*A*) and in the lung (*B*). Note that negligible amounts of CO_2 can form carbamino compounds with blood proteins other than hemoglobin and may also be hydrated in trivial amounts in the plasma to form carbonic acid and then bicarbonate (not shown in diagram). (*From Levitzky MG: Pulmonary Physiology, 4th ed. New York, McGraw-Hill, 1995, with permission.*)

in the plasma, and some of it then diffuses into the erythrocytes. Some of this carbon dioxide dissolves in the cytosol, some forms carbamino compounds with hemoglobin, and some is hydrated by carbonic anhydrase to form carbonic acid. At low PO_2's, the erythrocytes contain substantial amounts of deoxyhemoglobin, which is able to accept the hydrogen ion liberated by the dissociation of carbonic acid. Because bicarbonate ions diffuse out of the erythrocyte through the cell membrane much more readily than do hydrogen ions, an electrical imbalance within the cell should occur. However, electrical neutrality is maintained by the diffusion of chloride ions into the cell to match the movement of bicarbonate ions out of the cell. This is called the chloride shift. To maintain the osmotic equilibrium, small amounts of water also move into the cell.

At the lung, the PO_2 is high and the PCO_2 is low. As oxygen combines with hemoglobin, the hydrogen ions that had been absorbed when the hemoglobin was in the deoxyhemoglobin state are released. They combine with bicarbonate ions to form carbonic acid. The acid, in turn, breaks down into carbon dioxide and water. Coincidentally, carbon dioxide is also released from the carbamino compounds, the formation of which is less favorable at high PO_2's. Carbon dioxide then diffuses out of the erythrocytes and plasma and into the alveoli. A chloride shift also occurs in a direction opposite to that in the tissues to maintain electrical neutrality.

BIBLIOGRAPHY

Levitzky MG: *Pulmonary Physiology,* 4th ed. New York, McGraw-Hill, 1995, pp 142–162.

Levitzky MG, Cairo JM, Hall SM: *Introduction to Respiratory Care.* Philadelphia, Saunders, pp 129–136.

Nunn JF: *Nunn's Applied Respiratory Physiology,* 4th ed. Oxford, Butterworth-Heinemann, 1993, pp 219–231; 269–287.

Prange HD: *Respiratory Physiology: Understanding Gas Exchange.* New York, Chapman & Hall, 1996, pp 83–117.

18

CONTROL OF BREATHING

OBJECTIVES

The reader should be able to:

1   Describe the general organization of the respiratory control system, including the centers that generate the spontaneous rhythmicity of breathing, the groups of neurons that affect inspiration and expiration, and the other centers in the brain stem that may influence the spontaneous rhythmicity of breathing.
2   List the cardiopulmonary and other reflexes that influence the breathing pattern.
3   Describe the effects of alterations in body oxygen, carbon dioxide, and hydrogen ion levels on the control of breathing.
4   Describe the sensors of the respiratory system for oxygen, carbon dioxide, and hydrogen ion concentration.

PERSPECTIVE

Breathing must be initiated in the central nervous system. Neurons in the brain stem *automatically* generate a cycle of inspiration and expiration. This spontaneous breathing cycle can be altered or temporarily suppressed by reflexes and higher centers in the brain.

The respiratory centers in the brain stem control breathing via a *final common pathway* consisting of the spinal cord, the innervation of the muscles of respiration (such as the phrenic nerves), and the muscles of respiration themselves. The *interval* between successive groups of discharges of the respiratory neurons determines the breathing frequency. The *frequency* and *duration* of neural discharges to each respiratory muscle fiber and the *number of respiratory muscle fibers* and types of muscles activated determine the tidal volume.

GENERATION OF SPONTANEOUS RESPIRATORY RHYTHMICITY

The neurons that initiate breathing are located in an area in the reticular formation of the medulla, beneath the floor of the fourth ventricle, known as the *medullary*

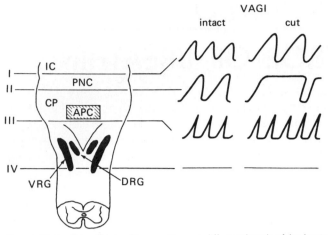

Figure 18-1 The effects of transections at different levels of the brain stem on the ventilatory pattern of anesthetized animals. At left is a diagram of the dorsal surface of the lower brain stem. At right is a diagram of the breathing patterns (inspiration is upward) corresponding to the transections with the vagus nerves intact or transected. (DRG = dorsal respiratory group; VRG = ventral respiratory group; APC = apneustic center; PNC = pneumotaxic center; IC = inferior colliculus; CP = cerebellar peduncle.) *(From Berger AJ, Mitchell RA, Severinghaus JW: Regulation of respiration. Reprinted by permission, New England Journal of Medicine, © 1977 Massachusettes Medical Society.)*

center (or medullary respiratory center). If the brain stem of an anesthetized animal is cut *above* this area, as shown in the transection labeled III in Fig. 18-1, a pattern of inspiration and expiration continues, even if all other nerves leading to this area, including the vagi, are also cut. If the brain stem is cut *below* this area, as seen in transection IV, breathing *stops*.

The medullary respiratory center consists of two dense bilateral aggregations of respiratory neurons known as the *dorsal respiratory groups* (DRG) and the *ventral respiratory groups* (VRG). Inspiratory and expiratory neurons are anatomically intermingled within these areas. The dorsal respiratory groups consist mainly of *inspiratory cells,* which project their fibers primarily to the contralateral spinal cord and innervate inspiratory muscles. They probably serve as the chief initiators of the activity of the phrenic nerves and are therefore responsible for the activity of the diaphragm. Although the dorsal respiratory group neurons send collateral fibers to neurons in the ventral respiratory groups, the latter sends very few collateral fibers to the dorsal respiratory groups.

The dorsal respiratory groups are located in the nuclei of the tractus solitarius, which are primary projection sites of afferent fibers of the ninth cranial nerve (the glossopharyngeal) and the tenth cranial nerve (the vagus). These nerves carry information about the arterial chemoreceptors and information about the systemic arterial blood pressure from the carotid and aortic baroreceptors. In addition, the vagus carries information from stretch receptors and other sensors in the lungs that may also profoundly influence the control of breathing. The location of the dorsal respiratory groups within the nuclei of the tractus solitarius suggests that

that group may be the site of integration of various inputs that can reflexly alter the spontaneous pattern of inspiration and expiration.

The dorsal respiratory groups have two populations of inspiratory neurons. One, called *alpha cells,* is inhibited by lung inflation; the second, the *beta cells,* is excited by lung inflation. These cells may play an important role in the Hering-Breuer reflexes discussed later in this chapter. The ventral respiratory group neurons include both inspiratory and expiratory cells. The major function of these cells is to drive either spinal respiratory neurons, innervating mainly the intercostal and abdominal muscles, or the auxiliary muscles of respiration innervated by the vagus nerves. Because the dorsal respiratory groups send many fibers to the ventral respiratory groups, but the ventral groups send few to the dorsal groups, the dorsal respiratory groups may drive the ventral respiratory groups, but reciprocal inhibition between the two groups is unlikely.

The exact mechanism by which the spontaneous rhythmicity of breathing is generated is as yet unknown. It now seems that cells in or near the dorsal respiratory groups act as pacemakers themselves and that their activity is modulated by information received from afferent nerves and higher brain centers.

MEDULLARY AND PONTINE RESPIRATORY CENTERS

Transection of the brain stem in the pons at the level denoted by the line labeled II in Fig. 18-1 results in a breathing pattern called *apneusis* if the vagus nerves have also been transected. Apneustic breathing is characterized by prolonged inspiratory efforts interrupted by occasional expirations. Afferent information reaching this *apneustic center* (labeled APC) via the vagus nerves must be important in preventing apneusis because apneusis does not occur if the vagus nerves are left intact, as shown in the figure.

Apneusis must involve a sustained discharge of medullary inspiratory neurons. Investigators believe that the apneustic center may be the site of the normal "inspiratory cutoff switch," that is, the site of projection of various types of afferent information, such as the information from receptors that respond to lung inflation, that can *terminate inspiration.* Apneusis results from the inactivation of the inspiratory cutoff mechanism. The specific group of neurons that functions as the apneustic center has not been identified.

If the brain stem is transected immediately below the inferior colliculus, as indicated by line I in Fig. 18-1, the balance between inspiration and expiration remains essentially normal—even if the vagus nerves are transected. A group of respiratory neurons known as the *pneumotaxic center* therefore acts to modulate the response of the apneustic center. These cells probably function to fine-tune the breathing pattern. Pulmonary inflation afferent information from stretch receptors in the lungs can inhibit the activity of the pneumotaxic center. The pneumotaxic center may also modulate the respiratory control system's response to other stimuli, such as hypercapnia or hypoxia.

SPINAL PATHWAYS

Axons from the dorsal respiratory groups, ventral respiratory groups, cortex, and other supraspinal sites project to the spinal white matter to affect the action of the diaphragm, and the intercostal and abdominal muscles. At the level of these spinal respiratory motor neurons, there is integration of descending influences as well as the presence of local spinal reflexes. In the spinal cord, ascending pathways carrying information from pain, touch, and temperature receptors, as well as from proprioceptors, can also affect breathing, as discussed in the next section. Inspiratory and expiratory fibers are apparently separated in the spinal cord.

REFLEX MECHANISMS OF RESPIRATORY CONTROL

A number of sensors in the lungs, cardiovascular system, muscles and tendons, and skin and viscera can affect the control of breathing by eliciting reflex changes, as shown in Table 18-1. Stimulation of pulmonary stretch receptors can elicit three respiratory reflexes: the Hering-Breuer inflation reflex, the Hering-Breuer deflation reflex, and the paradoxical reflex of Head.

The Hering-Breuer inflation reflex was originally believed to act to tonically limit the tidal volume because vagotomized, anesthetized animals breathe much more deeply and at a lower rate than they do before their vagus nerves are transected. However, more recent studies done on conscious adult humans have shown that the threshold of the Hering-Breuer inflation reflex occurs at tidal volumes greater than 800 to 1000 ml. The Hering-Breuer inflation reflex may help to minimize the work of breathing by inhibiting large tidal volumes and may prevent overdistention of the alveoli at high lung volumes. The reflex may also be important in the control of breathing in infants.

The Hering-Breuer deflation reflex may be responsible for the increased ventilation elicited when the lungs are deflated abnormally, as in pneumothorax, or it may play a role in the periodic spontaneous deep breaths (sighs) that help to prevent atelectasis. These sighs, which occur occasionally and irregularly during normal, quiet breathing, consist of a slow deep inspiration (larger than a normal tidal volume) followed by a slow expiration. The paradoxical reflex of Head may also be involved in the sigh response. Some investigators have suggested that the reflex is involved in generating the first breath of the newborn baby.

Other reflexes that can influence the respiratory cycle include the cough and sneeze reflexes, reflexes initiated by the pulmonary "J" receptors (for *juxtapulmonary capillary receptors,* which are stretch receptors and/or chemoreceptors probably located in the interstitium just outside the pulmonary capillaries), the arterial chemoreceptor and baroreceptor reflexes, and reflexes initiated by receptors in muscles and tendons and by pain receptors.

The arterial baroreceptors have a minor influence on the control of ventilation. Ventilation can be increased by stimulation of receptors in the muscles, tendons, and joints. Receptors in the muscles of respiration and rib cage may be important in compensating for elevated work loads and may help to minimize the work of breathing. Receptors in the limbs may participate in increasing ventilation during exercise. Somatic pain generally causes hyperpnea; visceral pain generally causes apnea or decreased ventilation. Pinching a patient whose breathing is depressed may increase ventilation via the ventilatory response to somatic pain.

INFLUENCES OF HIGHER CENTERS

The spontaneous rhythmicity generated by the medullary respiratory center can be altered voluntarily: A person can hyperventilate or hold the breath for several minutes. During speech, singing, or playing a wind instrument, higher brain centers automatically modify the normal breathing cycle.

CHEMICAL CONTROL OF BREATHING

The respiratory control system acts as a *negative feedback system*. Changes in the controlled variables—P_{O_2}, P_{CO_2}, and pH—normally result in adjustments of alveolar ventilation designed to return them to their normal levels. Chemoreceptors sensitive to their own local P_{O_2}, P_{CO_2}, and pH supply the central respiratory controller with the information necessary to properly adjust alveolar ventilation to change the whole-body P_{O_2}, P_{CO_2}, and pH.

Response to Carbon Dioxide

The arterial and cerebrospinal fluid partial pressures of carbon dioxide are probably the most important inputs to the central respiratory controller in establishing the breath-to-breath ventilatory rate and tidal volume. Elevated carbon dioxide levels are an extremely strong stimulus to ventilation. Only voluntary hyperventilation and exercise produce greater minute ventilations. The respiratory system normally regulates the arterial P_{CO_2} very precisely: During exercise, metabolic carbon dioxide production may be increased by a factor of 10, yet the arterial P_{CO_2} usually changes less than 1 torr.

Elevated levels of carbon dioxide in the inspired air (the $F_I{CO_2}$) usually increase alveolar ventilation. The greatest response is seen with about 5 to 10 percent carbon dioxide in the inspired gas, which corresponds to alveolar P_{CO_2}'s between about 40 and 70 torr. Above 10 to 15 percent carbon dioxide in inspired air, little further increase occurs in alveolar ventilation. Very high arterial P_{CO_2}'s (70 to 80 torr) may directly produce respiratory depression if they are encountered

Table 18-1 Reflex Mechanisms of Respiratory Control

Stimulus	Reflex name	Receptor	Afferent pathway	Effects
Lung inflation	Hering-Breuer inflation reflex	Stretch receptors with smooth muscle of large and small airways	Vagus	Respiratory: Cessation of inspiratory effort, apnea, or decreased breathing frequency Bronchodilation Cardiovascular: Increased heart rate, slight vasoconstriction
Lung deflation	Hering-Breuer deflation reflex	Possibly "J" receptors, irritant receptors in lungs, or stretch receptors in airways	Vagus	Respiratory: Hyperpnea
Lung inflation	Paradoxical reflex of head	Stretch receptors in lungs	Vagus	Respiratory: Inspiration
Negative pressure in the upper airway	Pharyngeal dilator reflex	Receptors in nose, mouth, upper airways	Trigeminal, laryngeal, glossopharyngeal	Respiratory: Contraction of pharyngeal dilator muscles
Mechanical or chemical irritation of airways	Cough	Receptors in upper airways, tracheobronchial tree	Vagus	Respiratory: Cough Bronchoconstriction
	Sneeze	Receptors in nasal mucosa	Trigeminal, olfactory	Sneeze Bronchoconstriction Cardiovascular: Increased blood pressure
Face immersion	Diving reflex	Receptors in nasal mucosa and face	Trigeminal	Respiratory: Apnea Cardiovascular: Decreased heart rate; vasoconstriction

Stimulus	Receptors	Afferent	Response
Pulmonary embolism	"J" receptors in pulmonary vessels	Vagus	Respiratory: Apnea or tachypnea
Pulmonary vascular congestion	"J" receptors in pulmonary vessels	Vagus	Respiratory: Tachypnea, possibly sensation of dyspnea
Specific chemicals in the pulmonary circulation	"J" receptors in pulmonary vessels	Vagus	Respiratory: Apnea or tachypnea, Bronchoconstriction
Low PaO_2, High $PaCO_2$, Low pHa — Arterial Chemoreceptor Reflex	Carotid bodies / Aortic bodies	Glossopharyngeal / Vagus	Respiratory: Hyperpnea, Bronchoconstriction; Cardiovascular: Decreased heart rate (direct effect), vasoconstriction
Increased systemic arterial blood pressure — Arterial Baroreceptor Reflex	Carotid sinus Stretch receptors / Aortic arch Stretch receptors	Glossopharyngeal / Vagus	Respiratory: Apnea, bronchodilation; Cardiovascular decreased heart rate, vasodilation, etc.
Stretch of muscles tendons, movement of joints	Muscle spindles, tendon organs, proprioreceptors	Various spinal pathways	Respiratory: Provide respiratory controller with feedback about work of breathing; stimulation of proprioreceptors in joints causes hyperpnea
Somatic pain	Pain receptors	Various spinal pathways	Respiratory: Hyperpnea; Cardiovascular: Increased heart rate, vasoconstriction, etc.

From Levitzky MG: *Pulmonary Physiology.* 4th ed. New York, McGraw-Hill, 1995, with permission.

acutely. Patients with hypercapnia resulting from chronic obstructive lung disease have secondary acid-base changes (renal and cerebrospinal fluid bicarbonate retention) and may have relatively normal arterial pH's and ventilation. Acutely encountered high carbon dioxide levels may result in dyspnea, severe headaches (partly from cerebral vasodilation), faintness, dulling of the consciousness, muscular rigidity, tremors, and ultimately convulsions.

Figure 18-2 shows the ventilatory response of a normal conscious person to physiologic levels of carbon dioxide. Inspired concentrations of carbon dioxide or metabolically produced carbon dioxide resulting in alveolar (and arterial) P_{CO_2}'s in the range of 38 to 50 torr increase alveolar ventilation linearly. The slope is rather steep; it varies from person to person, with young healthy adults having a slope of 2 to 5 liters/min/torr P_ACO_2 (mean = 2.0 to 2.5 liters/min/torr P_ACO_2).

Hypoxemia potentiates the ventilatory response to carbon dioxide, as shown in the figure. At lower arterial P_{O_2}'s (e.g., 35 to 50 torr) the response curve shifts to the left and the slope becomes steeper. That is, for any particular arterial P_{CO_2}, the ventilatory response becomes greater as the arterial P_{O_2} decreases. This increased ventilatory response may be an effect of the hypoxia at the chemoreceptors itself, or changes in the central acid-base status secondary to the hypoxia.

Many other factors can affect the carbon dioxide response curve, as shown in Fig. 18-3. Sleep shifts the curve slightly to the right. The arterial P_{CO_2} normally increases about 5 to 6 torr during slow-wave sleep. Narcotics and anesthetics may profoundly depress the ventilatory response to carbon dioxide. Respiratory de-

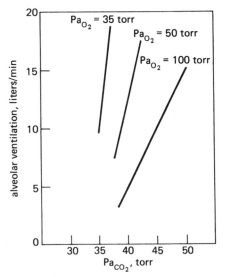

Figure 18-2 Diagram of ventilatory CO_2 response curves at three different levels of arterial PO_2. (From Levitzky MG: Pulmonary Physiology, 4th ed. New York, McGraw-Hill, 1995, with permission.)

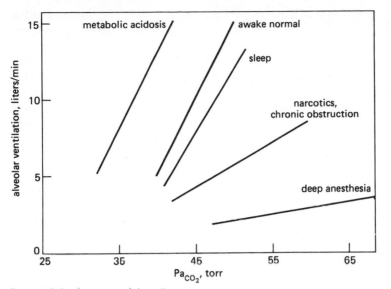

Figure 18-3 Diagram of the effects of sleep, narcotics, chronic pulmonary obstructive disease, deep anesthesia, and metabolic acidosis on the ventilatory response to carbon dioxide. (From Levitzky MG: Pulmonary Physiology, 4th ed. New York, McGraw-Hill, 1995, with permission.)

pression is the most common cause of death in cases of overdoses of opiate alkaloids and their derivatives, as well as barbiturates and most anesthetics. Hypoxic drive may be solely responsible for maintaining spontaneous breathing in patients with a depressed response to carbon dioxide. Chronic obstructive lung diseases depress the ventilatory response to hypercapnia, partly as a result of central acid-base changes and partly because the work of breathing may be so great that ventilation cannot be increased. Metabolic acidosis displaces the carbon dioxide response curve to the left, indicating that for any particular Pa_{CO_2} ventilation is increased during metabolic acidosis.

PERIPHERAL AND CENTRAL CHEMORECEPTORS

The *arterial chemoreceptors* (peripheral chemoreceptors) increase their firing rate in response to increased arterial P_{CO_2} or decreased arterial pH or P_{O_2}. The response of the receptors is sufficiently rapid and sensitive that they can relay information about breath-to-breath changes in the arterial blood composition to the medullary respiratory center.

The arterial chemoreceptors increase their activity *nearly linearly* with the arterial P_{CO_2} throughout the range of 20 to 60 torr. The exact mechanism by which the chemoreceptors work remains uncertain. A great amount of blood flows through the carotid body (per weight); the arteriovenous oxygen difference is extremely small (about 0.5 ml O_2/100 ml blood) despite the fact that it has one of the highest metabolic rates in the body. Certain drugs and enzyme poisons that block the formation of ATP stimulate the carotid body. For example, both cyanide and dinitrophenol directly stimulate the carotid body; this action may relate to the mechanism of the stimulatory effect of hypoxia on the arterial chemoreceptors.

Although the *central chemoreceptors* are in contact with cerebrospinal fluid (CSF), they are shielded from arterial blood by the blood-brain barrier. Carbon dioxide easily diffuses through the blood-brain barrier, but hydrogen ions and bicarbonate ions do not. Because of this difference, alterations in the arterial P_{CO_2} are rapidly transmitted to the CSF. In fact, in some circumstances, CSF may undergo changes in hydrogen ion concentration *opposite* to those in the blood, as discussed shortly.

The composition of CSF is considerably different from that of the blood. The pH of CSF is normally about 7.32, compared with a pH of 7.40 of arterial blood. The bicarbonate ion concentration is similar to that of the arterial blood, but the P_{CO_2} of the CSF is about 50 torr. The higher CSF P_{CO_2} is partly a result of the diffusion of metabolically produced carbon dioxide from cerebral tissue.

In CSF, the concentration of proteins is only in the range of 15 to 45 mg/ 100 ml, whereas in the *plasma* it normally ranges from 6.6 to 8.6 g/100 ml. This figure does not even include the hemoglobin in the red blood cells. Therefore, the only buffer of consequence in CSF is bicarbonate and there is much less ability to buffer hydrogen ions in the CSF. Arterial hypercapnia or metabolic acidosis in the brain thus leads to greater changes in hydrogen ion concentration in CSF than in the arterial blood. The central chemoreceptors are situated ventrolaterally at or just beneath the surface of the medulla. They respond to local increases in hydrogen ion concentration and/or P_{CO_2}. They are not stimulated by hypoxia and may even be depressed by it. Increases in their activity are thought to stimulate the medullary respiratory neurons in a manner similar to that of the peripheral chemoreceptors.

The relative contributions of the peripheral and central chemoreceptors in the ventilatory response to increased carbon dioxide levels is somewhat controversial. Experimental animals from which the fibers leading from the arterial chemoreceptors have been cut, or patients from whom carotid bodies have been removed, showed about 80 to 90 percent of the normal total *steady-state* response to increased inspired carbon dioxide concentrations (delivered in hyperoxic gas mixtures). This finding shows that the peripheral chemoreceptors contribute only about 10 to 20 percent of the steady-state response to hypercapnia. Other studies done on normoxic men show that up to one-third or one-half of the *transient response* can come from the arterial chemoreceptors when the arterial P_{CO_2} changes rapidly. That is, the central chemoreceptors may be mainly responsible for determining the resting ventilatory level or the long-term response to carbon dioxide inhalation; the peripheral chemoreceptors may be more important in short-term responses to carbon dioxide.

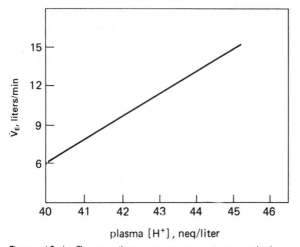

Figure 18-4 The ventilatory response to increased plasma hydrogen ion concentration. *(From Levitzky MG: Pulmonary Physiology, 4th ed. New York, McGraw-Hill, 1995, with permission.)*

Response to Hydrogen Ions

Changes in plasma hydrogen ion concentration over the range of 20 to 60 *nano-equivalents* per liter produce linear increases in ventilation as shown in Fig. 18-4. A metabolic acidosis that originates outside the brain results in hyperpnea coming almost exclusively from the peripheral chemoreceptors. Because hydrogen ions cross the blood-brain barrier so slowly, the central chemoreceptors are not affected at first. As acidotic stimulation of the peripheral chemoreceptors occurs, alveolar ventilation increases and the arterial P_{CO_2} falls. Because the CSF P_{CO_2} is in a kind of equilibrium with the arterial P_{CO_2}, carbon dioxide diffuses out of CSF and the CSF pH increases. Stimulation of the central chemoreceptor therefore decreases. If the situation persists (for hours or days), the bicarbonate concentration of CSF slowly declines, returning the pH of the cerebrospinal fluid toward normal (7.32). Investigators do not agree on how this occurs. The mechanism may be the slow diffusion of bicarbonate ions across the blood-brain barrier, the active transport of bicarbonate ions out of the CSF, or decreased *formation* of bicarbonate ions by carbonic anhydrase during formation of CSF. The bicarbonate concentration in the cerebrospinal fluid in patients having chronic respiratory acidosis (as in chronic obstructive lung disease) may be increased by similar mechanisms, because the pH of the cerebrospinal fluid is nearly normal.

Response to Hypoxia

The ventilatory response to hypoxia arises solely from the peripheral chemoreceptors. The carotid bodies are much more important in this response than the aortic bodies, which cannot sustain the ventilatory response to hypoxia by themselves. When no peripheral chemoreceptors are present, increasing degrees of hypoxia result in a progressive *depression* of the central respiratory controller. Therefore, when the peripheral chemoreceptors are intact, their excitation of the central respiratory controller must offset the direct depressant effect of hypoxia.

Figure 18-5 shows the response of the respiratory system to hypoxia. At a normal arterial PCO_2 of about 38 to 40 torr, little increase in ventilation occurs until the arterial PO_2 falls below about 50 to 60 torr. Note that the response to hypoxemia is potentiated at higher arterial PCO_2's.

Studies have shown that the respiratory response to hypoxia relates to the change in PO_2 rather than the change in *oxygen content*. In a person who has anemia (without acidosis), therefore, the condition does not stimulate ventilation inasmuch as the arterial PO_2 is normal and the arterial chemoreceptors are not stimulated.

Hypoxia alone, by stimulating alveolar ventilation, causes the arterial PCO_2 to decrease, which in turn may lead to respiratory alkalosis. This is part of the basis of the headache and many other symptoms associated with altitude sickness.

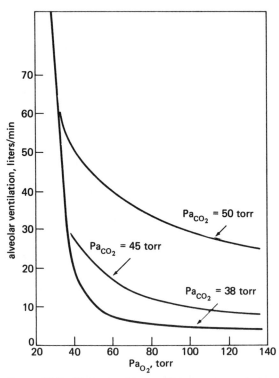

Figure 18-5   Diagram of the ventilatory response to hypoxia at three different arterial PCO_2 levels. *(From Levitzky MG: Pulmonary Physiology, 4th ed. New York, McGraw-Hill, 1995, with permission.)*

BIBLIOGRAPHY

Berger AJ: Control of breathing, in Murray JF, Nadel JA (eds): *Textbook of Respiratory Medicine,* 2d ed. Philadelphia, Saunders, 1994, pp 199–218.

Berger AJ, Mitchell RA, Severinghaus JW: Regulation of respiration. *N Engl J Med* 297: 92–97, 138–143, 194–201, 1977.

Bruce EN, Cherniack NS: Central chemoreceptors. *J Appl Physiol* 62:389–402, 1987.

Levitzky MG: *Pulmonary Physiology,* 4th ed. New York, McGraw-Hill, 1995, pp 187–197.

Murray JF: *The Normal Lung,* 2d ed. Philadelphia, Saunders, 1986, pp 233–260.

Nunn JF: *Nunn's Applied Respiratory Physiology,* 4th ed. Oxford, Butterworth-Heinemann, 1993, pp 90–116.

19

NONRESPIRATORY FUNCTIONS OF THE RESPIRATORY SYSTEM

OBJECTIVES
The reader should be able to:

1 Describe the mechanisms by which the lung is protected from the contaminants in inspired air and describe the "air-conditioning" function of the upper airways.
2 Describe the filtration and removal of particles from the inspired air.
3 Describe the removal of biologically active material from the inspired air.
4 Describe the reservoir and filtration functions of the pulmonary circulation.
5 List the metabolic functions of the lung, including the handling of vasoactive material in the blood.

PERSPECTIVE
The nonrespiratory functions of the respiratory system include its own defense against inhaled particulate matter; the storage and filtration of blood for the systemic circulation; the conversion, metabolism, and release of vasoactive agents in the blood; and the formation and release of substances used in the alveoli, airways, or systemic circulation.

PULMONARY DEFENSE MECHANISMS
Inspired air may contain dust, pollen, ash, and other products of combustion, microorganisms, particulate material, hazardous chemicals, and toxic gases. Each day, a person brings 8000 to 10,000 liters of air through the airways, and about two-thirds of that reaches the delicate alveolar surfaces.

"Air Conditioning"   The alveoli must be protected against cold and kept from drying out. The mucosa lining the nose, the nasal turbinates, and the oropharynx and nasopharynx has a large surface area and a rich blood supply. As inhaled air passes over these surfaces, it is warmed to body temperature and humidified, especially if breathing is done through the nose.

Olfaction   Because the olfactory receptors are positioned in the posterior nasal cavity and not in the trachea or alveoli, a person can *sniff* to detect the odors of hazardous gases or other material in the air. This quick, shallow inhalation through the nose brings gases into contact with the olfactory sensors without inspiring the possibly noxious gases into the lung.

Filtration   The filtration system works better if one is breathing through the nose. Air moving through the nose is first filtered as it passes through the nasal hairs, or *vibrissae*. This prevents most particles larger than 10 to 15 μm in diameter from moving farther toward the lung. Most particles greater than 10 μm in diameter are caught in the large surface area of the nasal septum and turbinates. The direction of the inspired airstream changes abruptly at the nasopharynx, and most particles of about 10 μm in diameter, because of their inertia, land on the back wall of the pharynx. The tonsils and adenoids, located near this impaction site, provide immunologic defense against biologically active material filtered at this point. Air entering the trachea usually has few particles larger than 10 μm, and most of these impact at the carina or within the bronchi

Most particles in the size range of 2 to 5 μm settle by gravity in the smaller airways, where the linear velocity is extremely low. Thus impaction or sedimentation removes most of the particles between 2 and 10 μm in diameter, which become trapped in the mucus lining the upper airways, trachea, bronchi, and bronchioles. Smaller particles and all foreign gases enter the alveolar ducts and alveoli. Some smaller particles (0.1 μm and smaller) are deposited by Brownian motion; other particles, between 0.1 and 0.5 μm in diameter, generally remain suspended as aerosols, and about 80 percent of them are exhaled.

Removal of Inspired or Aspirated Particles   Filtered material trapped in the mucus lining of the respiratory tract can be removed in several ways, including the *mucociliary escalator* and reflex coughing or sneezing.

A mucus-covered, ciliated epithelium lines the entire respiratory tract, from the upper airways to the terminal bronchioles. The only exceptions are parts of the pharynx and the anterior third of the nasal cavity. The mucus is produced by the goblet cells and mucus-secreting glands of the airways. In pathologic states, such as chronic bronchitis, the number of goblet cells may increase and the mucus glands may hypertrophy, causing mucus gland secretion and mucus viscosity to increase considerably.

The cilia lining the airways beat in such a way that the mucus covering them always is pushed up the airway, away from the alveoli and toward the pharynx. Several studies have shown that cigarette smoke inhibits or impairs ciliary function.

The mucociliary escalator is an important mechanism for removing inhaled particles that stick to the lining of the airways. Material trapped in the mucus is continuously moved toward the pharynx. When mucus reaches the pharynx, it is usually swallowed, expectorated, or removed by blowing one's nose. Patients who cannot clear their tracheobronchial secretions (such as an intubated patient, or one unable to cough adequately) must be cared for because they continue to produce secretions. If the secretions are not removed from the patient by suction or other means, airway obstruction develops.

Stimulation of receptors in the nose, trachea, larynx, or elsewhere in the respiratory tract, either mechanically or chemically, may cause bronchoconstriction, averting deeper penetration of the irritant into the airways. It may also evoke a cough or a sneeze. A *sneeze* results when receptors in the nose or nasopharynx are stimulated; a *cough* results from stimulation of receptors in the trachea. In both the sneeze and the cough, after a deep inhalation, often to almost total lung capacity, a forced expiration occurs against apposed vocal cords and a closed glottis. During this phase of the reflex, intrapleural pressure may rise to more than 100 mmHg. The vocal cords and glottis open suddenly, and pressure in the airways falls rapidly, causing the airways to be compressed and an explosive expiration with very great linear airflow velocities. These high airflow rates through the narrowed airways are likely to propel the irritant, along with some mucus, out of the respiratory tract. A sneeze, of course, propels the material through the nose; a cough propels it through the mouth. The cough or sneeze reflex is also useful in helping to move the mucus lining of the airways toward the nose and mouth.

Several mechanisms may be involved in the removal of inhaled material that reaches the terminal airways and alveoli, including ingestion by alveolar macrophages, nonspecific enzymatic destruction, entry into the lymphatics, and immunologic reactions.

Alveolar macrophages (alveolar type III cells) are large mononuclear ameboid cells found on the alveolar surface. The macrophages may engulf particles and, by lysosomal action, destroy them. Most bacteria are digested in this way. However, some material taken in by the macrophages, such as silica, is not degradable by these cells and may even be toxic to them. If the macrophages bearing such material are not removed from the lung, the material is redeposited on the alveolar surface when the macrophages die. The mean life span of alveolar macrophages is apparently 1 to 5 weeks. Macrophages carrying such nondigestable material are chiefly removed by migration to the mucociliary escalator. They may also migrate from the alveolar surface into the interstitium, from which they may enter the lymphatic system. Cigarette smoke has been shown to inhibit macrophage function. Alveolar macrophages are also important in the lung's immune and inflammatory responses. They secrete many enzymes, arachidonic acid metabolites, immune response components, and mediators that modulate the function of other cells such as lymphocytes.

Some particles reach the mucociliary escalator because the alveolar fluid lining itself is slowly moving upward toward the respiratory bronchioles. Others penetrate into the interstitial space or enter the blood, where they are phagocytized by interstitial macrophages or blood phagocytes or enter the lymphatics. Particles may be destroyed or detoxified by surface enzymes and factors in the serum and in airway secretions.

NONRESPIRATORY FUNCTIONS OF THE PULMONARY CIRCULATION

The normal pulmonary blood volume is about 250 to 300 ml of blood per square meter of body surface area. This would give a typical adult male a pulmonary blood volume of about 500 ml. The pulmonary circulation can therefore act as a *reservoir for the left ventricle*. If left ventricular output is transiently greater than systemic venous return, that output can be maintained for a few strokes by drawing on blood stored in the pulmonary circulation.

Because all mixed venous blood must pass through the pulmonary capillaries, the pulmonary circulation can serve as a *filter*, trapping materials that enter the blood and protecting the systemic circulation. The particles filtered may include small fibrin or blood clots, masses of platelets or leukocytes, fat cells, bone marrow, detached cancer cells, gas bubbles, agglutinated erythrocytes (especially in sickle cell anemia), and debris from stored blood or intravenous solutions. If such materials were to enter the arterial side of the systemic circulation, they could occlude vascular beds that have no collateral circulation. Such occlusion would be particularly disastrous if it happened in the vessels supplying blood to the central nervous system or the myocardium.

The lung is able to perform this valuable service because it has many more pulmonary capillaries than are necessary for gas exchange at rest, and because most of the trapped material is removed from the pulmonary circulation within 4 to 5 days. The materials trapped in the pulmonary vascular bed are removed by lytic enzymes in the vascular endothelium, ingestion by macrophages, and penetration to the lymphatic system. Blood administered to patients on cardiopulmonary bypass must be filtered for them because their pulmonary capillary filtration system is circumvented.

The hydrostatic pressure in the pulmonary capillaries, normally far lower than the colloid osmotic pressure of the plasma proteins, tends to draw fluid from the alveoli into the pulmonary capillaries and thus keep the alveolar surface free of liquids other than pulmonary surfactant. Fresh water that is inhaled into the lungs rapidly becomes absorbed into the blood. This quick absorption protects the gas exchange function of the lungs and acts against transudation of fluid from the capillaries to the alveoli.

Drugs or chemical substances that readily diffuse or otherwise pass through the alveolar-capillary barrier rapidly enter the systemic circulation. The lungs are frequently utilized as the route of administration of anesthetic gases.

Table 19-1   Uptake or Conversion by the Lungs of Chemical
Substrates in Mixed Venous Blood

Substance in mixed venous blood	Result of a single pass through the lung
Prostaglandins E_1, E_2, $F_{2\alpha}$	Almost completely removed
Prostaglandins A_1, A_2, I_2	Not affected
Leukotrienes	Almost completely removed
Serotonin	85–95% removed
Acetylcholine	Inactivated by cholinsterases in blood
Histamine	Not affected
Epinephrine	Not affected
Norepinephrine	Approximated 30% removed
Isoproterenol	Not affected
Dopamine	Not affected
Bradykinin	Approximately 80% inactivated
Angiotensin I	Approximately 70% converted to angiotensin II
Angiotensin II	Not affected
Vasopressin	Not affected
Oxytocin	Not affected
Gastrin	Not affected
ATP, AMP	40–90% removed

From Levitzky MG: *Pulmonary Physiology:* 4th ed. New York, McGraw-Hill, 1995, with permission.

METABOLIC FUNCTIONS OF THE LUNG

Many vasoactive substances are inactivated, changed, or removed from the blood as they pass through the lungs. The endothelium of the vessels of the pulmonary circulation, which has a tremendous surface area in contact with the mixed venous blood, is believed to be the site of this metabolic activity. Prostaglandins E_1, E_2, and $F_{2\alpha}$ and most leukotrienes are almost completely removed during a single pass through the lungs as shown in Table 19-1. On the other hand, prostaglandins A_1 and A_2 and prostacyclin are not affected by the pulmonary circulation. Similarly, about 30 percent of the norepinephrine and about 80 percent of the bradykinin in mixed venous blood is removed in one pass through the lungs, but epinephrine and isoproterenol are unaffected. Angiotensin I is converted to angiotensin II in the lung.

Several substances having effects in the lung are known to be synthesized and released by pulmonary cells. *Pulmonary surfactant* is synthesized in type II alveolar epithelial cells and released onto the alveolar surface. *Histamine, serotonin, lysosomal enzymes, prostaglandins, leukotrienes, platelet activating factor,* and *neutrophil and eosinophil chemotactic factors* can be released from mast cells in the lung in response to conditions like pulmonary emboli or anaphylaxis, causing bronchoconstriction and immune or inflammatory responses and possibly initiating other cardiopulmonary reflexes. Alveolar macrophages have also been shown to produce a number of substances. Whatever substance or substances are the *chemical mediators* involved in the hypoxic pulmonary vasoconstriction, they are produced and act in the lung. Many other substances are also produced by the lung cells and released into the alveoli and airways, including mucus and other tracheobronchial secretions, surface enzymes, proteins, immunologically active substances, and other factors. These substances are synthesized in the goblet cells, submucosal gland cells, Clara cells, or macrophages.

Bradykinin, histamine, serotonin, heparin, and prostaglandins E_2 and $F_{2\alpha}$ are all stored in the lung and, under certain circumstances, may be released into the general circulation. For example, heparin, histamine, serotonin, and prostaglandins E_2 and $F_{2\alpha}$ are released during anaphylactic shock.

The lung must be able to respond to injury as well as meet its own cellular energy requirements. Type II alveolar epithelial cells play a major role in the lung's response to injury of type I cells. Investigators have shown that after injury, the type II cells can proliferate and develop into type I cells.

BIBLIOGRAPHY

Clarke SW, Yeates D: Deposition and clearance, in Murray JF, Nadel JA (eds): *Textbook of Respiratory Medicine,* 2d ed. Philadelphia, Saunders, 1994, pp 345–369.

Fels AOS, Chon ZA: The alveolar macrophage. *J Appl Physiol* 60:353–369, 1986.

Fishman AP, Fisher AB (eds): *Handbook of Physiology,* sec 3: *The Respiratory System,* vol I: *Circulation and Nonrespiratory Functions.* Bethesda, MD, American Physiological Society, 1985.

Green GM, Jakab GJ, Low RB, Davis GS: Defense mechanisms of the respiratory membrane. *Am Rev Resp Dis* 115:479–514, 1977.

Levitzky MG: *Pulmonary Physiology,* 4th ed. New York, McGraw-Hill, 1995, pp 213–225.

Murray JF: *The Normal Lung,* 2d ed. Philadelphia, Saunders, 1986, pp 283–337.

Nunn JF: *Nunn's Applied Respiratory Physiology,* 4th ed. Oxford, Butterworth-Heinemann, 1993, pp 306–317.

Proctor DF: The upper airways. *Am Rev Resp Dis* 115:97–129, 315–342, 1977.

Proctor DF, Andersen I (eds): *The Nose: Upper Airway Physiology and the Atmospheric Environment.* Amsterdam, Elsevier Biomedical, 1982.

Part 3

EFFECTS OF ANESTHESIA

20

EFFECTS OF ANESTHESIA ON CIRCULATORY FUNCTION

Consideration of the effects of anesthesia on circulatory function includes several realms of perioperative influences: 1. preoperative and intraoperative anesthesia drugs; 2. mode of ventilation; 3. intravenous fluid therapy; 4. position of the patient; and 5. environmental factors (e.g., temperature). An important goal of anesthetic management is maintenance of normal physiology, which includes counteracting the effects of the surgical procedure. The surgical site can obviously have profound circulatory influences during cardiac or vascular surgery. Neurosurgery, especially involving the brainstem vasomotor areas, can also affect cardiovascular function.

Surgery can greatly affect venous return to the heart in ways other than hemorrhage and third-space loss. Surgical retractors can compress the inferior vena cava during upper abdominal surgery, reducing preload. Changes in intrathoracic pressure due to mechanical ventilation or loss of negative intrapleural pressure secondary to thoracotomy also compromise preload to the heart.

INHALATIONAL ANESTHETICS

The vasodilating effects of halothane, its cardiac depressant effects, and its sensitization of the myocardium to catecholamines, are well known. The risk of halothane hepatitis has led to a discontinuation of its use for adults. Cardiac depression occasionally follows inhalation induction of a pediatric patient with halothane, but adequate circulation is usually restored following prompt administration of atropine and reduction of the dose of halothane. Managed care and cost containment efforts have led to a resurgence in its popularity in pediatric anesthesia, because it is so inexpensive in comparison to other inhalant agents. Conversely, isoflurane does not predispose to ventricular ectopy in the presence of exogenous catecholamines. Inspired concentrations of isoflurane as well as desflurane greater than 1 MAC (minimal alveolar concentration) can increase the heart rate. Therefore, tachycardia may not indicate inadequate anesthesia. Additionally, desflurane produces a dose-dependent decrease in blood pressure. Inhalation anesthetics produce a titratable myocardial depression and blunt the sympathetic response to surgical stimulation. Volatile anesthetics are coronary vasodilators, with isoflurane producing the greatest effect. Research suggesting coronary "steal" and increased incidence of coronary ischemia have not been reproduced by subsequent clinical studies.

During pediatric surgery, the immature myocardium and vasomotor system are very sensitive to the depressant effects of volatile agents. Nitrous oxide tends to increase pulmonary vascular resistance in adults, but has less of this effect in pediatric patients. In any case, nitrous oxide can increase the size of systemic air emboli.

INTRAVENOUS INDUCTION AGENTS

Perioperative events produce varying and sometimes opposing effects on the cardiovascular system. Preoperative anxiety can stimulate the sympathetic nervous system causing tachycardia and hypertension and occasionally provoking an anginal episode in a susceptible individual. Most of the hypnotic drugs used during induction of anesthesia produce dose-dependent cardiovascular effects. Induction doses of thiopental, thiamylal, and methohexital produce a transient 10 to 20 mmHg decrease in blood pressure offset by a 15 to 20 beat-per-min increase in heart rate in normovolemic patients. This transient decrease in blood pressure is mainly due to peripheral vasodilation which is caused by depression of the medullary vasomotor center. Barbiturate induction agents directly depress the myocardium, but this is usually compensated for by increased sympathetic tone. High doses can cause dangerous myocardial depression. Hypovolemic patients are more vulnerable to marked blood pressure reduction by these drugs. Ketamine's cardiovascular effects normally resemble stimulation of the sympathetic nervous system, producing increased systemic and pulmonary arterial blood pressure, heart rate, cardiac output, and myocardial oxygen requirements. Ketamine possesses direct myocardial depressant effects which can be exhibited as hypotension and hypoperfusion in patients that are catecholamine depleted (as in some critically ill or septic patients). Etomidate produces minimal changes in heart rate and cardiac output, whereas mean arterial pressure may decrease up to 15 percent due to reduction in systemic vascular resistance. Propofol produces a greater reduction in blood pressure than comparable doses of thiopental. Exaggerated blood pressure effects of propofol may occur in elderly patients and in patients who are hypovolemic or who have poor left ventricular function. Benzodiazepines cause minimal depression of the cardiovascular system (although exaggerated effects can occur in elderly patients or certain susceptible individuals). In general, benzodiazepines produce minimal decreases in blood pressure, cardiac output, and systemic vascular resistance, as well as transient decreases in baroreceptor responses. The cardiovascular effects of midazolam are greater than they are for diazepam and occasionally produce marked hypertension.

Local Anesthetics

Local anesthetics act to decrease myocardial automaticity and decrease the slope of phase 4 of the pacemaker cell action potential by blocking cardiac sodium channels. Local anesthetic toxicity includes hypotension, dysrhythmias, and A-V heart block. Intravenous lidocaine (0.5 to 1 mg/kg) is commonly used perioperatively for treatment of acute ventricular ectopy. Additionally, it is sometimes used prophylactically during induction to reduce sympathetic stimulation, tachycardia, hypertension, ectopy, and bronchoconstriction. Accidental intravenous injection or systemic absorption of large doses of local anesthetics (e.g., during attempted regional anesthesia) can cause high plasma levels. Additionally, continuous infusions of amide local anesthetics in patients with decreased liver metabolism can produce profound cardiovascular depression to the point of cardiac standstill. The presence of epinephrine increases the maximum allowable dose of local anesthetic. Due to intense protein binding to myocardial protein by bupivacaine, protracted cardiovascular depression can result from excessive blood levels. For this reason bupivacaine is not used for intravenous regional (Bier) block.

Neuromuscular Blocking Drugs

Newer neuromuscular blocking drugs are characterized by minimal cardiovascular effects (except for the slight histamine release associated with atricurium and mivacurium). In contrast, older neuromuscular blockers were associated with histamine release and muscarinic and/or autonomic ganglia effects. Succinylcholine stimulates autonomic ganglia as well as cardiac muscarinics. Curare blocks autonomic ganglia and causes moderate histamine release. Metocurine weakly blocks autonomic ganglia and slightly releases histamine. Pancuronium and gallamine block cardiac muscarinic receptors.

Anticholinesterase Drugs

Anticholinesterase drugs are usually administered with antimuscarinics because undesirable muscarinic effects (bradycardia, salivation, broncoconstriction, miosis, and hyperperistalsis) are evoked at lower concentrations of acetylcholine than are needed to reverse neuromuscular blockade.

Narcotics

The cardiovascular effects of narcotics are generally related to decreased sympathetic tone. The newer lyophilic narcotics, such as fentanyl and sufentanyl, are characterized by bradycardia, sometimes resulting in hypotension if high doses are used. Meperidine produces the greatest negative inotropic effects of the commonly used narcotics, and causes tachycardia due to its antimuscarinic effects. Although meperidine is not useful for treatment of diarrhea and has weak antitussic effects, it is effective for reducing postoperative shivering. The histamine release associated with morphine is responsible for many of its cardiovascular effects. The use of nitrous oxide with high dose narcotics has been shown to cause cardiovascular depression, decreased cardiac output, decreased blood pressure, and increased filling pressure. Opiods predictably cause hypotension when combined with benzodiazepines.

CARDIOVASCULAR EFFECTS OF VENTILATION

Thoracotomy causes loss of the normally negative intrapleural pressure and reduces venous return. At the same time, positive pressure ventilation is required, which further raises intrapleural pressure while reducing venous return. Normally intrapleural pressure is approximately -3 to -5 cmH$_2$O. Peak airway pressure during mechanical ventilation of healthy lungs is about 20 cmH$_2$O with a mean airway pressure of about 8 cmH$_2$O. Mechanical ventilation during certain disease states can produce much higher mean and peak airway pressures. The relation between airway pressure and venous return has led to the development of formulas to predict the effects of changing airway pressures (e.g., continuous positive airway pressure) on pulmonary artery occlusion pressures. However, the relation between airway pressures and vascular pressures is unreliable especially in lung diseases that produce increased fluid in the alveoli and pulmonary interstitium. The effects of ventilation on the circulatory system pertain mainly to changes in the venous return. Different modes of ventilation produce varying levels of intrathoracic pressure during the ventilatory cycle, which result in a waxing and waning of venous return. Mechanical ventilation is associated with higher mean intrathoracic pressures than those associated with spontaneous ventilation. In a similar manner, continuous positive airway pressure decreases venous return. Pulmonary vasodilator tone is increased by acidosis, hypercapnia, atelectasis, and hypoxia. Hypoxic pulmonary vasoconstriction is decreased by alkalosis, nitroprusside, nitroglycerin, nitric oxide, volatile anesthetics, and certain prostaglandins.

INTRAVENOUS FLUID THERAPY

Intravenous fluid administration is usually managed intraoperatively by an anesthesia care provider. The volume and type of fluid can produce profound effects on hemodynamic status. The use of crystalloid-containing solutions is governed by the 3 : 1 ratio of fluid remaining intravascularly following intravenous infusion. The basis for only one-third of the crystalloid solution remaining intravascularly is due to the equilibration of the intravascular and interstitial spaces through the capillary walls. For a 70-kg adult, the volume of the intravascular space is about 5 liters while the interstitial space is about 12 liters and hence the ratio of 2 ml going interstitially while 1 ml remains intravascular.

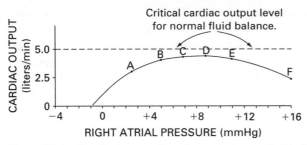

Figure 20-1 Greatly depressed cardiac output curve that indicates decompensated heart disease. Progressive fluid retention raises the right atrial pressure, and the cardiac output progresses from point A to point F *(From Guyton, with permission).*

Perioperative blood loss and fluid administration cause changes in the blood's hematocrit and viscosity. Viscosity plays a role in determining vascular resistance (see Poiseuille's law, in Chap. 5). Changes in vascular resistance affect blood pressure and tissue perfusion, with perhaps the most striking clinical example being sickle cell anemia during a sickle crisis.

The most graphic representation of the relation between intravascular volume status and cardiac function is demonstrated by Starling's curve of cardiac function (Fig. 20-1).

POSITIONING THE PATIENT

Head-up or head-down tilt of the surgical bed greatly influences venous return to the heart, especially for anesthetized patients under the influence of vasodilating anesthetic drugs. Additionally, anesthesia frequently blunts the baroreceptor reflex and other compensatory mechanisms that act to maintain preload.

Monitoring the cardiovascular status of the anesthetized patient is also complicated by changes in position. Changes in location of the patient's right atrium (phlebostatic axis) relative to pressure transducers can produce artifacts in cardiovascular pressure determination. Placement of the transducer at the midbrain level for a patient in the sitting position is useful for obtaining an approximation of cerebral perfusion pressure.

ENVIRONMENTAL AND SURGICAL FACTORS

The temperature of the operating room can greatly influence the body temperature, especially for pediatric patients. Hypothermia tends to produce a peripheral vasoconstriction as the body attempts to maintain core temperature. This can influence the function of monitors such as pulse oximeters. Furthermore, postoperative shivering increases oxygen demand and heart rate at a time when the patient's ventilation may be compromised. Partial airway obstruction from decreased tone of the tongue and pharynx, residual muscle relaxation, narcosis, and continued effects of inhaled agents tend to result in hypoventilation. Conversely, simple hyperthermia causes peripheral vasodilation and increased cardiac output. Pathologic hyperthermia (e.g., sepsis, thyrotoxicosis, and malignant hyperthermia) can be associated with dysrhythmias, electrolyte shifts, and alterations in cardiac metabolism leading to impaired myocardial function.

Vigilance of the anesthesia care provider can reduce the physiologic impact of surgery. The oculocardiac reflex can frequently be terminated by cessation of traction on the extraocular muscles. Likewise, runs of ventricular tachycardia during insertion of central lines usually stop if the guidewire or catheter is withdrawn or inserted further.

In summary, the drugs, intravenous fluid, and method of ventilation provided during anesthesia produce dramatic circulatory effects. Factors not completely under the control of the anesthesia care provider (room temperature, surgical site, and patient position) can be modified to reduce cardiovascular compromise.

BIBLIOGRAPHY

Hollinger IB, Diseases of the Cardiovascular System. In Katz J, and Steward DJ, (eds): *Anesthesia and Uncommon Pediatric Diseases.* Saunders, Philadelphia, 1989.

Kaplan JA, (ed): *Cardiac Anesthesia,* 2nd ed. Grune & Stratton, Orlando, Fl., 1987.

Rosow CE: Cardiovascular effects of opiod anesthesia. *Mt. Sinai J Med* 54:273, 1987.

Stoelting RK, *Pharmacology and Physiology in Anesthetic Practice.* Lippincott, Philadelphia, 2nd ed. 1991.

Stoelting RK, Dierdorf SF, and McCammon RL, *Anesthesia and Co-Existing Disease,* 2nd ed., Churchill Livingstone, New York, 1988.

Thomas SJ, & Kramer JL, (eds) *Manual of Cardiac Anesthesia,* 2nd ed. Churchill Livingstone, New York, 1993.

21

EFFECTS OF ANESTHESIA ON PULMONARY FUNCTION

OBJECTIVES

The reader should be able to:

1 Describe the effects of general anesthesia on the mechanics of the lung and chest wall.
2 Explain anesthetic effects on the volume and distribution of alveolar ventilation.
3 Describe anesthetic alterations on the cardiac output and the distribution of pulmonary blood flow.
4 Describe the effects of inhaled anesthetics on the matching of ventilation and perfusion.
5 Describe the effects of anesthesia drugs on the control of breathing.
6 Explain how general anesthesia can affect the airway.

PERSPECTIVE

General anesthesia can have profound effects on pulmonary function. Some of these are direct effects of anesthetic drugs on the respiratory system; others result from associated aspects of general anesthesia such as altered body position, intubation, mechanical ventilation, and the use of neuromuscular blocking agents and other drugs. Alterations in the cardiovascular system caused by general anesthesia can also affect pulmonary function by changing the amount and distribution of pulmonary blood flow.

It is difficult to generalize the effects of anesthesia on pulmonary function because of differences between anesthetics and the routes of administration employed, differences in the body positions and ventilatory modes used in various surgical procedures, the unavailability of some kinds of data from normal conscious and anesthetized human subjects, and differences in the age and cardiopulmonary status of the patients included in clinical studies. Nonetheless, there is agreement on a number of pulmonary consequences of general anesthesia, although the mechanisms responsible for these alterations frequently remain controversial because of difficulty obtaining data from human subjects and because conclusions drawn from animal experiments may not correspond exactly to human physiology.

General anesthesia may have major effects on the mechanics of the lung and the chest wall, the volume and distribution of alveolar ventilation, the cardiac output and the distribution of pulmonary blood flow, the matching of ventilation and perfusion, and the control of breathing. General anesthesia may also affect the airways, and the transport and diffusion of oxygen and carbon dioxide.

EFFECTS OF ANESTHESIA ON RESPIRATORY MECHANICS

There is no doubt that general anesthesia affects the mechanics of the respiratory system. It has significant effects on the functional residual capacity (FRC), the respiratory muscles, and the shape and motion of the lungs and chest wall. It may affect the diameter of the airways.

Effects on the FRC

As noted in a previous chapter, the FRC is determined by the balance between the inward recoil of the lungs and the outward recoil of the chest wall when the respiratory muscles are relaxed. When a normal conscious person changes from the upright to the supine position, the FRC decreases by about 33 percent. For a typical 70-kg person that would represent a decrease of about 1 liter, from an FRC of 3 liters in the upright position to an FRC of 2 liters in the supine position.

A number of studies have demonstrated a significant decrease in the FRC within a few minutes of the induction of almost any general anesthetic to a supine patient. With inhalant anesthetics this decrease is approximately 16 to 20 percent of the already reduced FRC of the supine individual and therefore represents an additional decrease of approximately 400 ml in a 70-kg person. Intravenous general anesthetics usually cause a slightly smaller decrease in FRC than the inhalant anesthetics. Ketamine has little effect on the FRC.

The decrease in FRC associated with general anesthesia does not appear to occur if the patient is anesthetized in an upright posture, although it does occur if the patient is prone. The FRC does not fall progressively and the decrease is not exacerbated by high F_IO_2's; therefore neither absorption atelectasis nor airway closure seems to be the primary cause of the decreased FRC. Although the FRC decreases nearly immediately after induction of general anesthesia, it does not return to normal for a few hours. The decrease in FRC occurs whether the patient is paralyzed or not, and it does not result from mechanical ventilation.

There is no single, simple explanation for the decrease in FRC caused by the induction of general anesthesia. As already discussed, absorption atelectasis seems unlikely to cause the decreased FRC. More likely potential explanations include a change in the position of the diaphragm, a change in the cross-sectional area of the rib cage, and an increased central blood volume.

The FRC is defined as the volume of air in the lungs at the end of a normal tidal expiration. It is usually described in elementary textbooks as representing the balance point between the inward recoil of the lungs and the outward recoil of the chest wall when the respiratory muscles are not contracting actively, with the implication that they are completely relaxed. However, a number of studies have demonstrated the presence of respiratory muscle tone at the FRC in subjects in the supine position. General anesthetics that alter or abolish this tone might be expected to alter the shape and movement of the chest wall and lungs, as would paralytic agents used during general anesthesia.

The diaphragm separates the thorax from the contents of the abdominal cavity. A loss of diaphragmatic tone with general anesthesia would be expected to cause the diaphragm of a recumbent spontaneously breathing patient to move toward the head, as the flaccid diaphragm responds to the gradient between the positive pressure in the abdominal cavity and the negative pressure in the thorax. Paralysis and mechanical ventilation, with or without positive end-expiratory pressure, would also be expected to have major effects on respiratory mechanics, as will be discussed later in this chapter.

Several investigators have attempted to determine whether the induction of general anesthesia causes such a cephalad displacement of the diaphragm at the FRC, and if it does occur, determine the magnitude of the effect on the FRC. There is agreement that the resting position of the diaphragm of a recumbent patient moves cephalad with the induction of most general anesthetics. However, estimates of the reduction of the FRC of supine subjects caused by this displacement range from about 100 to 500 ml. On the other hand, the study finding the least effect of the displacement of the diaphragm on the FRC of supine subjects (an average decrease of only 99 ml) demonstrated that the diaphragmatic displacement caused by the induction of general anesthesia to prone subjects resulted in an average decrease of 615 ml, as shown in Fig. 21-1.

General anesthesia also decreases the tone of the intercostal muscles, and combined with the decreased tone of the diaphragm, this results in a change in the cross-sectional shape of the thorax. As shown in Fig. 21-2, the anterior-posterior dimension of the chest of a supine subject is decreased slightly with the induction of anesthesia–paralysis, and the lateral dimension of the thorax increases slightly. Studies have attributed approximately 150 to 250 ml of the decrease in FRC that occurs with the induction of general anesthetics to this flattening of the thorax.

The third potential mechanism for the decrease in FRC seen with the induction of general anesthesia is an increase in intrathoracic blood volume. There is no agreement on whether this occurs, with some studies finding increases in central blood volume, others finding decreases, and at least one finding no change. Differences between these studies probably result from differences in the anesthetics and ventilatory modes used.

SUPINE   PRONE

Awake, spontaneous

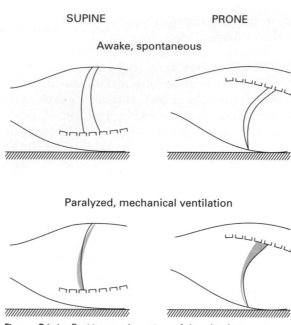

Paralyzed, mechanical ventilation

Figure 21-1   Position and motion of the diaphragm in supine and prone subjects during awake, spontaneous breathing and during anesthesia, paralysis, and mechanical ventilation. Shaded areas represent the movement of the diaphragm during mechanical ventilation. (*Reproduced with permission from Rehder K: Mechanics of the lung and chest wall. Acta Anaesthesiol Scand* 34, suppl 94:32–36, 1990.)

Regardless of the mechanisms of the reduced FRC, such a reduction in the shape and resting volumes of the chest wall and the lungs would be expected to cause secondary alterations in the physiology of the respiratory system. A decrease in lung volume would be expected to decrease the diameter of small airways because smaller alveoli would exert less traction on them. This, in turn, might decrease the anatomic dead space, in addition to causing increased airways resistance. However, because most of the commonly used inhalant anesthetics are bronchodilators, decreases in the diameters of small airways do not usually contribute to increased airways resistance or decreased anatomic dead space with general anesthesia. However, airways resistance may increase with the induction of general anesthesia because of changes in the upper airways, particularly the pharynx. Intubation with a relatively small diameter endotracheal tube or collapse of pharyngeal structures during mask ventilation can increase airways resistance.

General anesthesia has been reported to decrease the activity of the genioglossus muscle, which can cause the tongue to fall against the posterior wall of the pharynx (if the patient is supine) and partially obstruct the pharyngeal airway. The soft palate may move posteriorly and obstruct the nasopharynx; the epiglottis also moves posteriorly. The result of these alterations is significantly increased resistance to airflow through the upper airway.

   The reduction in the FRC is most likely responsible for another consistent result of general anesthesia, which is decreased static compliance of the respiratory system. This decrease in respiratory system compliance is almost entirely a result of decreased lung compliance because the compliance of the chest wall is largely unchanged. Several studies have found decreases in lung compliance of approximately 50 percent with the induction of general anesthesia. Paralysis has little additional effect. Although a decrease in pulmonary surfactant production or activity secondary to general anesthesia has been suggested to contribute to this decrease in pulmonary compliance, there is little evidence for this. The most reasonable current explanation for the decreased lung compliance is that it represents atelectasis resulting from the altered mechanics of the chest wall and the consequent reduction in FRC. This "compression atelectasis" would also partly explain the decrease in arterial PO_2 and the increase in the alveolar-arterial oxygen difference that frequently accompany general anesthesia. Other explanations will be discussed later in this chapter. Ketamine administration does not appear to decrease lung compliance. This is consistent with its not causing a decrease in FRC and supports the concept that the decrease in lung compliance is a result of the factors that decrease the FRC.

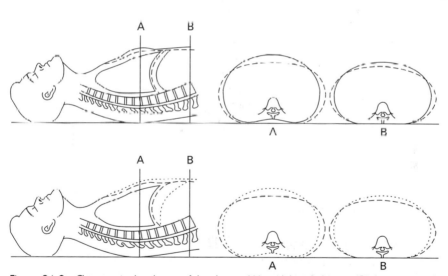

Figure 21-2   Changes in the shape of the thorax (A) and the abdomen (B) that occur with anesthesia paralysis (top) and with anesthesia–paralysis and mechanical ventilation (bottom) of supine patients. *Top:* Solid line = awake; dashed line = anesthesia–paralysis. With anesthesia–paralysis the anterior-posterior dimensions of both thorax and abdomen decrease and the lateral dimensions increase. *Bottom:* dashed line = FRC; dotted line = FRC + V, generated with mechanical ventilation. The anterior-posterior dimensions of both the thorax and abdomen increase with the tidal volume while the lateral dimensions decrease. *[Reproduced with permission from Rehder K, Marsh HM: Respiratory mechanics during anesthesia and mechanical ventilation, in Macklem PT, Mead J (eds): Handbook of Physiology, sec 3: The Respiratory System, vol III: Mechanics of Breathing, part 2. Bethesda, MD, American Physiological Society, 1986, pp 737–752.]*

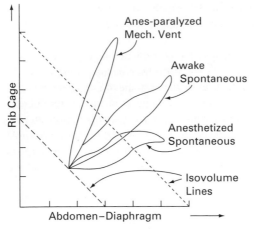

Figure 21-3 Contributions of rib cage movement and diaphragm-abdomen movement to the tidal volume in supine awake spontaneously breathing, anesthetized spontaneously breathing, and anesthetized-paralyzed mechanically ventilated human subjects. A breath with equal contributions from the diaphragm-abdomen and rib cage movement would produce a loop with a slope of 1. Anesthesia decreases rib cage movement during spontaneous breathing but increases it with paralysis and mechanical ventilation. *[Reproduced with permission from Froese AB: Effects of anesthesia and paralysis on the chest wall, in Covino BG,Fozzard HA, Rehder K, Strichartz G (eds): Effects of Anesthesia, Bethesda, MD, American Physiological Society, 1985, pp 107–120.]*

Effects on Chest Wall and Lung Motion

Diaphragmatic motion is usually considered to be responsible for at least two-thirds of the tidal volume of an awake person in the supine position and breathing normally. The remaining portion of the tidal volume is attributed to rib cage motion. However, such determinations of the relative contributions of the motion of the diaphragm and the rib cage are difficult to interpret, because the data are difficult to obtain and because the diaphragm, rib cage, and abdominal muscles are mechanically interdependent. Furthermore, changes in body position, changes in the magnitude of the tidal volume, or differences in body configurations may alter the proportion of rib cage and diaphragmatic motion in generating the tidal volume. For example, rib cage motion may contribute more to the tidal volume when a person is standing or seated upright than when he or she is supine.

General anesthesia can have profound effects on the relative contributions of rib cage and diaphragmatic motion to the tidal volume. In one study, the results of which are summarized in Fig. 21-3, rib cage motion contributed 43 percent of the resting tidal volume in awake supine subjects. In spontaneously breathing supine subjects anesthetized with halothane, rib cage motion accounted for only 19 percent of the tidal volume. In contrast, in anesthetized-paralyzed subjects maintained with mechanical ventilation, the rib cage contribution to the tidal volume predominates.

The most reasonable explanation for the decreased contribution of rib cage motion to the tidal volume of anesthetized spontaneously breathing supine subjects is that general anesthesia appears to suppress or even abolish the activity of the intercostal muscles at levels that do not affect the activity of the diaphragm. The predominance of rib cage motion over diaphragmatic motion during the passive expansion of the thorax in supine, mechanically ventilated anesthetized-paralyzed subjects likely results from the necessity for the flaccid diaphragm to displace the largely incompressible contents of the abdomen. Putting this another way, the transdiaphragmatic pressure gradient during positive-pressure ventilation is less than the pressure gradient across the rib cage because the abdominal pressure is positive. The passive tension of the diaphragm may also play a role in this difference.

The effects of the contents of the abdomen on the transdiaphragmatic pressure gradient and the motion of the diaphragm may also help explain alterations in the regional distribution of alveolar ventilation with anesthesia−paralysis and mechanical ventilation, as discussed in the next section.

Effects on the Distribution of Alveolar Ventilation

As discussed in Chap 13, when a person is breathing tidally from the FRC in the upright, supine, or even lateral decubitus position, there is relatively more alveolar ventilation in gravity-dependent than in nondependent regions. The usual explanation for this gradient of alveolar ventilation is that there is also a gradient of pleural pressure, which is more negative in nondependent than in gravity-dependent regions. This results in larger alveoli in nondependent regions than in dependent regions. These larger alveoli are less compliant than those in dependent regions, so they have smaller volume changes for similar changes in transpulmonary pressure.

This difference in ventilation between gravity-dependent and nondependent alveoli is decreased or even abolished during anesthesia−paralysis and mechanical ventilation of subjects in the supine and lateral decubitus positions, as shown in Fig. 21-4. A plausible explanation for this is that alveolar ventilation follows the motion of the diaphragm, which is shown in Fig. 21-5. Note that in the awake spontaneously breathing supine subject, most of the diaphragmatic movement is in the gravity-dependent dorsal region. This probably results from the normal mechanics of the diaphragm, which functions differently ventrally and dorsally. The dorsal portions of the diaphragm are inserted into the spinal column by the two crura; the ventral portions of the diaphragm are inserted into the lower ribs and the sternum.

With anesthesia−paralysis and mechanical ventilation, in subjects in the supine position, the diaphragm moves differently, with some studies showing fairly uniform motion ventrally and dorsally and others showing most of the motion in the ventral, nondependent regions. This preferential movement of the nondependent diaphragm of supine anesthetized-paralyzed subjects seems reasonable be-

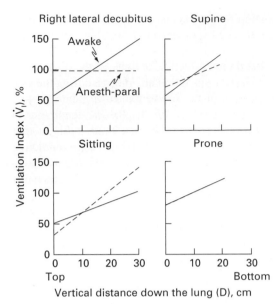

Figure 21-4 Effect of anesthesia–paralysis on regional ventilation in four different body positions. Solid line = awake; dashed line = anesthesia–paralysis. Regional ventilation became more uniform in the supine and right lateral decubitus positions, became less uniform in the sitting position, and did not change with anesthesia–paralysis in the prone position. *(Reproduced with permission from Rehder K, Knopp TJ, Sessler AD: Regional intrapulmonary gas distribution in awake and anesthetized-paralyzed prone man. J Appl Physiol 45:528–535, 1978.)*

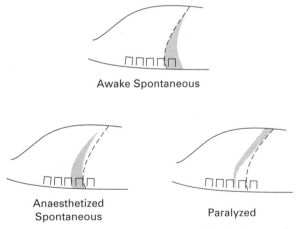

Figure 21-5 Position and movement of the diaphragm during tidal breathing in a supine subject in the awake spontaneously breathing, anesthetized spontaneously breathing, and anesthetized-paralyzed mechanically ventilated states. Dashed lines = movement of the diaphragm during tidal breathing. *(Reproduced with permission from Froese AB, Bryan AC: Effects of anesthesia and paralysis on the diaphragmatic mechanics in man. Anesthesiology 41:242–255, 1974.)*

cause the contents of the abdomen are mainly incompressible liquids and would be expected to result in a hydrostatic pressure gradient in the gravity-dependent dorsal regions opposing movement of the diaphragm. This would be similar for subjects in the lateral decubitus position.

Unfortunately this simple explanation does not appear to completely account for the regional distribution of alveolar ventilation because, as seen in Fig. 21-1, in awake spontaneously breathing subjects in the prone position, most of diaphragmatic motion is in the nondependent dorsal region, but there is more alveolar ventilation in the gravity-dependent ventral regions. With anesthesia–paralysis and mechanical ventilation, there is little change in either diaphragmatic motion (Fig. 21-5) or the distribution of alveolar ventilation (Fig. 21-4). Furthermore, in both the supine and prone positions, rib cage motion is responsible for more of the tidal volume during anesthesia–paralysis and mechanical ventilation. Intraoperative mechanical ventilation is usually at larger tidal volumes (10 to 12 ml/kg) than during spontaneous ventilation (6 to 7 ml/kg). Subsequent increases in airway pressure during mechanical ventilation may play a role in the compliance changes. It is not yet clear what other factors may be involved in the more uniform distribution of alveolar ventilation in anesthetized-paralyzed mechanically ventilated subjects in the supine or lateral decubitus position. This more uniform distribution of alveolar ventilation may have important consequences in the matching of ventilation and perfusion during general anesthesia, as will be discussed shortly.

Effects on Cardiac Output and the Distribution of Pulmonary Blood Flow

General anesthesia usually causes a significant decrease in the cardiac output, even in patients with normal cardiovascular systems. The decrease in cardiac output is exacerbated by positive-pressure ventilation, especially if it is accompanied by positive end-expiratory pressure (PEEP). There are many potential explanations for this decreased cardiac output.

Many general anesthetics decrease cardiac output by direct depression of the myocardium. Halothane, or enflurane in normal anesthetic concentrations, depresses cardiac output 20 to 50 percent from that of an awake individual; the main mechanism appears to be a direct negative inotropic effect. Other inhalant anesthetics and most intravenous anesthetic agents have somewhat less direct effects on the heart, although thiopental does have a significant negative inotropic effect on the myocardium. Any anesthetic agent that directly or reflexly decreases heart rate decreases the cardiac output.

General anesthesia may also decrease the cardiac output by changing the left ventricular afterload or preload. Agents that increase the afterload by directly or reflexly causing arteriolar constriction would be expected to decrease cardiac output in the absence of other effects. Agents that cause venodilation would decrease the cardiac output by decreasing venous return and thus decreasing the preload.

There are a number of proposed mechanisms for the decreased cardiac output caused by positive-pressure ventilation with positive end-expiratory pressure. Positive intrapleural pressure could, by decreasing the transmural pressure gradient, cause compression of the intrathoracic great veins, and therefore decrease venous return. Similarly, positive-pressure ventilation with positive end-expiratory pressure causes compression of both the alveolar and extraalveolar vessels of the pulmonary circulation, thus increasing pulmonary vascular resistance and increasing the afterload of the right ventricle. This could decrease the flow of pulmonary venous blood to the left atrium. Positive intrapleural pressure could also impede right ventricular filling by decreasing the transmural pressure gradient during diastole. An increased right ventricular afterload could decrease right ventricular emptying, leading to *increased* right ventricular diastolic volume and therefore displacing the interventricular septum toward the left ventricle and decreasing left ventricular filling. Finally, stretch receptors in the lungs or the heart may cause reflex inhibition of the myocardium or cause the release of mediators that affect the heart or blood vessels.

Effects on the Distribution of Pulmonary Blood Flow

It is widely accepted that general anesthesia does not alter the gradient of blood flow from the upper to lower regions of the lung. That is, there is more blood flow per unit volume in gravity-dependent regions of the lung than in nondependent regions, as was shown in Fig. 15-2. As discussed previously, this gradient results from greater intravascular pressures causing more recruitment and distention of pulmonary vessels in gravity-dependent lung regions. This results in less resistance to blood flow in lower regions of the lung.

Although increasing blood flow per unit volume with distance down the lung is maintained with general anesthesia, the low cardiac outputs described above usually result in decreased or even absent perfusion in the uppermost portions of the lung. Thus increased physiologic dead space is usually seen as a consequence of general anesthesia. This increase in physiologic dead space is almost entirely due to increased alveolar dead space, which could be explained by the development of zone 1 (in which alveolar pressure exceeds pulmonary artery pressure) or overventilation of underperfused alveoli, or both. There is no clear evidence that the alveolar dead space results from the development of zone 1 in hypoperfused nondependent lung regions, which would be unlikely in supine patients exposed to moderate airway pressures and levels of PEEP. Therefore, overventilation of poorly perfused alveoli seems a more likely explanation. Whatever the explanation, general anesthesia usually increases alveolar dead space by 50 to 100 ml and may introduce an arterial-alveolar PCO_2 gradient of 5 mmHg (measured as arterial PCO_2 minus the end-tidal PCO_2).

Effects on Hypoxic Pulmonary Vasoconstriction and the Intrapulmonary Shunt

Most determinations of the intrapulmonary shunt during general anesthesia show a significant increase from that in the awake state. The intrapulmonary shunt of awake normal subjects is approximately 2 to 4 percent of the cardiac output; various studies on anesthetized subjects have determined the intrapulmonary shunt to be 6 to 14 percent of the cardiac output. Determinations of the intrapulmonary shunt using the shunt equation (see Chap. 15) represent a total of true shunt ($\dot{V}/\dot{Q} = 0$) plus shuntlike alveolar-capillary units (those with low $\dot{V}/\dot{Q}$'s). Thus these calculations of intrapulmonary shunts represent the total perfusion of unventilated alveoli and poorly ventilated alveoli, and possibly even hyperperfusion of normally ventilated alveoli. Any increase in the intrapulmonary shunt would be expected to decrease the arterial PO_2 and increase the alveolar-arterial PO_2 difference.

Several of the effects of general anesthesia combine to increase the intrapulmonary shunt. The first of these, compression atelectasis, was discussed earlier in this chapter. Changes in the tone of the respiratory muscles, the position of the diaphragm, and the shape of the rib cage combine to decrease the thoracic volume, decreasing the FRC and causing atelectasis. A second effect is greater ventilation of alveoli in the upper lung regions, possibly caused by preferential movement of the diaphragm in nondependent lung regions, in patients in the supine or lateral decubitus positions. If greater perfusion of gravity-dependent lung regions persists in these patients, as described above, then low $\dot{V}/\dot{Q}$ units will develop in lower parts of the lungs.

One mechanism that would be expected to reduce the effects of atelectasis and regional alterations in the matching of ventilation and perfusion is hypoxic pulmonary vasoconstriction. However, hypoxic pulmonary vasoconstriction is not completely effective in diverting blood flow away from poorly ventilated, unventilated, or atelectatic lung regions in awake normal healthy subjects. There is general agreement that most inhalant anesthetics further decrease the effectiveness of hypoxic pulmonary vasoconstriction, although most intravenous agents do not. The inhibition of hypoxic pulmonary vasoconstriction by the inhalant anesthetics contributes to the decreased arterial PO_2 and increased alveolar-arterial PO_2 difference usually seen with general anesthesia with inhaled agents.

Effects on Ventilation-Perfusion Relationships and Oxygen and Carbon Dioxide Transport

As discussed in the previous sections, general anesthesia increases the proportion of the lung with high ventilation-perfusion ratios and may even cause the development of areas of alveolar dead space, which have infinite ventilation-perfusion ratios. This would be expected to lead to an arterial-alveolar PCO_2 difference. General anesthesia also increases the intrapulmonary shunt (true shunt plus shuntlike units), which increases the alveolar-arterial PO_2 gradient.

A more specific graphic method of assessing ventilation-perfusion relationships in human subjects, called *the multiple inert gas elimination technique,* can be used to monitor the effects of general anesthesia on pulmonary gas exchange. The technique uses the concept that the elimination via the lungs of different gases dissolved in the venous blood will be affected differently by variations in the ventilation-perfusion ratios of alveolar-capillary units, according to the solubility of each gas in the blood. At a ventilation-perfusion ratio of 1.0, a greater volume of a relatively soluble gas would be retained in the blood than would that of a relatively insoluble gas. Thus the retention of any particular gas by a single alveolar-capillary unit is dependent on the blood-gas partition coefficient of the gas and the ventilation-perfusion ratio of the unit. Gases with very low solubilities in the blood would only be retained in the blood by units with very low (or zero) ventilation-perfusion ratios. Gases with very high solubilities in the blood would be mainly eliminated in the expired air of units with very high ventilation-perfusion ratios.

In the standard multiple inert gas elimination technique for assessing ventilation-perfusion relationships, a mixture of six gases dissolved in saline is infused into a peripheral arm vein at a constant rate of 2 to 5 ml/min, until a steady state of gas exchange is established. This usually takes about 20 min. The six gases, sulfur hexafluoride, ethane, cyclopropane, halothane, diethyl ether, and acetone, were chosen to represent a wide range of solubilities in blood, with acetone the most soluble and sulfur hexafluoride the least soluble. Samples of expired air and arterial blood are analyzed by gas chromatography to determine the concentrations of each of the six gases. Other data usually obtained include cardiac output by indicator dilution, minute ventilation, and arterial and mixed venous blood gases.

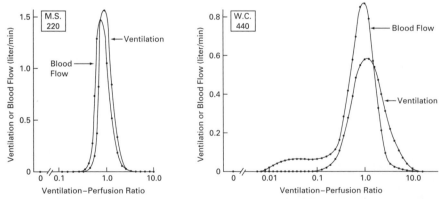

Figure 21-6 Distributions of ventilation and perfusion ratios, obtained with the multiple inert gas elimination technique, in normal men, 22 (A) and 44 (B) years of age. *(Reproduced from Wagner PD, Laravuso RB, Uhl RR, West JB: Continuous distributions of ventilation-perfusion ratios in normal subjects breathing air and 100 per cent O₂. (Reprinted from* **The Journal of Clinical Investigation,** *1974, 54:54–68, by copyright permission of The American Society for Clinical Investigation.)*

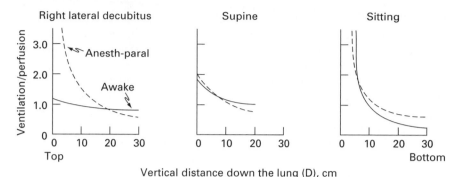

Figure 21-7 The effect of anesthesia–paralysis on regional ventilation-perfusion ratios determined with radioactive xenon in human subjects in three different body positions. Solid line = awake, spontaneously breathing; dashed lines = anesthesia–paralysis. Ventilation-perfusion relationships were altered significantly by anesthesia–paralysis only when subjects were in the right lateral decubitus position. (*Reproduced with permission from Rehder K: Anaesthesia and the respiratory system. Can Anaesth Soc J 26:451–462, 1979.*)

Graphs plotting the blood-gas partition coefficients for each of the six gases versus their retentions and excretions are constructed. A computer is then used to convert these data into graphs like the one shown in Fig. 21-6A. The graph, which shows the distribution of ventilation-perfusion ratios in a young healthy male subject, can be read as a frequency histogram. The x axis is the spectrum of ventilation-perfusion ratios from 0 to 100, displayed as a logarithmic scale. The y axis shows the amount of ventilation or blood flow going to alveolar-capillary units with ventilation-perfusion ratio on the x axis. The figure demonstrates that almost all of the blood flow and ventilation go to alveolar-capillary units with ventilation-perfusion ratios near 1 in this young, healthy subject. There is no ventilation or perfusion of units with ratios below 0.3 or above 3.0. Figure 21-6B shows the distribution of ventilation and perfusion in a healthy middle-aged subject. Note the wider dispersion of ventilation and perfusion, with more perfusion going to units with ratios above 3.0 and much more going to units with ratios below 0.3. Similarly, the ventilation is also more widely distributed. Note that there was no true intrapulmonary shunt in either subject, that is, no blood flow to alveolar-capillary units with ventilation-perfusion ratios of zero.

Investigations of the effects of general anesthesia on the distribution of ventilation-perfusion ratios have yielded results that are only partly consistent. Although there are a number of reasons for this, including differences in the anesthetics and ventilatory modes used and the body positions and the medical status of the subjects or patients involved, the age of the subjects appears to be the most important variable from study to study.

Figure 21-7 shows the changes in regional ventilation-perfusion relationships for young, healthy subjects in three different body positions. As might be expected from the discussion in previous sections of this chapter, there is little effect of general anesthesia on the distribution of $\dot{V}/\dot{Q}$'s from the top of the lung to bottom in the sitting or supine positions. However, there is a major effect in the lateral decubitus position, with a significant development of high ventilation-perfusion ratios in upper parts of the lung and the development of some lower ventilation-perfusion ratios in lower regions of the lung.

The multiple inert gas elimination technique gives another perspective on changes in the distribution of ventilation and perfusion that occur with general anesthesia in a young, healthy adult. Figure 21-8 shows the ventilation and perfusion profiles of a 29-year-old healthy male before and after the induction of general anesthesia. They are typical of those of a number of subjects who were studied, whose ages ranged from 24 to 33 years. Note that in the awake state, all of this subject's ventilation and perfusion went to units with $\dot{V}/\dot{Q}$'s between 0.1 and 1.0. The mean $\dot{V}/\dot{Q}$ of the ventilation distribution in this study was 0.81 in the supine position in the awake state; the mean $\dot{V}/\dot{Q}$ of the perfusion distribution was 0.58. There was no intrapulmonary shunt. Although several of the gases in the multiple inert gas elimination technique have anesthetic properties, they are used in such low concentrations that they do not affect the subjects in the awake state. General anesthesia was induced with thiopental and maintained with methoxyflurane. Pancuronium bromide was also used. As shown in the figure, anesthesia–paralysis had moderate effects on the distribution of ventilation and perfusion. The perfusion distribution was somewhat wider, with some perfusion of units with $\dot{V}/\dot{Q}$'s above 1.0. The ventilation distribution was both much wider and bimodal, with significant ventilation of units with $\dot{V}/\dot{Q}$'s between 10 and 100, corresponding to alveolar dead space–like areas. The mean $\dot{V}/\dot{Q}$ of the ventilation distribution was increased to 1.17 after anesthesia–paralysis; the mean $\dot{V}/\dot{Q}$ of the perfusion distribution was unchanged at 0.59. Intrapulmonary shunt remained at zero in this subject; it did not increase significantly in the subjects in the study.

Another study used the multiple inert gas elimination technique on middle-aged healthy subjects ranging in age from 37 to 64 years (average age of 51 years) to show the effects of anesthesia, mechanical ventilation, and positive end-expiratory pressure on the distribution of ventilation and perfusion. As seen in

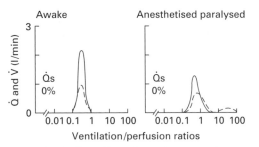

Figure 21-8   The effect of anesthesia paralysis on ventilation (dashed lines) and perfusion (solid lines) distribution in a young, healthy supine subject. (*Reproduced with permission from Nunn JF: Nunn's Applied Respiratory Physiology, 4th ed. London, Butterworth-Heinemann, 1993, pp 384–417; and Rehder K, Knopp TJ, Sessler AD, Didier EP: Ventilation-perfusion relationship in young healthy awake and anesthetized-paralyzed young man. J Appl Physiol 47:745–753, 1979.*)

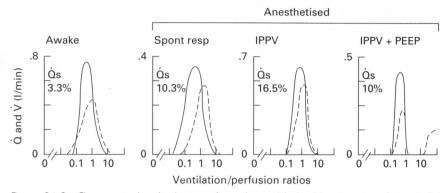

Figure 21-9 Changes in the distribution of ventilation (dashed lines) and perfusion (solid lines) distribution caused by a general anesthesia with spontaneous breathing, mechanical ventilation without positive end-expiratory pressure (IPPV), and mechanical ventilation with positive end-expiratory pressure (IPPV + PEEP). (*Reproduced with permission from Nunn JF: Nunn's Applied Respiratory Physiology, 4th ed. London, Butterworth-Heinemann, 1993, pp 384–417; and Bindslev L, Hedenstierna G, Santesson J, Gottlieb I, Carvallhas A: Ventilation-perfusion distribution during inhalation anesthesia; Effects of spontaneous breathing, mechanical ventilation and positive end-expiratory pressure. Acta Anaesthesiol Scand 25:360–371, 1981.*)

the example shown in Fig. 21-9, these older subjects had somewhat wider distributions of ventilation and perfusion in the awake state in the supine position, with the mean $\dot{V}/\dot{Q}$ of the ventilation distribution equal to 0.81 and the mean $\dot{V}/\dot{Q}$ of the perfusion distribution equal to 0.47. The mean intrapulmonary shunt was 1.6 percent of the cardiac output. (It was 3.3 percent in the subject shown in the figure.) Anesthesia with spontaneous breathing widened the distributions slightly, if at all, but the ventilation mean $\dot{V}/\dot{Q}$ increased to 1.30. The perfusion mean $\dot{V}/\dot{Q}$ was relatively unchanged at 0.51. The mean shunt increased to 6.2 percent of the cardiac output. (It was 10.3 percent in the subject shown in the figure.) Mechanical ventilation without positive end-expiratory pressure (labeled IPPV in the figure) increased the mean $\dot{V}/\dot{Q}$ of the ventilation distribution to 2.2, but it did not widen the distribution profile significantly. The mean $\dot{V}/\dot{Q}$ of the perfusion distribution increased to 0.83, with no change in the width of the distribution profile. Mean shunt increased to 8.6 percent of the cardiac output. (It was 16.5 percent in the subject shown in the figure.) Mechanical ventilation with positive end-expiratory pressure (IPPV + PEEP in the figure) increased the mean $\dot{V}/\dot{Q}$ of the ventilation distribution to 3.03 and decreased the mean $\dot{V}/\dot{Q}$ of the perfusion distribution to 0.55. The ventilation distribution became bimodal, with significant ventilation of alveolar dead space–like units; the width of the perfusion distribution decreased slightly. Intrapulmonary shunt decreased to 4.1 percent of the cardiac output.

In summary, in supine middle-aged subjects, general anesthesia with spontaneous ventilation, which decreased the mean cardiac output from 6.1 to 5.0 liters/min, increased the intrapulmonary shunt and increased the ventilation of units with higher $\dot{V}/\dot{Q}$'s. Mechanical ventilation without PEEP, which further decreased the cardiac output to 4.5 liters/min, increased the intrapulmonary shunt, and increased the ventilation of units with high $\dot{V}/\dot{Q}$'s. Mechanical ventilation with PEEP, which decreased cardiac output to 3.7 liters/min, decreased the shunt but greatly increased the ventilation of units with very high $\dot{V}/\dot{Q}$'s, thus increasing the alveolar dead space-like regions in the lung.

A third study using the multiple inert gas elimination technique was done with supine patients whose ages ranged from 52 to 72 years (mean age 60 years). These older patients included smokers and some with chronic obstructive pulmonary disease. Halothane or halothane and nitrous oxide was used as the anesthetic. As shown in Fig. 21-10, the perfusion responses of the 10 patients fell into three patterns: increased perfusion of low $\dot{V}/\dot{Q}$ units, with little increase in shunt; increased shunt, with little increase in perfusion of shuntlike areas; or both.

In conclusion, the age and cardiopulmonary status of patients are important determinants of the effects of general anesthesia on the distribution of ventilation and perfusion. As these effects of ventilation-perfusion relationships on the PaO_2 and oxygen content of the blood are considered, remember that oxygen delivery to the tissues is determined by both the O_2 content of the arterial blood and the cardiac output. Thus the addition of PEEP may increase the PaO_2, but if it is already high, little additional O_2 will be carried in the blood and the delivery may decrease if cardiac output is decreased by the PEEP. Finally, there is no evidence that the inhalant anesthetics alter the P_{50} of blood.

Effects of General Anesthesia on the Control of Breathing

The effects of general anesthesia on the control of breathing are of concern during anesthesia without assisted ventilation and also as postsurgical patients are weaned from mechanical ventilation. General anesthesia is almost always associated with decreased spontaneous alveolar ventilation. Although this is partly

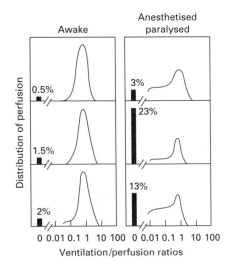

Figure 21-10 Three patterns of alterations in perfusion caused by anesthesia paralysis in elderly surgical patients. (Reproduced with permission from Nunn JF: Nunn's Applied Respiratory Physiology, 4th ed. London, Butterworth-Heinemann, 1993, pp 384–417; and Dueck R, Young I, Clausen J, Wagner PD: Altered distribution of pulmonary ventilation and blood flow following induction of inhalational anesthesia. Anesthesiology 52:113–125:1980.)

accounted for by a usual decrease in the metabolic rate of approximately 15 percent below the basal metabolic rate during general anesthesia, much of the decrease results from respiratory depressant effects of the anesthetic used.

Effects on the Responses to Carbon Dioxide and Metabolic Acidosis

Almost all general anesthetics depress the response to carbon dioxide, as was shown in Fig. 18-3. This results in lower minute ventilation and higher arterial Pco_2's, as well as less of an increase in ventilation per increase in Pco_2. All of the commonly used inhalant anesthetics depress the response to CO_2 in a dose-dependent manner, with halothane having somewhat less effect than enflurane and isoflurane. Diethyl ether is much less depressant than halothane. Barbiturate anesthetics all depress the response to carbon dioxide, as do the opiates. Ketamine does not appear to depress the response to carbon dioxide. The respiratory depression caused by anesthesia is partly reversed by surgical manipulation, probably by stimulation of pain receptors. General anesthesia also depresses the response to metabolic acidosis in a dose-dependent manner.

Effects on the Response to Hypoxia

Most inhalant anesthetics also depress the response to hypoxia, possibly by a direct effect on the arterial chemoreceptors. This depressed response to hypoxia has the unfortunate consequence of not maintaining the ventilation of patients whose ventilatory response to carbon dioxide is also depressed by general anesthesia, chronic obstructive pulmonary disease, or both.

Effects on the Response to Increased Resistance

Although the preceding discussion would suggest that the ventilatory response to increased airways resistance would be impaired by general anesthesia, anesthetized patients can usually respond to increased resistive loads with little problem.

BIBLIOGRAPHY

Barnas GM, Green MD, MacKenzie CF, et al: Effect of posture on lung and regional chest wall mechanics. *Anesthesiology* 78:251–259, 1993.

Bendixen HH, Laver MB: Hypoxia in anesthesia: A review. *Clin Pharmacol Ther* 6:510–539, 1965.

Bindslev L, Hedenstierna G, Santesson J, et al: Ventilation-perfusion distribution during inhalation anaesthesia. *Acta Anaesthesiol. Scand.* 25:360–371, 1981.

Eisenkraft JB: Effects of anaesthetics on the pulmonary circulation. *Br J Anaesth* 65:63–78, 1990.

Fletcher R: Dead space during anaesthesia. *Acta Anaesthesiol Scand* 34, suppl 94:46–50, 1990.

Fletcher R: The arterial–end tidal CO_2 difference during cardiothoracic surgery. *J Cardiothorac Anesth* 4:105–117, 1990.

Froese AB: Effects of anesthesia and paralysis on the chest wall, in Covino BG, Fozzard HA, Rehder K, Strichartz G (eds): *Effects of Anesthesia.* Bethesda, MD, American Physiological Society, 1985, pp 107–120.

Gal TJ: *Respiratory Physiology in Anesthetic Practice.* Baltimore, Williams & Wilkins, 1991.

Hedenstierna G: Gas exchange during anaesthesia. *Br J Anaesth* 64:507–514, 1990.

Hedenstierna G: Gas exchange during anaesthesia. *Acta Anaesthesiol Scand* 34, suppl 94: 27–31, 1990.

Hedenstierna G: Ventilation-perfusion relationships during anaesthesia. *Thorax* 50:85–91, 1995.

Hirschman CA, Bergman NA: Factors influencing intrapulmonary airway calibre during anesthesia. *Br J Anaesth* 65:30–42, 1990.

Hornbein TF: Anesthetics and ventilatory control, in Covino BG, Fozzard HA, Rehder K, Strichartz G (eds): *Effects of Anesthesia.* Bethesda, MD, American Physiological Society, 1985, pp 75–90.

Krayer S, Rehder K, Vettermann J, et al: Position and motion of the human diaphragm during anesthesia-paralysis. *Anesthesiology* 70:891–898, 1989.

Marshall BE: Hypoxic pulmonary vasoconstriction. *Acta Anesthesiol Scand* 34, suppl 94: 37–41, 1990.

Marshall BE, Marshall C: Anesthesia and Pulmonary Circulation, in Covino BG, Fozzard HA, Rehder K, Strichartz G (eds): *Effects of Anesthesia,* Bethesda, MD, American Physiological Society, 1985, pp 121–136.

Marshall BE, Wyche MQ Jr: Hypoxemia during and after anesthesia. *Anesthesiology* 37: 178–209, 1972.

Milic-Emili J, Robatto FM, Bates JHT: Respiratory mechanics in anaesthesia. *Br J Anaesth,* 65:4–12, 1990.

Nunn JF: *Nunn's Applied Respiratory Physiology,* 4th ed. Butterworth-Heinemann, London, 1993, pp 384–417.

Nunn JF: Anesthesia and pulmonary gas exchange, in Covino BG, Fozzard HA, Rehder K, Strichartz G (eds): *Effects of Anesthesia.* Bethesda, MD, American Physiological Society, 1985, pp 137–147.

Rehder K: Anaesthesia and the respiratory system, *Can Anaesth Soc J* 26:451–462, 1979.

Rehder K: Anesthesia and the mechanics of respiration, in Covino BG, Fozzard HA, Rehder K, Strichartz G (eds): *Effects of Anesthesia.* Bethesda, MD, American Physiological Society, 1985, pp 91–106.

Rehder K: Mechanics of the lung and chest wall, *Acta Anaesthesiol Scand* 34, suppl 94: 32–36, 1990.

Rehder K, Marsh HM: Respiratory mechanics during anesthesia and mechanical ventilation, in Macklem PT, Mead J (eds): *Handbook of Physiology,* sec 3: *The Respiratory System,* vol III: *Mechanics of Breathing,* part 2. Bethesda, MD, American Physiological Society, 1986, pp 737–752.

Rehder K, Sessler AD, Marsh HM: General anesthesia and the lung. *Am Rev Respir Dis* 112:541–563, 1975.

Schmid ER, Rehder K: General anesthesia and the chest wall. *Anesthesiology* 55:668–675, 1981.

Versprille A: The pulmonary circulation during mechanical ventilation. *Acta Anaesthesiol Scand* 34, suppl 94:51–62, 1990.

Wagner PD, Laravuso RB, Uhl RR, West JB: Continuous distributions of ventilation-perfusion ratios in normal subjects breathing air and 100 percent O_2. *J Clin Invest* 54:54–68, 1974.

Warner DO, Warner MA, Ritman EL: Human chest wall function while awake and during halothane anesthesia: I. Quiet breathing. *Anesthesiology* 82:6–19, 1995.

West JB: Ventilation-perfusion relationships. *Am Rev Respir Dis* 116:917–943, 1977.

West JB: *Ventilation/Blood Flow and Gas Exchange,* 5th ed. Oxford, Blackwell, 1990, 95–109.

22

ANESTHETIC MANAGEMENT OF THE PATIENT WITH HEART DISEASE

Generally, anesthetic management of the patient with heart disease differs depending on whether cardiac or noncardiac surgery is planned. Anesthesia for cardiac surgery encompasses many surgical procedures including coronary revascularization, valvular repair or replacement, correction of congenital defects, and palliative procedures. Extensive cardiovascular monitoring is usually employed (frequently including intraoperative echocardiography), and direct visualization of the heart can give information on cardiac status. The surgical procedure usually improves cardiac function or reserve, although cardiopulmonary bypass and hypothermia can transiently reduce contractility. In contrast, patients with cardiac disease anesthetized for noncardiac surgery are monitored in proportion to the physiologic implications of the surgery and the severity of the cardiovascular disease. The surgery usually produces no improvement in cardiac function while the anesthesia drugs, mechanical ventilation, and postoperative restrictive pulmonary defects can produce further cardiovascular compromise.

CORONARY ARTERY DISEASE

Management of the patient with coronary artery disease focuses on the balance between myocardial oxygen supply and demand. Preoperative anxiety and tachycardia (greater than 110 beats per minute) increase the incidence of ischemia, but hypertensive and hypotensive episodes are not as significant. The rate-pressure product (systolic pressure × heart rate), triple index (systolic pressure × heart rate × pulmonary capillary wedge pressure), and the tension time index (heart rate × area under the systolic portion of the aortic pressure curve) have been used to estimate myocardial oxygen demand. Continuous monitoring of multiple electrocardiogram (ECG) leads can accurately demonstrate the occurrence of myocardial ischemia in patients with multivessel disease. The use of ST-segment trending has also improved the detection of perioperative ischemia. Benefits of pulmonary artery catheterization remain controversial, although complications associated with its use are well documented. Intraoperative two-dimensional transesophageal echocardiography (2 D-TEE) can reveal signs of ischemia such as changes in ejection and symmetry of chamber contraction. Additionally, intraoperative 2 D-TEE can detect the success of valvular replacement and repair of congenital heart disease. Interpretation of echocardiography to guide surgery usually involves a cardiologist with the anesthesiologist's involvement influenced by personal interest and departmental reimbursement patterns. Prospective studies have shown that the choice for anesthetics has little bearing on the outcome following coronary artery bypass grafting (CABG) or valvular heart surgery. A "fast-track" early extubation (less than 12 h) anesthetic technique has been recommended for selected CABG patients, resulting in decreased length of intensive care unit stay and hospital cost while mortality was unchanged.

Cardiopulmonary Bypass

Cardiopulmonary bypass provides perfusion and gas exchange via an oxygenator, that also eliminates carbon dioxide (sometimes so successfully that carbon dioxide must be added before the blood is returned to the body). The two main types of oxygenators in use today are the *bubble oxygenator*, which provides a gas interface, and the more expensive *membrane oxygenator*, which has no gas interface and is less damaging to red blood cells.

Before the patient is put on bypass, heparin should be administered via a central line through which blood can easily be aspirated or the heparin should be given by the surgeon (usually intracardiac). Sufficient prolongation of the activated clotting time must be present before the patient is put on bypass.

Abnormal heart rate and rhythm are common at the end of cardiopulmonary bypass and can require the use of a pacemaker. Persistent poor contractility, arterial hypotension, and low cardiac output are managed by manipulation of preload and (sometimes multiple) infusions of vasoactive and inotropic drugs. Failure to successfully terminate cardiopulmonary bypass after administration of various drug combinations may necessitate insertion of an intraaortic balloon pump or ventricular assist device.

Cardiac Pacemakers   If time permits, a cardiologist can be called to the operating room to assist with pacemaker placement management. Occasionally, however, pacemaker failure, profound bradycardia, or other conduction abnormalities can so seriously compromise cardiac function that immediate pacing may be necessary.

Cardiac glycosides are used for the treatment of cardiac tachydysrhythmia and congestive heart failure. Digoxin may be useful in the treatment of atrial fibrillation, atrial flutter, PAT, and PSVT. Cardiac glycosides inhibit the sodium potassium pump and reduce the transport of sodium and calcium out of the cell. The increased intracellular calcium is believed to be responsible for the increased contractility. Digoxin also causes sensitization of the carotid sinus reflex and increases parasympathetic activity. The increased vagal tone slows sinoatrial node activity and delays conduction through the atrioventricular (AV) node causing a slower heart rate. Digoxin can decrease the ventricular rate when there has been a rapid ventricular response to atrial fibrillation or flutter. This allows more time for ventricular filling and coronary perfusion.

Digoxin toxicity produces prolonged PR interval, AV block, and atrial or ventricular dysrhythmia (due to increased automaticity), which includes ventricular fibrillation. Treatment of digoxin toxicity includes correction of electrolyte abnormalities (potassium, calcium, and magnesium). Phenytoin and lidocaine are helpful in reducing automaticity. Atropine may be useful in treating bradycardia, but a temporary pacemaker may be needed if complete AV block is present. Digoxin immune Antigen Binding Fragment (FAB) contains antibodies specific to digoxin and, following intravenous administration, symptoms of digoxin toxicity improve within one-half hour or less.

Temporary epicardial pacemaker lead placement commonly is performed in conjunction with cardiac surgery. Placement of permanent epicardial pacemaker leads requires general anesthesia, while insertion of transvenous pacing systems can be performed under local anesthesia and sedation. Transcutaneous pacing (using large thoracic patches anterior and posterior to the heart) can be useful for emergency treatment of severe bradycardia.

Certain cardiac anomalies or prior cardiac surgery can prevent transvenous lead placement. Tricuspid atresia or a Fontan operation (anastomoses of right atrium to the pulmonary artery) prevents placement of ventricular placing leads. A Glenn shunt (anastomoses of the right pulmonary artery to the superior vena cava) makes it impossible to pass a lead from the superior vena cava into the heart.

Pacing to Terminate Tachydysrhythmia   As an alternative to pharmacologic treatment of supraventricular or ventricular tachydysrhythmia, overdrive pacing is sometimes used. When tachycardia is detected, the pacemaker delivers pulses at a rate faster than the tachycardia rate. The pacing burst captures the atrium and frequently when the burst ends so does the tachycardia.

Pulse Generator   Pulse generators can be temporary external generators or permanent implantable pacers. The pacemaker first senses the intrinsic activity of the heart. It must be set to avoid oversensing, which is sensing the contraction of skeletal muscles or activity of the other cardiac chambers (e.g., an atrial pacer sensing ventricular activity).

The pulse generator must determine when to pace the heart, based on the timing of previously sensed and paced events.

Pacing Leads   The electrodes can be sewn or inserted into the epicardial surface of the heart. These epicardial leads can be attached to either the atrium, the ventricle, or both. Transvenous leads are in contact with the endocardial surface of the heart and likewise can be in contact with the atrium, the ventricle, or both. Both epicardial and transvenous leads may be temporary for short-term pacing (such as the immediate postoperative period) or can be permanent.

CARDIAC PATIENTS FOR NONCARDIAC SURGERY

More than one-quarter of the patients anesthetized in the United States are at risk for or have clinically significant cardiovascular disease. Patients for noncardiac surgery usually do not have as extensive a cardiovascular workup as the open heart surgical patient. In addition, they tend not to be as well prepared medically and usually lack the extensive monitoring and treatment resources available during and following cardiac surgery. Coronary artery disease is the cardiovascular disease with the highest morbidity and mortality rate, affecting nearly 7 million patients per year. Determination of the severity of the coronary artery disease is based on several factors including age (greater than or less than 70 years old), prior myocardial infarction, prior angina, previous congestive heart failure (CHF), ventricular arrhythmias, diabetes mellitus requiring treatment, and the presence of Q-waves on the ECG. The two preoperative factors most associated with postoperative morbidity are myocardial infarction within 6 months of surgery and current CHF, especially in the presence of a S_3 gallop. Certain surgical procedures including vascular, intraabdominal, and intrathoracic operations are associated with increased risk of perioperative ischemia. A comprehensive patient history is a crucial first step in determining the extent of additional preoperative workup, the extensiveness of intra- and postoperative monitoring, and the necessity for postoperative intensive care admission. Early aggressive management of the patient with cardiac disease undergoing noncardiac surgery appears to have beneficial effects on morbidity and mortality rates.

ANESTHESIA FOR PEDIATRIC CARDIAC SURGERY

Identifying and understanding the pathophysiology of a patient's heart defect is an essential starting point for planning anesthesia management. Congenital heart defects traditionally are divided into three categories:

1. Obstructive lesions that impede ventricular emptying, such as coarctation of the aorta, aortic or subaortic stenosis, and pulmonic stenosis
2. Lesions producing left-to-right (acyanotic) shunting, such as atrial septal defect, ventricular septal defect, PDA, and AV canal
3. Lesions causing right-to-left (cyanotic) shunting, such as Tetralogy of Fallot, pulmonary atresia, tricuspid atresia, double outlet right ventricle, and total anomalous venous return

In actuality, many shunts are bidirectional with the direction of flow through the shunt changing during the different phases of the cardiac cycle. Changes in pulmonary vascular resistance (PVR) (such as those accompanying airway pressure changes during the ventilatory cycle), variations in systemic vascular resistance (SVR), and the relative resistances in the pulmonary and systemic circulations determine the direction of shunt flow. Reversal of an acyanotic shunt can result in severe arterial desaturation and increased risk of systemic embolization. Increased PVR due to increased hypoxic pulmonary vasoconstriction (resulting from acidosis, atelectasis, and alveolar hypoxia and hypercarbia) can be caused by loss of airway patency and hypoventilation. Anesthesia techniques for repair of bidirectional shunting congenital heart defects tend to lower PVR and maintain SVR favoring slightly increased left-to-right shunting.

Tetralogy of Fallot is one of the more common bidirectional shunting congenital heart defects. Before repair, increases in PVR can cause marked cyanosis (a "tet" spell). Adequate preoperative sedation, minimal stimulation, continuation of beta antagonist (used to reduce right ventricular outflow obstruction), avoidance of hypovolemia, and maintenance of adequate anesthetic depth can help prevent these episodes. Relief of airway obstruction, hyperventilation with 100% oxygen, increased anesthetic depth, 5 to 10 mcg/kg of phenylephrine intravenously, 100 to 200 mcg/kg/min of esmolol, and aortic compression are useful in treating these spells. It should be noted that while mechanical hyperventilation with 100% oxygen reduces hypoxic pulmonary vasoconstriction, the increased airway pressure can produce increased PVR and persistence of cyanosis. Following tetralogy repair, residual pulmonary insufficiency, right bundle branch block, and right ventricular dysfunction (secondary to right ventriculotomy and cardiopulmonary bypass) can contribute to postoperative cardiovascular instability.

Much attention is given to the fact that patients with right-to-left shunting have slower inhalation induction than normal patients, while patients with left-to-right shunting "breathe down" more rapidly than patients with normal hearts. Left-to-right shunting causes recirculation of blood through the lungs and a rapid rise in blood partial pressures of agents, while right-to-left shunting diverts blood away from the alveoli delaying the rise of blood levels of volatile anesthesia gases. However, in clinical practice, the use of premedication, intravenous narcotics, muscle relaxants, and newer less soluble volatile agents make these differences less significant. Furthermore, a "pure" intravenous technique frequently is used in patients with the most severe heart disease. Many pediatric cardiac surgeons and anesthesiologists avoid the use of inhaled anesthetics because of their cardiac depressant effects in the presence of the reduced contractility associated with many congenital defects. The use of high inspired oxygen concentrations, controlled ventilation, and, in some cases, avoidance of nitrous oxide (which can increase pulmonary vascular resistance and enlarge air emboli) is desirable for patients with cyanotic shunting and those with pulmonary hypertension, to help avoid worsening the shunt.

Ketamine given intramuscularly or intravenously is a useful induction agent for most patients with congenital heart disease (except perhaps for those with coronary insufficiency) because it usually maintains a favorable relationship between systemic and pulmonary vascular resistances. An increase in PVR that is sometimes seen with ketamine is probably secondary to loss of airway patency and hypoventilation. It is also not a direct effect of the drug because it does not occur when adequate ventilation is maintained.

Conditions with a large left-to-right shunt (such as a large ventricular septal defect) can cause volume overload of the left ventricle, congestive heart failure, and failure to thrive. The increased pulmonary blood flow and pressure can produce Eisenmenger's physiology of increased PVR resulting in intractable pulmonary hypertension.

Certain congenital cardiovascular defects require the patency of a communication between the systemic and pulmonary circulations. In some cases (such as pulmonary atresia and severe Tetralogy of Fallot), this communication provides blood flow to the lungs. In other defects, systemic blood flow is provided via the shunt, such as with coarctation of the aorta. Infusions of the prostaglandin PGE_1 can help maintain patency of the ductus arteriosus until a surgical anastomosis can be made. Surgical anastomoses are discussed in Chap. 10.

Patients with severe cyanotic heart disease tend to be polycythemic due to high levels of erythropoietin from the kidneys. If the hematocrit is greater than 60, then preoperative hydration and sometimes pre- and postoperative erythropheresis may be indicated to decrease blood viscosity and enhance oxygen delivery to the tissues. Additionally, reducing the hematocrit reduces cardiac work and oxygen demand.

Use of air traps in combination with careful removal of bubbles from intravenous (especially if the patient has right-to-left shunting) and intraarterial lines is necessary to avoid embolization to vital organs. It is important to note that if intravenous lines are prepared ahead of time and then placed in refrigeration, small bubbles (which may be hard to detect) present in the tubing upon removal from refrigeration will enlarge as the tubing reaches room temperature.

In most pediatric patients with minimal vascular disease on bypass, even high flows (up to 150 ml/kg/min) can produce fairly low systemic mean arterial pressures. When putting a patient on bypass, it is important to be sure that there is no venous obstruction to the superior vena cava because high venous pressure in the brain during bypass when mean arterial pressures are low can result in dangerous decreased cerebral perfusion. On bypass, a venous PO_2 of 40 mmHg or greater helps assure adequate tissue oxygenation.

Radial arterial lines, especially for neonates and infants, are by necessity of such small diameter that arterial pressure traces are very diminished following bypass (especially if vasoconstrictors are administered). For this reason, femoral arterial lines are frequently used instead.

Transport of the patient from the operating room to the intensive care unit is an interval during which cardiovascular instability often occurs. Hypoventilation at this time (especially if the patient was extubated at the end of surgery) can produce markedly elevated PVR. Vasoactive and inotropic infusions are fre-

Table 22-1   Endocarditis Antibiotic Prophylaxis

Drug	Dosage
Dental and respiratory tract procedures	
Standard oral regimen	
Amoxicillin	50 mg/kg PO 1 h before procedure, then 25 mg/kg PO 6 h later
Oral regimen for patients allergic to penicillin	
Erythromycin	20 mg/kg PO 2 h before procedure, then 10 mg/kg PO 6 h later
	or
Clindamycin	10 mg/kg PO 1 h before procedure, then 5 mg/kg PO 6 h later
Standard IV regimen	
Ampicillin	50 mg/kg IM or IV 30 min before procedure, then 25 mg/kg IM or IV 6 h later or 25 mg/kg amoxicillin PO 6 h after initial ampicillin dose
For patients allergic to penicillin	
Clindamycin	10 mg/kg IV 30 min before procedure, then 5 mg/kg IV 6 h later
For patients allergic to penicillin and considered high risk	
Vancomycin	20 mg/kg IVPB over 1 h (to avoid red man syndrome) starting 1 h before procedure; no repeat dose necessary
Gastrointestinal, genitourinary, and other high risk procedures	
Standard regimen	
Ampicillin, gentamicin, and amoxicillin	50 mg/kg ampicillin plus 2.0 mg/kg gentamicin (not to exceed 80 mg) IM or IV 30 min before procedure, then parenteral dose can be repeated 8 h after initial dose or amoxicillin 25 mg/kg PO 6 h after the initial dose
For patients allergic to penicillin	
Vancomycin and gentamicin	20 mg/kg vancomycin IVPB over 1 h (to avoid red man syndrome) starting 1 h before procedure, plus 2.0 mg/kg gentamicin (not to exceed 80 mg) and repeated once 8 h after initial dose

PO, by mouth; IV, intravenous; IM, intramuscular; (IVPB), intravenous piggy back.

quently interrupted while the patient is being moved. Cardiac tamponade can rapidly develop even in the presence of apparently properly working pericardial drainage tubes. Also, hypovolemia frequently develops immediately postoperatively so blood and blood products such as albumin must be available during transport. Adequate transport monitoring is essential, especially if the surgery affects the heart's conducting system.

Prevention of Bacterial Endocarditis

Certain dental and medical procedures are frequently associated with transient bacteremia. Antibiotic prophylaxis (see Table 22-1) is recommended if certain cardiac conditions are present. These include most congenital cardiac malformations, rheumatic and other acquired valvular dysfunction (including mitral valve prolapse with regurgitation), prosthetic valves, surgically constructed systemic-pulmonary shunts or conduits, hypertrophic cardiomyopathy, and previous bacterial endocarditis. Characteristics that these cardiac conditions share include the presence of excessive turbulence, prosthetic implants, and/or an irregular endocardial surface that favors bacterial adherence and the development of bacterial endocarditis. Endocarditis antibiotic prophylaxis is recommended for dental or medical procedures associated with the likely development of bacteremia. Prophylaxis is not recommended for patients with isolated secundum atrial septal defects and mitral valve prolapse with regurgitation, as well as previous Kawasaki disease or rheumatic fever without valvular dysfunction. Additionally, prophylactic antibiotics are not necessary following coronary artery bypass graft surgery, implantation of cardiac pacemakers and defibrillators, and after 6 months following uncomplicated repair of secundum atrial septal defect, ventricular septal defect, or patent ductus arteriosus (PDA).

Procedures that are unlikely to cause bacteremia do not require endocarditis prophylaxis. Such procedures include endotracheal intubation, flexible bronchoscopy, endoscopy, cardiac catheterization, cesarean section, and dental procedures not likely to cause gingival bleeding. In the absence of infection prophylaxis is not needed for urethral catheterization, dilatation and curettage, uncomplicated vaginal delivery, therapeutic abortion, sterilization procedures, and insertion or removal of intrauterine contraceptive devices. Endocarditis prophylaxis is recommended for the following procedures: vaginal delivery in the presence of infection, vaginal hysterectomy, prostatic surgery, and urinary tract surgery or catheterization if urinary infection is present. Additionally, urethral dilatation, cystoscopy, gall bladder surgery, esophageal dilatation, sclerotherapy for esophageal varices, and rigid bronchoscopy necessitate prophylaxis. Also, antibiotic prophylaxis is recommended for tonsillectomy and/or adenoidectomy, surgery involving intestinal or respiratory mucosa, incision and drainage of infected tissue, and dental procedures (including cleaning) that commonly cause gingival or mucosal bleeding.

For most routine pediatric surgery in this country, the patient has an inhalational induction and then the IV is started. Intravenous antibiotic prophylaxis can then be carried out at that time because there is usually about a 30-minute interval of prepping and draping (especially at academic institutions). Additionally, tissue drug levels are more rapidly attained when the drugs are administered intravenously rather than orally. Also, reactions to the antibiotics can be more effectively detected and treated in the operating room than in the preoperative holding area. However, preoperative oral antibiotics are the more cost effective choice.

Noncardiac Surgery for Pediatric Patients with Heart Disease

Approximately 25 percent of children with congenital heart disease have an associated noncardiac congenital anomaly which often requires surgical intervention. Conversely, patients for surgical repair of noncardiac congenital anomalies must be evaluated for the presence of congenital heart disease. Pediatric patients with heart disease for noncardiac surgery require individualized care. Not only is there a vast array of congenital heart defects (although the ten most common congenital anomalies encompass 90 percent of the total number of cases), each syndrome can range from mild to severe in its presentation. Also, the child may have already undergone a palliative procedure or surgical correction with subsequent cardiac function ranging from normal to severely impaired. Although most children with heart disease tolerate anesthesia and noncardiac surgery without problems, their decreased cardiac reserve renders them more susceptible to serious problems secondary to hypoventilation, inappropriate choice and dosage of anesthetic drugs, over- or undertransfusion of intravenous fluids, and the physiologic effects of major surgery. The use of high inspired oxygen concentrations and controlled ventilation is desirable for patients with cyanotic shunting and those with pulmonary hypertension to help prevent increased PVR and worsening of cyanosis. Meticulous removal of bubbles from intravenous lines and injections is mandatory.

BIBLIOGRAPHY

Campbell FW, Schwartz AJ: Problems in the anesthetic management in children with congenital heart disease for noncardiac surgery. *Problems in Anesthesia,* Philadelphia, Lippincott, 1987, pp. 411–433.

Committee on Rheumatic Fever, Endocarditis, and Kawasaki Disease of the Council on Cardiovascular Disease in the Young of the American Heart Association: Prevention of Bacterial Endocarditis. Recommendations by the American Heart Association. *JAMA* 264:2919–2922, 1990.

Fleisher LA, Barash PG: Preoperative cardiac evaluation for noncardiac surgery: a functional approach. *Anesth Analg* 74:586–598, 1992.

Goldman L, Cladera DL, Nussbaum SR, et al: Multifactorial index of cardiac risk in noncardiac surgical procedures. *N Engl J Med* 297:845–850, 1977.

Hollenberg M, Mangano DT, Browner WS, et al: Predictors of postoperative myocardial ischemia in patients undergoing noncardiac surgery. The Study of Perioperative Ischemia Research Group. *JAMA* 268:205–209, 1992.

Shah KB, Kleinman BS, Rao T, et al: Angina and other risk factors in patients with cardiac diseases undergoing noncardiac operations. *Anesth Analg* 70:240–247, 1990.

23

ANESTHETIC MANAGEMENT OF THE PATIENT WITH PULMONARY DISEASE

Patients with preexisting pulmonary disease present a number of perioperative challenges. Management of patients with restrictive lung disease is quite different from that of those with obstructive lung disease.

Patients with restrictive lung disease tend to respond better to mechanical ventilation with relatively small tidal volumes (10 to 12 ml/kg), high ventilator rates, and increased inspiratory time (even to the point of reversed I : E ratio). Increased airway resistance can be acute (e.g., due to a foreign body in the airway or stimulation of airway irritant receptors) or chronic, such as obstructive pulmonary disease (emphysema, bronchitis, or asthma). With obstructive lung disease, short inspiratory times and prolonged expiratory times are useful. Bronchodilator therapy is a mainstay for treatment of reversible airway obstruction. The use of continuous positive airway pressure in patients with obstructive lung disease is relatively contraindicated. However, it is occasionally useful to treat the temporary hypoinflation caused by the restrictive defects due to anesthesia and surgery. Pulmonary embolism occurring during or shortly before surgery can make anesthetic management much more difficult. Perioperative care of the patient with pulmonary disease is complicated by the respiratory effects of anesthesia, including stimulation of airway irritant receptors, reductions in functional residual capacity (FRC) and compliance, and changes in chemoreceptor sensitivity.

INTRATHORACIC VERSUS EXTRATHORACIC AIRWAY STENOSIS

Narrowing of the airway in the neck (e.g., tracheomalacia or airway compression that is caused by a tumor) causes increased stridor during inspiration. Exhalation dilates the extrathoracic airways decreasing resistance. The opposite is true concerning intrathoracic airway narrowing. During inspiration the tethering effect of lung parenchyma (and more negative intrapleural pressure in spontaneous breathing) dilates the conducting airways. Expiration reduces the airway's diameter, increasing resistance especially during forced exhalation. Mediastinal tumors, such as those associated with lymphoma, produce serious anesthetic risks including total airway obstruction. Patients with intrathoracic lesions that produce significant airway narrowing and dyspnea tolerate surgery with local anesthesia, sedation, and spontaneous ventilation much better than they do with general anesthesia and controlled ventilation. When general anesthesia is mandatory, for example, during open lung biopsy, loss of spontaneous ventilation can result in complete airway obstruction. Advancing the endotracheal tube past the narrowed portion of the airway can restore ventilation, although endobronchial intubation may result (with resultant atelectasis of the nonventilated lung). Fortunately, these tumors are usually very responsive to treatment and shrink rapidly, relieving the airway compromise and allowing extubation after just a few days.

ANESTHESIA AND RESTRICTIVE LUNG DISEASE

Usually, perfusion goes to dependent alveoli (due to the effects of gravity) and ventilation goes to dependent alveoli (because they are more compliant than nondependent alveoli when the FRC is normal). Thus, there is good matching of ventilation and perfusion. With restrictive lung disease, lung compliance is reduced causing decreases in all lung volumes. When this occurs, the dependent alveoli exhibit a greater reduction in volume than the nondependent alveoli. Atelectatic and nearly deflated alveoli are less compliant than alveoli that are closer to their midinflation volume. Therefore, when FRC is reduced, nondependent alveoli are more compliant than dependent ones. A greater portion of ventilation will go to the nondependent regions of the lung, while perfusion proportionately is increased in the dependent lung regions. This results in a ventilation and perfusion mismatch with a shuntlike effect. Chronic restrictive disease such as scoliosis can result in severe hypoinflation of the lungs, atelectasis (one of the triggers for hypoxic pulmonary vasoconstriction), pulmonary hypertension, and failure of the right side of the heart (cor pulmonale).

By reducing tidal volume and increasing ventilatory rate, the patient with restrictive disease can usually be ventilated mechanically to normocapnia without excessive peak airway pressure (which increases the risk of barotrauma). Adult respiratory distress syndrome is a restrictive condition that can be treated by mechanical ventilation with low tidal volume, reversed I:E ratio, and elective hypercapnia so that minute ventilation and airway pressure can be reduced. Normally, the I:E ratio is 1:2 with the three phases of the ventilatory cycle—inspiration, expiration, and expiratory pause—being of approximately equal duration. Reversal of the I:E ratio to 2:1 produces a slow, prolonged inspiration which helps reduce peak inspiratory pressure, while the expiratory recoil of the poorly compliant lung produces rapid exhalation. Thoracic, as well as abdominal, surgery produces restrictive-like reductions in FRC that can persist for several weeks postoperatively. An upper abdominal incision can reduce vital capacity (VC) by 60 percent while a lower abdominal incision is associated with approximately a 30 percent reduction in VC. The reduction in VC associated with restrictive lung disease can result in an inability to cough effectively to clear the airway of secretions. Prolonged postoperative intubation may be necessary for adequate bronchopulmonary hygiene.

ANESTHESIA AND OBSTRUCTIVE LUNG DISEASE

Obstructive lung disease produces increased resistance to airflow, which is sometimes reversible (responsive to bronchodilator therapy). Time for exhalation must be maximized to allow deflation of the lung. Hyperinflation produces the classic findings of barrel chest, flattened diaphragms, and increased work of breathing. Although emphysema is associated with loss of elastic tissue in the lungs' parenchyma, high pressures are needed to move the tidal volume (due to decreased compliance). This is because the FRC is so large due to the increased residual volume (because of trapped gas behind collapsed airways). Even though the lungs of emphysematous patients are more compliant than lungs of healthy patients during VC measurements, tidal volume is exchanged on top of such a large FRC that compliance is decreased (because the lungs are less compliant at very high and at very low lung volumes). Mechanical ventilation with relatively large tidal volumes and low ventilatory rates maximize the time for exhalation. Additionally, increasing inspiratory flow rate decreases inspiratory time while prolonging exhalation. The I : E ratio can be decreased as much as 1 : 6 and even 1 : 8, although excessively high peak airway pressures should be avoided to reduce the risk of barotrauma. The large residual volume present in emphysema patients can be due to the presence of pulmonary blebs (bullae), which are pockets of trapped gas that can expand and rupture if nitrous oxide is used.

The increased work of breathing associated with chronic obstructive pulmonary disease can result in hypoventilation and hypercapnia. Chronic hypercapnia can desensitize the chemoreceptors to the ventilatory stimulating effects of carbon dioxide. Hypoxic drive can then become the primary controller of ventilation. Maintenance of normocapnia by mechanical ventilation intraoperatively can result in prolonged periods of apnea (and desaturation), while attempting to reestablish spontaneous ventilation at the end of surgery. Furthermore, the use of increased inspired oxygen concentration can also blunt the hypoxic drive resulting in greater hypoventilation. Patients with obstructive lung disease are especially sensitive to the ventilatory depressant effects of anesthesia drugs. Even fairly low concentrations of inhaled agents can decrease the ventilatory response to carbon dioxide, acidosis, and hypoxemia. Similarly, narcotics are more likely to cause ventilatory depression in these patients.

Perioperative bronchoconstriction (Table 23-1) is associated with increased pulmonary morbidity (e.g., desaturation, hospital admission following outpatient surgery, intensive care unit admission, prolonged intubation, and mechanical ven-

Table 23-1 Conditions Causing Elevations in Peak Inspiratory Pressure (with Normal Baseline Pressure)

Mechanical obstruction of the endotracheal tube
  Kinking
  Secretion or foreign body in airway
  Overinflation of the cuff
Bucking, loss of muscle relaxation, or endobronchial intubation
Pulmonary edema
Tension pneumothorax
Pulmonary embolism
Bronchoconstriction
  Aspiration of gastric contents
  Asthma or viral upper respiratory infection
  Stimulation of irritant receptors or carina
Excessive tidal volume or peak flow rates
Inadequate expiration time or "stacking of breaths"

tilation). Bronchospasm following induction of anesthesia, laryngoscopy, and endotracheal intubation can be reduced by insuring therapeutic levels of preoperative bronchodilators and adequate depth of anesthesia. Use of intravenous narcotics and/or lidocaine intravenously or endotracheally can blunt airway irritant reflexes. Because perioperative bronchospasm is mediated largely by vagal reflexes, pretreatment with antimuscarinic drugs can help decrease bronchoconstriction during induction. Preexisting upper respiratory tract viral infection (persisting for 3 to 4 weeks following infection) is associated with increased risk of perioperative bronchospasm. Elevated peak airway pressure and bronchoconstriction are also associated with aspiration of gastric contents. The normal tone of the bronchial smooth muscle balances the volume of the anatomic dead space and airway resistance. These opposing forces affect the work of breathing. Reduction of the anatomic dead space improves the efficiency of breathing by better matching ventilation and perfusion. Conversely, reduction in airway diameter tends to increase the work of breathing. Clinical spirometry has been underutilized as a technique to evaluate abnormalities in airways resistance and responsiveness to bronchodilators. Increases in FEV_1 must be greater than 15 percent to be considered a significant response to bronchodilation.

Delivery of sympathomimetic drugs (such as albuterol) by aerosol to the endotracheal tube via the anesthesia circuit provides rapid and effective bronchodilation. Metered-dose inhalers are convenient to administer, but nebulizers are also useful.

PULMONARY EMBOLISM

Pulmonary emboli most commonly arise from thrombi in the deep veins of the legs, the pelvic veins, and the right atrium (during atrial fibrillation). Following embolization, alveolar dead space acutely increases but local bronchoconstriction may serve as a compensatory mechanism to reduce ventilation to the unperfused area (thus returning ventilation-perfusion ratios toward normal). Pulmonary vascular resistance acutely increases due to mechanical obstruction of blood flow as well as by local release of vasoconstrictors such as serotonin. Excessive increases in pulmonary vascular resistance can result in right ventricular failure.

Clinical signs of pulmonary embolism are nonspecific, especially under general anesthesia. They include dyspnea, tachypnea (30 to 50 breaths per minute), tachycardia, elevated central venous pressure, hypotension, and wheezing. Arterial blood gases may reveal hypoxemia, which can be explained by the ventilation-perfusion mismatch. Although alveolar dead space is the primary defect created by a pulmonary embolism, the subsequent relative overperfusion of nonembolized alveoli (by the extra blood diverted from the obstructed vessels) can produce a shuntlike state. Although alveolar dead space decreases the efficiency of elimination of CO_2 from the body, hypocapnia is reflected by the blood gases. This is most likely due to the hypoxic drive to ventilation and stimulation of the pulmonary vascular (type J) stretch receptors.

Management of pulmonary embolism during anesthesia includes increased inspired oxygen concentration. Isoprotenol, dopamine, and dobutamine can help treat the low cardiac output. Aminophylline is useful to reduce bronchoconstriction (if present) and also can help reduce pulmonary vascular resistance. Heparin prevents extension of venous thrombi and embolization of additional thrombi as well. Heparin also blocks serotonin release (which is believed to cause pulmonary vasoconstriction). Embolectomy or thrombolysis (with drugs such as urokinase or streptokinase) is sometimes necessary, especially for large emboli. Placement of an umbrella filter (Greenfield) in the inferior vena cava can help prevent subsequent pulmonary embolization.

In summary, perioperative care of the patient with pulmonary disease requires diligent preoperative evaluation to determine the characteristics and extent of the defect. Intraoperative considerations include ventilatory management, administration of bronchodilators, and regard for respiratory effects of the anesthetic drugs and techniques. Postoperative concerns center mainly on return of adequate spontaneous ventilation.

BIBLIOGRAPHY

Bemunof, JL: *Anesthesia for Thoracic Surgery.* WB Saunders, Philadelphia, 1987.

Bemunof, JL, Alfrey, DD: Anesthesia for thoracic surgery. In Miller RE (Ed): *Anesthesia.* 3rd ed. Churchill Livingstone, New York, 1990.

Eisenkraft, J, Cohen, E, Neustein, SM: Anesthesia for thoracic surgery, p. 943–988. In Barash PG, Cullen, BF, Stoelting, RK: *Clinical Anesthesia.* 2 ed JB Lippincott, Philadelphia, 1992.

Gal, TJ: *Respiratory Physiology in Anesthetic Practice.* William & Wilkins, Baltimore, 1991.

Kaplan J: *Thoracic Surgery.* 2nd ed. New York: Churchill Livingstone, 1991.

Marshall, BE, Longnecker, SE, Fairley, HB: *Anesthesia for Thoracic Procedures.* 2nd ed. Churchill Livingstone, New York, 1991.

24

CARDIOPULMONARY CHANGES THROUGH LIFE

OBJECTIVES

The student knows the cardiopulmonary alterations that occur with fetal and neonatal development, childhood growth, and aging. Specifically, the student can do the following:

1 Describe the major concepts of embryologic development of the cardiovascular and pulmonary systems.
2 Describe the anatomy and physiology of the fetal circulation.
3 Discuss the cardiopulmonary alterations that occur at birth.
4 Describe the cardiopulmonary developmental changes that occur during childhood.
5 Discuss the physiologic effects of aging on the cardiopulmonary system.

A thorough understanding of the differences in normal cardiovascular function, respiratory mechanics, and gas exchange at different stages of life is essential to the practice of anesthesiology.

FETAL DEVELOPMENT OF THE CARDIOVASCULAR AND PULMONARY SYSTEMS

The embryologic development of the cardiovascular and respiratory systems is briefly summarized in this section as background for the morphology, physiology, and pathophysiology of prematurely born infants and many congenital and perinatal problems.

Development of the Heart

The cardiovascular system may be the first system in the embryo to function as it does as an adult, with blood flow beginning after only the third week of development. The heart starts to form 18 to 19 days after fertilization. Two endo-cardial *heart tubes* develop and then start to fuse at about day 21. During the next 2 days, this heart tube grows much faster than the developing blood vessels to which it is attached. It then dilates and begins to form constrictions that separate it into chambers and vessels: *the atrium, ventricle, truncus arteriosus, sinus ve-nosus, and the bulbus cordis* (Fig. 24-1A and B). At this stage, blood flows upward from the sinus venosus to the atrium and then to the ventricle, which is located above the atrium. The heart tube then doubles over on itself, forming the U-shaped bulboventricular loop shown in Fig. 24-1C approximately 24 days after fertilization. As heart growth continues, the atrium is pushed upward and the ventricle is pushed downward, as shown by the arrows in Fig. 24-1C, so that the atrium is positioned above the ventricle.

The single atrium and the single ventricle of the developing heart each divide into left and right chambers during the period between the middle of the fourth week and the end of the fifth week after fertilization (Fig. 24-2). The opening between the atrium and ventricle, which is called the *atrioventricular canal* at this stage, is divided into left and right atrioventricular canals by the development of *endocardial cushions* that then fuse (Fig. 24-3A). The atrial septum begins to form as a membrane called a *septum primum* and grows from the upper part of the atrium toward the fused endocardial cushions (Fig. 24-3B and C). The opening remaining between the septum primum and the endocardial cushions is called the *foramen primum.* The septum primum eventually fuses with the endocardial cush-ions, closing the foramen primum. However, during this time perforations appear in the upper part of the septum primum, forming a new opening called the *foramen secundum* (Fig. 24-3C and D). Another membrane, the *septum secundum,* then grows from the upper part of the atrium, eventually covering the foramen secun-

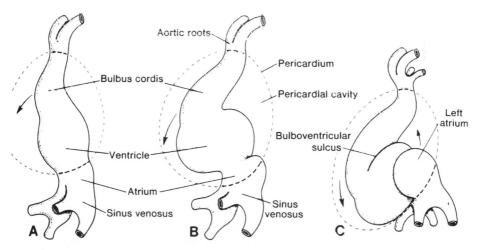

Figure 24-1 Development of the fetal heart during the fourth week of life. **A.** Approxi-mately 22 days after conception. **B.** Approximately 23 days after conception: **C.** Approxi-mately 24 days after conception. (*Reproduced with permission from Sadler TW:* Langman's Medical Embryology, *7th ed. Williams & Wilkins, Baltimore, 1995.*)

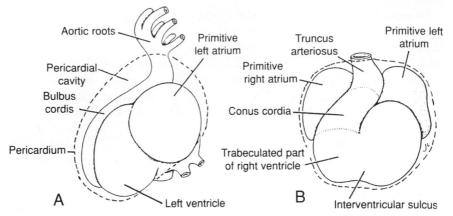

Figure 24-2 The fetal heart at approximately 28 days after conception. **A.** View from the left side. **B.** Frontal view. (*Reproduced with permission from Sadler TW:* Langman's Medical Embryology, *7th ed, Williams & Wilkins, Baltimore, 1995.*

dum. An orifice remaining in the septum secundum is called the *foramen ovale*. Although it is covered by the septum secundum, the thin lower part of the septum primum is not fused to the septum secundum. The septum primum, therefore, acts as the valve of the foramen ovale until after birth. During this period, the coronary sinus starts to form from the left side of the sinus venosus, while the right side becomes part of the wall of the right atrium.

The ventricular septum forms as a ridge of muscle that projects from the lower part of the single ventricle (Fig. 24-3B through D). This *interventricular septum* grows toward the fused endocardial cushions. An *interventricular foramen* exists until there is complete fusion of the septum and the endocardial cushions, which occurs at about the end of the seventh week of gestation. During this period, spirally arranged ridges appear in the truncus arteriosus. These truncal ridges, shown in Fig. 24-4B and C, fuse to form the aorticopulmonary septum that separates the pulmonary trunk from the aorta (Fig. 24-4E). Closure of the interventricular foramen and separation of the pulmonary artery from the aorta establishes the configuration of the right ventricle connected with the pulmonary artery and the left ventricle connected with the aorta. The bulbus cordis is ultimately incorporated into the ventricular walls. Figures 24-4G and H demonstrate how the spiral arrangement of the aorticopulmonary septum causes the aorta and pulmonary trunk to twist about each other as they originate from the heart.

Development of the Systemic Arteries

The systemic arteries develop from six pairs of *aortic arch arteries* (also called *brachial arch arteries*), which arise from the truncus arteriosus and terminate in the dorsal aorta of the same side. Figure 24-5 shows that these aortic arch arteries do not exist at the same time. During the sixth to eighth week of development, the first and second pairs of aortic arch arteries (Fig. 24-5A) disappear, and the

LATER HEART DEVELOPMENT

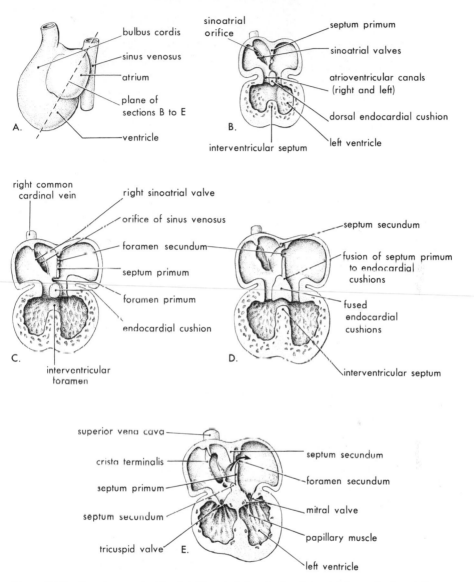

Figure 24-3 Development of the fetal heart during the fourth to eighth week of gestation, showing the fusion of the endocardial cushions to separate the atria from the ventricles and the development of the interatrial and interventricular septas to separate the left and right hearts. **A.** Dotted line shows the plane of the sections **B** to **E. B.** Heart at about 28 days of gestation. **C.** Heart at about 30 days. **D.** Heart at about 35 days. **E.** Heart at about 8 weeks. (*Reproduced with permission from Moore KL: Before We Are Born: Basic Embryology and Birth Defects, 2nd ed. Saunders, Philadelphia, 1983.*)

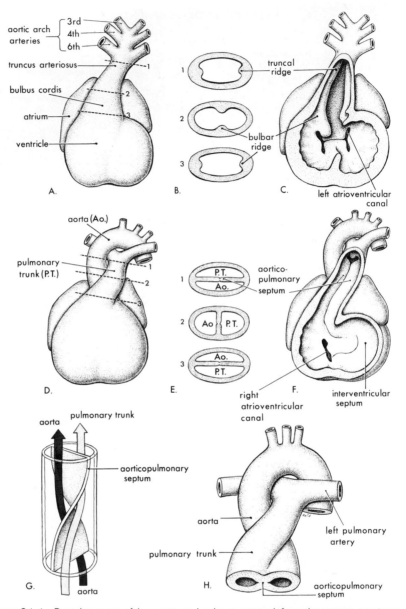

Figure 24-4   Development of the aorta and pulmonary trunk from the truncus arteriosus and bulbus cordis. **A** to **C.** The fetal heart at 5 weeks of gestation. **A.** Ventral view of the heart. **B.** Transverse sections through the truncus arteriosus and bulbus cordis at sites indicated in **A.** **C.** The heart at 5 weeks of development, shown with the ventral wall removed. **D** to **F.** The fetal heart at 6 weeks of development. **D.** Ventral view of the heart. **E.** Transverse sections through the aorta and pulmonary trunk showing the aorticopulmonary septum at sites indicated in *D; F,* the heart at 6 weeks of development shown with the ventral wall removed. *G,* Illustration of the spiral development of the aorticopulmonary septum. *H,* Final form of the aorta and pulmonary artery. *(From Moore, K.L.: Before We Are Born: Basic Embryology and Birth Defects, 2nd ed. Philadelphia, Saunders, 1983, with permission.)*

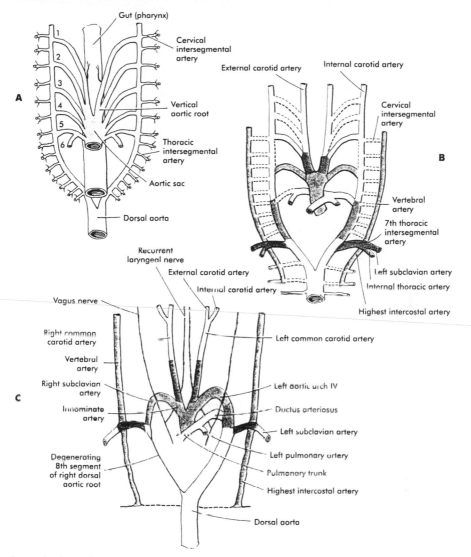

Figure 24-5 *A,* The embryonic aortic arch system. *B* and *C,* Later steps in the transformation of the aortic arch system in the human. Disposition of the recurrent laryngeal nerve in relation to the right fourth and left six arch is also shown in *C. (Reproduced with permission from Carlsen, B.M.: Human Embryology and Developmental Biology. Mosby, St. Louis, 1994, with permission.)*

proximal parts of the third pair become the common carotid arteries. These join the dorsal aorta to form the internal carotid arteries (Fig. 24-5B and C). The left fourth aortic arch artery becomes part of the arch of the aorta; the right becomes the initial portion of the right subclavian artery. The fifth aortic arch artery disappears. The left part of the sixth aortic arch artery develops into part of the left pulmonary artery. Part of the sixth aortic arch artery remains as a connection between the aorta and the pulmonary artery, called the *ductus arteriosus* (Fig. 24-5C). The right pulmonary artery develops from part of the right sixth aortic arch artery.

Development of the Lungs

Unlike the heart, the lungs are not ready to assume their main adult function until late in fetal development. Lung development is usually divided into three stages based on histological appearance: the *pseudoglandular stage,* the *canalicular stage,* and the *alveolar stage.*

The Pseudoglandular Stage (5 to 16 weeks)   The airways of the respiratory system are derived from the *laryngotracheal groove* of the embryo, which begins as an outpouching of the primitive pharynx during the fourth week of gestation. This outpouching, or *diverticulum,* grows away from the pharynx forming a separate lung bud (Fig. 24-6A). The folds in the tracheoesophageal structure grow toward each other, ultimately fusing to form the tracheoesophageal septum (also shown in Fig. 24-6A). The septum thus separates the developing larynx and tracheobronchial tree from the esophagus. The lung splits into the two *bronchial buds* (Fig. 24-6B and C) during the end of the fourth week of development. These buds extend into the pleural cavities and become the two mainstem bronchi. During the fifth week after conception, the right bronchopulmonary bud gives rise to three secondary buds which ultimately develop into the right upper, middle, and lower lobes. The left bronchopulmonary bud gives rise to the two secondary buds, which develop into left upper and lower lobes. (See Fig. 24-6D and E.) The tertiary buds shown in Fig. 24-6F develop into the bronchopulmonary segments. As the lungs continue to grow they are covered by the visceral pleura; at the same time the thoracic cavity is lined with the parietal pleura.

The histology of the tracheobronchial tree develops during this same period generally beginning with the trachea and progressing peripherally. Mesenchymal cells surrounding the endodermal lining of the laryngotracheal tube give rise to the connective tissue, cartilage, and smooth muscle of the larynx and the trachea; the columnar epithelium and glands of the tracheobronchial tree are derived from the endoderm. The tracheal cartilage begins to appear during the eighth week after conception, and the tracheal lining begins to become ciliated by about the tenth week. Mucous glands appear in the upper part of the tracheobronchial tree in the twelfth week of development and are seen farther down the tree shortly thereafter. Cartilage is present in the main-stem bronchi by the tenth week of development and in the segmental bronchi by the twelfth week. Cilia appear in the main-stem bronchi at the twelfth week and in segmental bronchi at the thirteenth week. Mucous glands appear in the bronchi at the thirteenth week and begin to produce mucus a week later.

The pulmonary arteries develop from the sixth aortic arch artery during the fifth and sixth weeks after conception (Fig. 24-5C). The pulmonary arteries grow

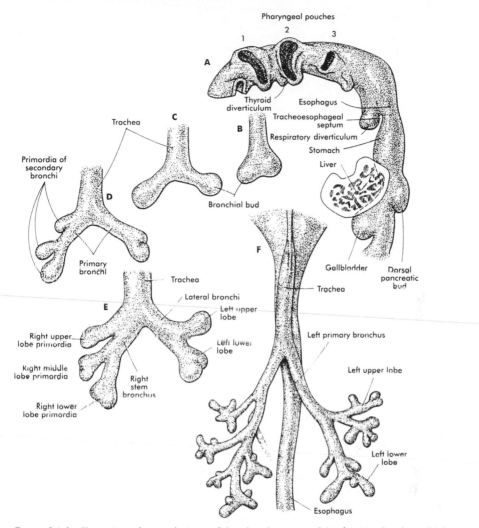

Figure 24-6 Illustration of ventral views of the development of the fetal tracheobronchial tree at about 4 weeks of development: **A.** Lateral view of the pharynx. **B.** At 4 weeks. **C.** At about 32 days. **D.** At about 33 days. **E.** At the end of the fifth week. **F.** Early in the seventh week. (*Reproduced with permission from Carlson BM:* Human Embryology and Developmental Biology. *Mosby, St. Louis; 1994.*)

and branch parallel to the growth of the branches of the two main-stem bronchi. Pulmonary veins develop from the wall of the left atrium, starting at about four weeks after conception. Bronchial arteries develop from dorsal aorta, starting in the seventh to eighth week, and form many connections with the pulmonary circulation.

Development of the lower portions of the tracheobronchial tree and the alveolar-capillary gas exchange units occurs during the second and third stages of

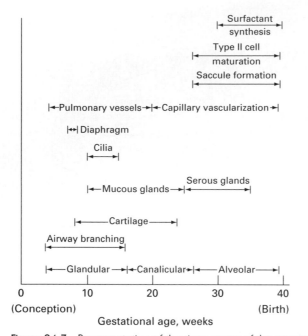

Figure 24-7 Representation of the time course of the aspects of fetal lung development. (*Reproduced with permission from Brody JS: Lung Development, Growth and Repair, in Fishman AP (ed)* Pulmonary Diseases and Disorders, *McGraw-Hill, New York, 1980.*)

fetal lung development, the *canalicular stage* and the *alveolar stage*. All three stages are indicated at the bottom of Fig. 24-7, which summarizes the time course of the important aspects of lung development.

The Canalicular Stage (16 to 26 weeks)   The glandular or pseudoglandular stage ends during the fifteenth to sixteenth week of fetal development. Up to this point the lungs resemble glands because they consist of small branching airways lined with a large number of mucous glands. During the canalicular stage, the lumens of the airways enlarge and the terminal bronchioles give rise to respiratory bronchioles. The respiratory bronchioles divide into alveolar ducts and *terminal air sacs*, which later develop into alveolar cells. Epithelial cells begin to differentiate into two populations: one gradually becoming thin squamous cells and the other becoming cuboidal secretory cells (Fig. 24-8). Pulmonary capillaries and lymphatics begin to form during this period.

The Alveolar Stage (26 weeks to birth)   During this final stage, the pulmonary capillary network proliferates around the developing alveoli. The epithelial alveolar cells continue to differentiate into flattened (squamous) type I alveolar epithelial cells or cuboidal type II alveolar epithelial cells (Fig. 24-8B).

These type II cells begin to produce functional pulmonary surfactant after about the seventh month of gestation.

Therefore, after seven to eight months of normal development, the fetal lungs are capable of their main adult function of gas exchange between the blood and the external environment. At the end of the normal gestation period of nine months almost all 23 branchings (or generations) of the airways appear to have occurred, resulting in a number of alveolar ducts approximately one-tenth that of the adult and a number of alveoli approximately one-fifteenth that of the adult. The pulmonary circulation has developed, and pulmonary capillaries have proliferated around the alveoli, forming a surface area for gas exchange approximately one-twentieth that of the adult. Furthermore, pulmonary surfactant is produced by the type II alveolar epithelial cells.

At birth, the lungs are partly filled with a mixture of amniotic fluid and secretions from the glands of the tracheobronchial tree. The lungs must be inflated with the neonate's first breath, and the fluid must also be removed. Before a discussion of the events associated with the neonate's first breath can occur,

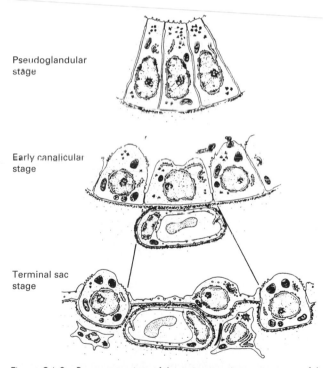

Pseudoglandular
stage

Early canalicular
stage

Terminal sac
stage

Figure 24-8 Representation of the microscopic appearance of the fetal lung. **A.** The pseudoglandular stage (about 17 weeks of gestation). **B.** Early in the canalicular stage (about 18 weeks of gestation). **C.** The terminal sac stage (about 26 weeks of gestation). (*Reproduced with permission from Burri PH, Weibel ER: The ultrastructure and morphology of the developing lung, in Hodson WA (ed):* Development of the Lung, *Marcel Dekker Inc., New York, 1977.*)

however, a review of the anatomy and physiology of fetal circulation must take place.

FETAL CIRCULATION

The fetal circulation differs from that of the adult because of the presence of the placenta, the ductus venosus, the foramen ovale, and the ductus arteriosus. The two ventricles of the fetus pump in parallel; in the adult the two ventricles pump in series.

The Placenta

Gas exchange between the fetus and mother occurs in the placenta, as does the exchange of nutrients from the mother's blood for waste products from the fetus. The placenta weighs about one-half kg at birth.

After the fertilized ovum is implanted in the wall of the uterus, blood-filled sinuses develop between the endometrium of the uterus and the surface of the embryo. These sinuses are supplied with arterial blood from the *uterine artery* of the mother and are drained by the *uterine veins*. As the embryo grows, fetal capillaries project into the sinuses, forming the *chorionic villi,* which interdigitate with the maternal blood sinuses. The chorionic villi increase the area of contact between the fetal and maternal circulations, which is helpful because the thickness of the diffusion barrier is much greater in the placenta than it is in the adult lung.

Fetal blood entering the placenta via the umbilical arteries is low in oxygen (the partial pressure of oxygen (PO_2) is about 25 mmHg) and high in carbon dioxide (the partial pressure of carbon dioxide (PCO_2) is about 50 torr). As this blood travels through the placental capillaries of the fetus, it equilibrates with the maternal blood, which has a PO_2 of about 100 mmHg and a PCO_2 of about 36 mmHg (pregnant women hyperventilate because of elevated progesterone levels). Blood returning to the fetus from the placenta has a PO_2 of only about 35 mmHg and a PCO_2 of about 45 mmHg. This is partly a result of the thick diffusion barrier between the maternal and fetal portions of the placenta and partly due to the high oxygen consumption of the placenta itself.

Two factors assist in oxygen transfer between the fetus and the mother and oxygen transport by fetal blood. Fetal hemoglobin concentration is higher than in that of the adult, so the oxygen carrying capacity of fetal blood may be greater than that of the adult. The oxyhemoglobin dissociation curve of fetal blood is shifted to the left, as shown in Fig. 24-9, probably because 2,3 DPG has little affinity for fetal hemoglobin. Thus fetal hemoglobin (HbF) has a greater affinity for oxygen than does adult hemoglobin (HbA) at the same PO_2. This helps remove oxygen from the maternal hemoglobin while maintaining a partial pressure gradient for diffusion from the maternal to the fetal blood. Fetal hemoglobin concentration may be as high as 18 to 20 g Hb per 100 ml of blood and its P_{50} as

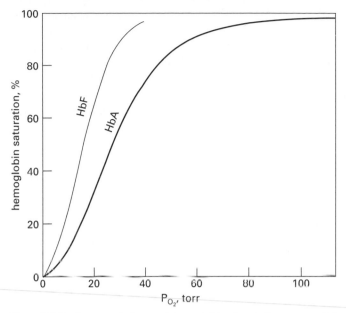

Figure 24-9 Representation oxyhemoglobin dissociation curves of blood from a fetus (HbF) and blood from an adult (HbA). (*Reproduced with permission from Levitzky MG:* Pulmonary Physiology, *4th ed. McGraw-Hill, New York, 1995.*)

low as 19 mmHg. Fetal oxygen consumption is about 7 ml/min/kg or about 20 to 25 ml/min near term.

Anatomy and Physiology of the Fetal Circulation

The *umbilical vein* transports "arterial" blood (PO_2 is 30 to 35 mmHg) from the placenta to the fetus (Fig. 24-10). After giving rise to branches that supply the left two-thirds of the liver, the umbilical vein joins a branch of the portal vein called the *portal sinus* to form the *ductus venosus*. Portal sinus blood flow is from the umbilical vein to the portal vein. The right third of the liver, which is supplied by branches of the portal vein, therefore receives a mixture of umbilical vein blood and portal venous blood with a lower PO_2. The ductus venosus runs along the underside of the liver and joins the *inferior vena cava*. The blood in the inferior vena cava drains the abdominal viscera and the lower extremities so *below* its connection with the ductus venosus its PO_2 is very low (about 14 mmHg). *Above* the ductus venosus, blood from the inferior vena cava has a higher PO_2 because of the blood in the ductus venosus coming from the umbilical vein.

Blood coming into the heart from the inferior vena cava is divided into two streams by a projection of the atrial septum called the *crista dividens*. Most of the blood passes through the *foramen ovale* and enters the left atrium, bypassing the lungs. (In the fetus the atrium extends dorsally beneath the rest of the heart to join the inferior vena cava at the foramen ovale.) The rest of the blood from the inferior vena cava joins *superior vena cava* blood draining the head and upper extremities and *coronary sinus* blood draining the myocardium. This blood passes into the right ventricle and is pumped to the lungs via the pulmonary artery. Pulmonary arterial blood P_{O_2} is approximately 20 mmHg, because it is a mixture of relatively well oxygenated inferior vena cava blood and blood low in oxygen from the head, upper extremities, and myocardium. Aortic blood is 25 to 30 mmHg, because it is mainly inferior vena cava blood, with only a small contribution from the pulmonary veins.

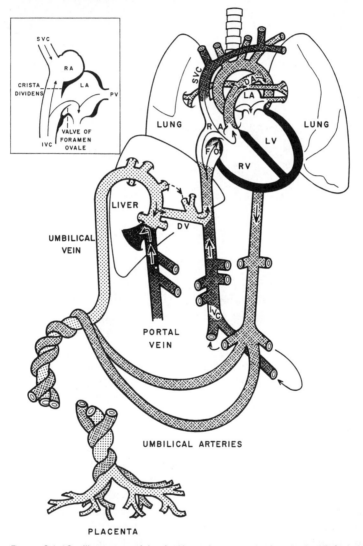

Figure 24-10   Illustration of the fetal circulation just before birth. (*Reproduced with permission from Dawes GS: Physiological changes in the circulation after birth, in Fishman AP, Richards DW (eds): Circulation of the Blood: Men & Ideas. Oxford Univ Press, New York, 1964.*)

In the fetus, the two ventricles pump in parallel, rather than in series. In contrast to the situation in the adult, they are similar in size and muscular development and pulmonary artery pressure is several millimeters of mercury greater than aortic pressure. Only 5 to 15 percent of the right ventricular output passes through the as yet uninflated lungs because they offer much greater resistance to blood flow than they do in the adult. Instead, most of the right ventricular output passes from the pulmonary artery to the aorta through the open *ductus arteriosus*.

Because the arteries supplying the heart, brain, and upper extremities originate from the aorta proximal to its connection with the pulmonary artery at the ductus arteriosus, the brain and heart are supplied with blood that has a relatively high PO_2 of 25 to 30 mmHg. Blood in the descending (or abdominal) aorta is a mixture from both ventricles, and so it has a lower PO_2 (20 to 23 mmHg). More than half of the combined output of the two ventricles perfuses the placenta via the umbilical arteries, with the remainder supplying the abdominal viscera and lower extremities.

The mean arterial blood pressure of the fetus increases during the last third of normal pregnancies to about 55 mmHg. Heart rate decreases during that period. These changes are associated with the development of the autonomic nervous system, especially the arterial baroreceptor and chemoreceptor reflexes.

CARDIOPULMONARY ALTERATIONS AT BIRTH

At birth, the neonate must assume the gas exchange function of the placenta by initiating the first breath, aerating the lungs, and reabsorbing fluid from the airways and air spaces. A number of changes in the neonate's cardiovascular system occurs to put the outputs of the two ventricles in series, with the output of the right ventricle perfusing the lungs.

Alterations in the Respiratory System

In order to inflate the lungs and begin breathing, the neonate must generate intrapleural pressures estimated to be from -30 to -70 cmH_2O to overcome the surface tension of the alveoli, the tissue resistance of the lungs and the chest wall, and the viscosity of the liquid in the airways. The fetus begins to make respiratory movements in utero during the later stages of gestation. These movements are believed to be important in the development of the strength of the respiratory muscles. Chemical and physical factors may combine to initiate the neonate's first breath, including stimulation of the arterial and central chemoreceptors, caused by hypoxia, hypercapnia, or both; the sensation of the reduction in ambient temperature; and tactile sensations, including pain.

Alveoli open serially, that is one after the other, because of both Laplace's law and the structural interdependence of the alveolar septa. Inflation of the alveoli is probably nearly complete within a few breaths, especially if the baby cries. Prenatal liquids appear to be removed from the lungs by several mechanisms, including osmosis into the capillaries, removal by lymphatic drainage after diffusion into the interstitium, and pinocytosis.

Alterations in the Circulation

Umbilical blood flow continues after delivery, but decreases rapidly even if the umbilical cord is not clamped and tied. The mechanism by which umbilical blood flow decreases is not known, but it may involve compression of the umbilical cord in the uterus during delivery, catecholamines from the neonate's adrenal medulla, or exposure to the cold ambient air.

The foramen ovale closes a few minutes after delivery, partly because cessation of umbilical venous blood flow following umbilical cord clamping decreases venous return and lowers right atrial pressure; and partly because lung inflation increases pulmonary blood flow, leading to increased pulmonary venous return to the left atrium, which increases left atrial pressure. These two factors tend to reverse the pressure gradient across the foramen ovale, and the valve closes. The valve usually adheres to the edge of the foramen ovale within a few days of birth. Elimination of the low resistance pathway for blood flow through the placenta increases systemic vascular resistance and ends blood flow through the ductus venosus. Fibrosis and closure of the ductus venosus occur within about seven days after birth.

Inflation of the neonate's previously collapsed lungs decreases pulmonary vascular resistance and pulmonary artery pressure and increases pulmonary blood flow six- to tenfold. Mechanisms that cause the decrease in pulmonary vascular resistance may include mechanical effects of the expanding alveoli, which should lengthen vessels and pull some open by traction; increased alveolar surface tension caused by the establishment of an air-liquid interface; relief of pulmonary vasoconstriction caused by alveolar hypoxia and, possibly, hypercapnia; and by release of pulmonary vasodilators, such as prostacyclin.

Aortic pressure increases at birth because of increased sympathetic stimulation and because cessation of perfusion of the placenta removes a large parallel pathway for blood flow. Increased aortic blood pressure, coupled with decreased pulmonary artery pressure, reverses the pressure gradient for blood flow through the ductus arteriosus so that blood begins to flow from the aorta to the pulmonary artery within an hour after birth. The ductus arteriosus begins to constrict within a few hours after birth, but does not close completely for one to eight days.

The elevated systemic P_{O_2} that occurs after birth is believed to be the stimulus that initiates constriction of the ductus arteriosus. The mechanism causing the constriction may involve decreased release of vasodilators such as prostacyclin, PGE_1, nitric oxide, or acetylcholine; or increased release of catecholamines, constrictor prostaglandins, or bradykinin. After the ductus arteriosus is occluded by contraction of its vascular smooth muscle, its wall is replaced by fibrous tissue. This usually occurs within two or three weeks after birth.

DEVELOPMENT OF THE CARDIOPULMONARY SYSTEM DURING CHILDHOOD

At birth, the cardiovascular system is normally far more developed than the respiratory system, so the changes in the respiratory system during childhood are more striking than those in the cardiovascular system.

Postnatal Cardiovascular Development

After the cardiovascular alterations normally associated with birth have occurred (cessation of blood flow to the placenta; increased pulmonary blood flow, and closure of the foramen ovale, ductus venosus, and ductus arteriosus), the developmental changes seen in the cardiovascular system are mainly related to changes in body mass and configuration and organ growth and function.

The heart, especially the left ventricle, matures and increases its ability to generate pressure and pump greater stroke volumes. This is important because the neonate has little ability to increase the stroke volume and therefore must increase cardiac output by increasing the heart rate. Bradycardic neonates may have difficulty maintaining their cardiac output. Resting cardiac output increases with age from about 750 ml/min at birth to the sixteenth or eighteenth year when it is about 5 liters/min. If it is expressed per kilogram of body weight, however, it falls from about 200 ml/kg/min at birth to about 100 mg/kg/min in teenagers. This decrease in cardiac output per body weight is especially rapid during the first few years. If cardiac output is expressed in square meter of *body surface area*, it stays fairly constant during postnatal growth and development. Heart rate decreases from about 150 beats per minute at birth to approximately 70 beats per minute in the young adult. Stroke volume therefore increases with age and does so somewhat faster than does cardiac output. Mean systemic blood pressure increases from about 60 mmHg at birth to the normal adult mean pressure of approximately 96 mmHg. Systemic vascular resistance decreases with growth and development, if expressed per square meter of body surface area.

Pulmonary artery pressure and pulmonary vascular resistance both decrease during the first year of life, as the smooth muscle of the medial layer of the pulmonary vessels decreases in thickness. Mean pulmonary artery pressure falls from about 50 mmHg at birth to nearly the adult mean pressure of approximately 15 mmHg within about a year after birth. Pulmonary blood flow stays relatively constant, if expressed per square meter of body surface area. As the pressure work done by the right ventricle decreases, the relative thickness of the right ventricular wall also decreases.

Postnatal Pulmonary Physiology

The mechanics of breathing in the normal newborn or infant differ considerably from those of the adult. However, measurements of pulmonary function and mechanics in neonates and infants are difficult, and results vary widely from study to study. At birth, the alveoli are smaller, fewer in number, and have greater total elastic recoil than those of the adult, as will be discussed later in this section. This greater inward elastic recoil results in much lower lung compliance in the neonate. If expressed per kilogram of body weight, determinations of the pulmonary compliance of the neonate range from approximately one-half that of the adult to a value comparable with that of the adult. Conversely, although the compliance of the chest wall of the newborn is much less than that of the adult, it is greater than that of the adult if expressed per kilogram of body weight. Thus, the relative inward recoil of the lungs is greater and the outward recoil of the chest wall is less in the neonate than they are in the adult. As would be expected from this, the functional residual capacity (FRC) is less in the neonate than it is in the adult. Expressed per kilogram of body weight, the FRC of the normal newborn is approximately one-half to two-thirds that of the adult. However, the FRC per kilogram of body weight of the neonate is much greater than predicted based on the relative elastic recoil of the lungs and chest wall. Therefore, the FRC of the neonate may be actively maintained by a reflex (possibly one of the Hering-Breuer reflexes) causing a diaphragmatic and intercostal muscle contraction at end expiration, as well as by glottic closure ["auto PEEP" (positive end-expiratory pressure)]. Thus, the depression of respiratory muscle activity caused by most general anesthetics (see Chap. 21) would be expected to further decrease the FRC in the neonate. This, combined with the newborn's high oxygen consumption (approximately twice that of the adult), leads to more rapid desaturation during hypoventilation or apnea.

Another consequence of the relatively low outward elastic recoil of the chest wall of the neonate is that the "residual volume" (RV) is more likely determined by airway closure than by the outward recoil of the chest wall. Expressed in kilograms of body weight, the neonate's RV is a little more than one-half that of the adult. The relatively weaker inspiratory muscles of the newborn, combined with the greater inward alveolar elastic recoil, result in neonate "total lung capacity" (TLC) per kilogram of body weight of about three-fourths that of the adult. (Note that in the earlier discussion *TLC* and *RV* are in quotation marks because they cannot be determined by the conventional methods of giving instructions to the subject. They are obtained from the newborn or infant during a "crying vital capacity," basically, a maximum scream.)

In addition to the relatively greater compliance of the neonate's chest wall, there are several differences between the mechanics of the chest wall of the neonate and those of the adult. Contraction of the external intercostals and accessory muscles of inspiration of the adult pull the rib cage up and out and make it more circular than those of the neonate during deep inspirations. The newborn's ribs extend more horizontally from the vertebral column than they do in the adult, and the configuration of the ribs is also more circular in the neonate. These differences make the actions of the newborn's rib cage less effective in generating inspiratory volume. The intercostal muscles are not well developed in the neonate and, combined with the relatively greater compliance of the rib cage, the stabilizing effect of intercostal muscle contraction during diaphragmatic contraction is much less effective in the neonate than in the adult. This is especially significant when this stabilizing effect of intercostal muscle contraction is inhibited, such as during REM sleep.

The diaphragm is flatter and less dome-shaped in the neonate than it is in the adult. This makes the diaphragm a less effective inspiratory muscle because of the effect of Laplace's law. As noted previously in this book, according to Laplace's law, tension is proportional to pressure times the radius of curvature ($T \propto P \times r$). Thus, a flatter diaphragm with a greater radius of curvature would have to develop greater tension to produce a given transdiaphragmatic pressure gradient.

The total resistance of the respiratory system is much greater in the newborn than it is in the adult. A somewhat greater proportion of the total resistance results from tissue resistance in the neonate, and there is much less resistance to airflow in the nasal passages of the newborn. For this reason some neonates may be obligate nose breathers.

Many important changes in the structure and function of the upper airways occur during infancy and the first four or five years of life. These result from the tissue growth or the development of neural mechanisms and reflexes, or both. In the neonate, the larynx and the epiglottis are structurally higher with respect to the cervical vertebrae than are those of the adult. Most of the time, especially when nursing, the epiglottis and uvula of the neonates make contact with the soft palate, allowing the neonate to swallow and breathe through the nose at the same time. This is why infants less than 3 to 5 months of age appear to be able to breathe through their mouths only when they are crying. As the infant grows, the larynx and epiglottis gradually move downward, so that by age five the epiglottis hardly makes contact with the uvula. In the adult, the larynx opens into the lowest part of the pharynx, so the lower pharynx is the pathway for both food and air. The relatively large epiglottis, tonsils, and adenoids of the infant and small child appear to be particularly sensitive to certain kinds of bacterial infections and may seriously impede airflow when they are inflamed. This problem may be exacerbated by the relatively soft laryngeal cartilages of the infant because they may collapse on aspiration. Dilation of the nares and much of the pharyngeal muscle contraction associated with inspiration also gradually decrease during the first few months of life. Reflexes and complex coordinated activities such as the cough reflex and speech develop during the first years of life.

The tracheobronchial tree continues to grow and develop after birth, and the number of alveoli increases exponentially for at least the first eight years. The diameter, length, and cross-sectional areas of the airways all increase from infancy to adulthood, with greater increases in the diameter and cross-sectional area than in the length of the individual larger airways. By 3 months of age, 21 of the 23 generations of airways have already developed. The total number of respiratory airways increases from about 1.5 million at birth to the adult figure of about 14 million by age 8.

The total number of alveoli increases from about 24 million at birth to about 280 million at age 8. Therefore, by the eighth year of life approximately 90 percent of the adult alveoli have developed. Alveoli increase in size as well as number during this period, a mean of about 50 μ in diameter at birth to 150 to 250 μ in diameter by the early teenage years, with little further increase thereafter. This increase in alveolar size may represent growth of alveolar septal tissue, changes in the distribution of alveolar elastin and collagen, and increased outward elastic recoil of the chest wall.

Pulmonary capillaries proliferate along with the increased number and size of the alveoli and continue to increase in number after the alveoli stop. The alveolar-capillary interface is believed to be about 2.8 m^2 in the newborn, about 6.5 m^2 at 3 months, and about 32 m^2 by age 8. Because the adult alveolar-capillary surface area is about 70 m^2, the continued increase in the number of pulmonary capillaries doubles the surface area available for gas exchange after the eighth year of age. The lungs of a newborn weigh about 50 g; those of a 12 to 14 year old weigh about 400 g; and those of an adult, 800 g.

The FRC increases with the growth and development of the lungs and alterations in the mechanics of the chest wall. The increase is linearly related to the length of the infant or the height of the child. The tidal volume stays fairly constant (expressed per weight) at 7 to 10 ml/kg from birth to adulthood, as does the anatomic dead space, which is about 2 ml/kg throughout the same period, and the ratio of dead space to tidal volume. Oxygen consumption decreases from 6 to 8 ml/kg/min in the neonate to about 3.2 ml/kg/min in the adult. The newborn's alveolar ventilation is 100 to 150 ml/kg/min, which is about twice that of the adult; the respiratory rate is about 40 breaths per minute compared with 13 breaths per minute for the adult.

The standard lung volumes and capacities, which, as noted, cannot be determined by conventional (voluntary) means in infants and young children, increase linearly with height between ages 6 and 18. Total lung capacity and vital capacity (VC) increase slightly more rapidly than does residual volume (RV).

CARDIOPULMONARY CONSEQUENCES OF AGING

Changes in the Cardiovascular System

There is little decrease with aging in the cardiovascular function of normal healthy adults at rest. However, the ability of adults to increase their cardiovascular performance during stresses such as exercise decreases progressively with age. This progressive decrease in maximal cardiovascular function is a result of structural alterations in the cardiovascular system that are similar to those that occur in the respiratory system with aging.

Structural Alterations   The ratio of collagen to elastin in the walls of arteries and veins increases progressively as people get older. Because collagen is much less distensible than elastin, this results in *decreased compliance* (or increased stiffness) of the aorta and the large arteries and veins, both radially and longitudinally. The walls of the ventricles probably also become less compliant.

Functional Alterations at Rest   The decrease in vascular distensibility, along with some degree of atherosclerotic alteration of the arterial tree, increases systemic vascular resistance and systemic diastolic blood pressure with age. The decreased distensibility of the aorta will cause a greater increase in the aortic systolic pressure above the diastolic pressure for the same stroke volume. Thus, the pulse pressure increases with age. The valves of the heart may also stiffen with age.

These increases in systolic and diastolic pressure elevate the afterload on the left ventricle and increase stroke work of the left ventricle. As the pressure work increases, the left ventricle is less able to generate stroke volume (especially *increases* in stroke volume), so the resting cardiac output, cardiac index, and stroke index all decrease progressively with age. The increased afterload also usually results in some degree of cardiac enlargement, resulting both from dilation during diastole and from muscular hypertrophy. Hypertrophy of the left ventricle causes slowing of contraction and relaxation.

Functional Alterations during Exercise   The aging-related structural changes in the cardiovascular system have a much greater effect on the response to physiologic stresses such as exercise than they do at rest. The maximum work capacity, as determined by the maximal oxygen uptake, decreases linearly after about 20 years of age. This is mainly a result of a diminished ability to increase the cardiac output (or index) by increasing stroke volume and heart rate. This diminished ability to increase the cardiac output may be a consequence of the increased stiffness of the aorta, arterial tree, and cardiac valves; the increased systemic vascular resistance; a decreased contractility of the ventricles; a decreased response to sympathetic stimulation; or a decreased effectiveness of the Frank-Starling mechanism.

Changes in the Respiratory System

Growth and development of the respiratory system end at about 20 years of age. Maximum performance levels on pulmonary function tests are usually achieved between ages 20 and 25 and decline progressively thereafter.

Structural Alterations   The structural changes that occur in the respiratory system with age affect the alveoli and the alveolar ducts, the rib cage and respiratory muscles, and the pulmonary blood vessels.

Alveoli and Alveolar Ducts   Alveolar ducts and respiratory bronchioles begin to enlarge around the age of 40, resulting in a larger fraction of the lung volume consisting of alveolar ducts and a smaller volume of the lung consisting of alveoli. The *alveolar surface area* decreases with age; it is not known whether this reflects a decrease in the number of alveolar septa or changes in their configuration. At the same time the elastic fibers in the walls of the alveoli and alveolar ducts that provide much of the structural support of the alveoli begin to degenerate. There are also changes in the cross-linking between collagen fibers, elastin fibers, and each other. These alterations in structure appear to be the source of *increased lung compliance* and *decreased pulmonary elastic recoil*. Age-related changes in the composition and turnover of pulmonary surfactant may also occur.

Chest Wall   Calcification of the *costal cartilages* occurring with aging results in decreased compliance and mobility of the rib cage. The spaces between *spinal vertebrae* also decrease and the degree of kyphotic spinal curvature increases, leading to a shorter thorax with an increased antero-posterior diameter. A greater deposition of abdominal and thoracic adipose tissue may also contribute to the decreased chest wall compliance of many elderly people. The strength of the muscles of breathing also decreases with age.

Pulmonary Vasculature   Larger pulmonary arteries thicken with age, especially the intimal and medial layers. Although resting mean pulmonary artery pressure and pulmonary vascular resistance do not usually decrease with age, the pulmonary vasculature becomes less distensible and there may be fewer unopened capillaries to recruit. Therefore, during exercise mean pulmonary artery pressure may increase more and pulmonary vascular resistance may decrease less than they do in young individuals. Pulmonary capillary blood volume decreases with age, because of loss or changes in the configuration of alveoli and alveolar septa, as well as a decreased cardiac index.

Larger Airways   Bronchial cartilages may calcify with aging. This may cause a slight increase in anatomic dead space in elderly people.

Functional Alterations   Aging causes changes in the lung volumes and capacities: the mechanics of breathing; gas exchange, the diffusing capacity, and the PaO_2; the control of breathing; exercise capacity; and the pulmonary defense mechanisms.

Lung Volumes and Capacities   Age-related changes in the standard lung volume and capacities are shown in Fig. 24-11. Although several studies have shown that the *TLC* decreases with age, there is no change in TLC if the data are normalized for the decrease in height that is seen in the elderly. The decreased height of the elderly is a result of the decrease in the size of the intervertebral spaces, as well as the fact that when compared at the same age, subjects from younger generations are taller than those from older generations probably as a result of better nutrition. The RV increases with age, as does the ratio of the RV

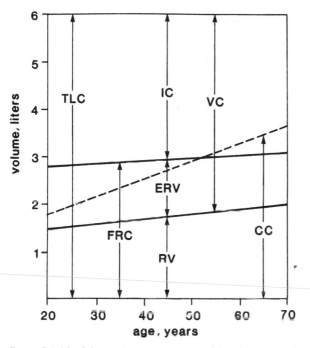

Figure 24-11   Schematic representation of the alterations of the standard lung volumes and capacities occurring with age. (TLC, total lung capacity; FRC, functional residual capacity; ERV, expiratory reserve volume; RV, residual volume; IC, inspiratory capacity; VC, vital capacity; CC, closing capacity.) (*Reproduced with permission from Levitzky MG: Effects of aging on the respiratory system. The Physiologist 27:102–107, 1984. American Physiological Society, Bethesda, MD*).

to the TLC. Because the TLC is unchanged by aging (if normalized for height) and the RV increases, the VC decreases with age. Studies of the effects of aging on the *FRC* have shown either no change in the FRC or that the FRC and FRC/TLC increase, but not as much as the RV and RV/TLC, respectively. These differences may reflect the way the FRC was determined in different studies, because the helium dilution and nitrogen washout techniques do not include gas trapped behind closed airways. However, the body plethysmograph technique does. As we will discuss shortly, there may be appreciable gas trapping at the FRC in elderly people. Studies have shown that the FRC increases with age, but there are even greater increases in RV; therefore, the *expiratory reserve volume* (ERV) decreases with age. The inspiratory capacity (IC) decreases with age in those studies showing an increasing FRC.

Mechanics of Breathing   As already noted, *the elastic recoil of the lungs* decreases with age, especially at higher lung volumes. *Static pulmonary compliance,* which is the inverse of the elastic recoil, therefore increases with age. Although *dynamic pulmonary compliance* becomes more frequency dependent with age, this probably reflects increased resistance to airflow in small airways more than it does decreased compliance of alveolar units. The increased resistance to airflow in small airways probably results from decreased alveolar elastic recoil leading to decreased support of small airways. The *compliance of the chest wall* decreases with age, and chest wall elastic recoil shifts from outward to inward at a much lower lung volume. The *closing capacity* (CC), often (incorrectly) called the closing volume, increases from about 30 percent of TLC at age 20 to about 55 percent at age 70 (Fig. 24-11). The CC may exceed the FRC in elderly people, which suggests that they may have airway closure and poorly ventilated or unventilated alveoli at resting lung volumes.

As discussed in Chap. 13, airway closure usually begins to occur in the lower regions of the lung of a normal young person who is standing or sitting in a upright posture. Small airways in lower regions of the lung are more likely to collapse than those in upper lung regions. This occurs because alveoli are at lower volumes and therefore have less elastic recoil helping to hold small airways open and because intrapleural pressure is greater (less negative at FRC and more positive during a forced expiration) than it is in upper regions. The pattern of greater ventilation in lower lung regions that is seen in normal young subjects therefore does not occur in the elderly. This may result in less efficient matching of pulmonary ventilation and perfusion and contributes to the decreasing PaO_2 seen with aging.

The *dynamic measurements of lung volume* decrease with age. The maximal expiratory flow rate, the maximal mid-expiratory flow rate, the forced expiratory volume in 1 second (FEV_1), and the ratio of the FEV_1 to the forced vital capacity (FVC) all decrease with age. This results from the diminishing strength of the expiratory muscles, decreasing chest wall compliance, and an increasing tendency for airways to close during forced expiratory efforts, causing gas to be trapped in the lungs. These factors also explain the increase in RV. The maximum voluntary ventilation (MVV), which is the maximum volume of air that can be breathed in and out in 12 to 15 s (expressed in liters per min), also decreases with age.

Pulmonary gas exchange   The PaO_2 decreases progressively and linearly with age, falling from approximately 95 torr at age 20 to about 75 torr at age 70. The PO_2 of well-ventilated alveoli, or P_AO_2, calculated using the alveolar air equation, does not change, so the *alveolar-arterial oxygen partial pressure gradient,* or (A-a) DO_2, increases progressively with age by the same amount. The factors that determine the (A-a)DO_2 include the physiologic shunt, which increases slightly from less than 5 percent at age 20 to approximately 15 percent at age 70; the matching of ventilation and perfusion; and the diffusing capacity.

Ventilation and perfusion are not matched as well in the lungs of the elderly as they are in the lungs of younger subjects. Alveolar ventilation becomes less uniform with age, because airway closure in the lower lung regions results in relatively more ventilation of upper lung regions, as discussed previously. However, studies have shown only slightly increased blood flow to upper lung regions in the elderly. The alveolar dead space increases in the elderly, probably because of a decreased cardiac index, leading to unrecruited pulmonary capillaries. Age-related structural alterations of pulmonary vessels may attenuate the strength of the hypoxic pulmonary vasoconstriction.

The *pulmonary diffusing capacity* (D_{LCO}) decreases progressively and linearly with age, falling approximately 20 percent over the course of adult life. This decrease probably results from a decreased alveolar surface area, as well as a decreased pulmonary capillary blood volume. The decreased diffusing capacity may not have as great an effect on the (A-a)DO_2 as does the increased $\dot{V}/\dot{Q}$ mismatch. There are no consistent age-related alterations to arterial partial pressure of carbon dioxide in blood (PaCO_2), probably because of the greater diffusivity of CO_2 through the alveolar-capillary barrier and the differences in the O_2 and CO_2 dissociation curves.

Control of Breathing The *ventilatory responses to hypoxia and hypercapnia* decrease with age. These decreased responses could result from several alterations in the respiratory system that occur with age, including decreased sensitivity of the central and arterial chemoreceptors or alterations in the central respiratory controller. However, it is much more likely that the attenuated responses to hypoxia and hypercapnia reflect decreased strength of the respiratory muscles and alterations in the mechanics of the lung and the chest wall. The occurrence of snoring and obstructive sleep apnea increases with aging, especially in men.

Exercise Capacity The ability to perform exercise, as indicated by the maximal oxygen uptake ($\dot{V}O_{2\,max}$), decrease progressively and linearly with age, falling about 35 percent between the ages of 20 and 70. The main cause of the decreased ability to exercise is probably a decreased ability to increase the cardiac output, although many of the alterations discussed earlier also contribute.

Pulmonary Defense Mechanisms The elderly have fewer cilia lining their airways than are seen in the lungs of younger individuals, which probably leads to a decreased efficiency of the *mucociliary escalator*. Elderly people also show decreased *reflex responses* to mechanical or chemical stimulation of the upper airways or tracheobronchial tree.

The alterations of the respiratory system that occur with aging are summarized in Table 24-1. The functional alterations are listed according to the structural changes thought to be responsible for them.

Table 24-1   Summary of the Effects of Aging on the Respiratory System:
Relationship of Changes in Structure to Changes in Function

Loss of alveolar elastic recoil:
  Increased static pulmonary compliance
  Decreased pulmonary elastic recoil pressure
  Increased FRC
  Decreased support of small airways
  Greater effect of dynamic compression
  Decreased dynamic lung volumes
  Increased RV
  Increased CC, gas trapping
  Decreased dynamic pulmonary compliance
  Less uniform alveolar ventilation
  Ventilation-perfusion mismatch
  Decreased response to hypoxia and hypercapnia

Alterations in chest wall structure and decreased respiratory muscle strength:
  Decreased chest wall compliance
  Increased RV
  Decreased VC, dynamic lung volumes
  Decreased MVV
  Decreased response to hypoxia and hypercapnia

Loss of alveolar surface area and changes in the pulmonary circulation:
  Ventilation-perfusion mismatch
  Increased alveolar dead space
  Decreased diffusing capacity
  Decreased P_aO_2
  Increased (A-a) PO_2

FRC, functional residual capacity; RV, residual volume; CC, closing capacity; VC, vital capacity; MVV, maximum voluntary ventilation; PaO_2, partial pressure of oxygen in arterial blood; (A-a)PO_2, alveolar-arterial oxygen partial pressure gradient.
    Adapted with permission from Levitzky MG: Effects of aging on the respiratory system. *The Physiologist* 27:102–107, 1984. American Physiological Society, Bethesda, MD.

BIBLIOGRAPHY

American Thoracic Society/European Respiratory Society: Respiratory mechanics in infants: Physiologic evaluation in health and disease. *Am Rev Respir Dis* 147:474–496, 1993.

American Thoracic Society/European Respiratory Society: Respiratory function measurements in infants: Measurement conditions. *Am J Respir Crit Care Med* 151:2058–2064, 1995.

Avery ME, Fletcher BD, Williams RG: *The Lung and its Disorders in the Newborn Infant*, 4th ed. Saunders, Philadelphia, 1981.

Brody, JS: Lung development, growth, and repair, in Fishman AP (ed): *Pulmonary Diseases and Disorders.* McGraw-Hill, New York, 1980, pp 298–314.

Burri PH: Development and regeneration of the lung, in Fishman AP (ed): *Pulmonary Diseases and Disorders,* 2nd ed. McGraw-Hill, New York, 1988, pp 61–78.

Burri PH, and Weibel ER: The ultrastructure and morphology of the developing lung, in Hodson WA (ed): *Development of the Lung.* Marcel Dekker Inc., New York, 1977, pp 215–268.

Carlson BM: *Human Embryology and Developmental Biology.* Mosby, St. Louis, 1994.

Comroe JH, Jr: Premature science and immature lungs, Parts I, II, and III. *Am Rev Resp Dis* 116:127–135, 311–323, 497–518, 1977.

Dawes GS: Physiological changes in the circulation after birth, in Fishman AP, and Richards DW (eds): *Circulation of the Blood: Men & Ideas.* Oxford Univ Press, New York, 1964, pp 743–816.

Duara S: Structure and function of the upper airway in neonates, in Polin RA, Fox WW (eds): *Fetal and Neonatal Physiology.* Saunders, Philadelphia, 1992, pp 823–828.

Fisher BJ, Carlo WA, Doershuk CF: Pulmonary function from infancy through adolescence, in Scarpelli EM (ed): *Pulmonary Physiology; Fetus, Newborn, Child, Adolescent,* 2nd ed. Lea & Febiger, Philadelphia, 1990, pp 421–445.

Gaultier C: Respiratory muscle function in humans. *Eur Respir J* 8:150–153, 1995.

Gupta SK, Wagener JS, Erenberg A: Pulmonary mechanics in healthy term neonates: Variability in measurements obtained with a computerized system. *J Pediatrics* 117:603–606, 1990.

Hand IL, Krauss AN, Auld PAM: Pulmonary physiology of the newborn infant, in Scarpelli EM (ed): *Pulmonary Physiology: Fetus, Newborn, Child, Adolescent,* 2nd ed. Lea & Febiger, Philadelphia, 1990, pp 405–420.

Hershenson MB: The respiratory muscles and the chest wall, in Beckerman RC, Brouillette RT, Hunt CE (eds): *Respiratory Control Disorders in Infants and Children.* Williams & Wilkins, Baltimore, 1992, pp 28–46.

Hershenson MB, Colin AA, Wohl MEB, Stark AR: Changes in the contribution of the rib cage to tidal breathing during infancy. *Am Rev Respir Dis* 141:922–925, 1990.

Hodson WA: Normal and abnormal structural development of the lung, in Polin RA, Fox WW (eds): *Fetal and Neonatal Physiology.* Saunders, Philadelphia, 1992, pp 771–782.

Jansen AH, Chernick V: Fetal breathing and development of control of breathing, *J Appl Physiol* 70:1431–1446, 1991.

Keele CA, Neil E, Joels N: *Samson Wright's Applied Physiology,* 13th ed. Oxford Univ Press, 1982, pp 585–587.

Levitzky MG: The effect of aging on the respiratory system. *The Physiologist* 27:102–107, 1984.

Levitzky MG: *Pulmonary Physiology,* 4th ed. McGraw-Hill, New York, 1995.

Lodrup Carlsen KC, Magnus P, Carlsen K-H: Lung function by tidal breathing in awake healthy newborn infants. *Eur Respir J* 7:1660–1668, 1994.

Moore KL: *Before We Are Born: Basic Embryology and Birth Defects,* 2nd ed. Saunders, Philadelphia, 1983.

Moore KL: *The Developing Human: Clinically Oriented Embryology,* 3rd ed. Saunders, Philadelphia, 1982.

Mortola JP: Measurements of respiratory mechanics, in Polin RA, Fox WW (eds): *Fetal and Neonatal Physiology.* Saunders, Philadelphia, 1992, pp 813–822.

Murray JF: *The Normal Lung,* 2nd ed. Saunders, Philadelphia, 1986, pp 1–59.

Netter FH: *The Ciba Collection of Medical Illustrations,* vol 5: Heart. Ciba, Summit, NJ, 1969, pp 112–164.

Netter FH: *The Ciba Collection of Medical Illustrations,* vol 7: Respiratory System. Ciba, Summit, NJ, 1979, pp 34–43, 107–115.

Pack AI, Millman RP: The lungs in later life, in Fishman AP (ed): *Pulmonary Diseases and Disorders,* 2nd ed. McGraw-Hill, New York, 1988, pp 79–90.

Plopper CG, Thurlbeck WM: Growth, aging, and adaptation, in Murray JF, Nadel JA (eds): *Textbook of Respiratory Medicine,* 2nd ed. Saunders, Philadelphia, 1994, pp 36–49.

Polgar G: Lung development and subsequent function in the adult, in Scarpelli EM (ed): *Pulmonary Physiology: Fetus, Newborn, Child, Adolescent,* 2nd ed. Lea & Febiger, Philadelphia, 1990, pp 473–487.

Polgar G, Weng TR: The functional development of the respiratory system: From the period of gestation to adulthood. *Am Rev Respir Dis* 120:625–695, 1979.

Rabbette PS, Costeloe KL, Stocks J: Persistence of the Hering-Breuer reflex beyond the neonatal period. *J Appl Physiol* 71:474–480, 1991.

Rigatto H: Maturation of breathing control in the fetus and newborn infant, in Beckerman RC, Brouillette RT, Hunt CE: *Respiratory Control Disorders in Infants and Children.* Williams & Wilkins, Baltimore, 1992, pp 61–75.

Rigatto H: Control of breathing in fetal life and onset and control of breathing in the neonate, in Polin RA, Fox WW (eds): *Fetal and Neonatal Physiology.* Saunders, Philadelphia, 1992, pp 790–801.

Rushmer RF: *Cardiovascular Dynamics,* 4th ed. Saunders, Philadelphia, 1976, pp 446–496.

Sadler TW: *Langman's Medical Embryology,* 7th ed. Williams & Wilkins, Baltimore, 1995.

Scarpelli EM (ed): *Pulmonary Physiology: Fetus, Newborn, Child, Adolescent,* 2nd ed. Lea & Febiger, Philadelphia, 1990.

Shepherd JT, Vanhoutte PM: *The Human Cardiovascular System: Facts and Concepts,* Raven, New York, 1979, pp 269–279.

Smith JJ, Kampine JP: *Circulatory Physiology—The Essentials,* 3rd ed. Williams & Wilkins, Baltimore, 1990, pp 242–248.

Stalcup SA, Mellins RB: Acute respiratory distress in the newborn infant, in Fishman AP (ed), *Pulmonary Diseases and Disorders.* McGraw-Hill, New York, 1980, pp 1653–1666.

Thach BT: Neuromuscular control of the upper airway, in Beckerman RC, Brouillette RT, Hunt CE (eds): *Respiratory Control Disorders in Infants and Children.* Williams & Wilkins, Baltimore, 1992, pp 47–60.

Weibel ER: *The Pathway for Oxygen: Structure and Function in the Mammalian Respiratory System.* Harvard Univ Press, Cambridge, Mass, 1984, pp 211–230.

Williams PL, Warwick R (eds): *Gray's Anatomy,* 36th Brit ed. Saunders, Philadelphia, 1980, pp 180–196, 207–210.

Woodrum D: Respiratory muscles, in Polin RA, Fox WW (eds): *Fetal and Neonatal Physiology.* Saunders, Philadelphia, 1992, pp. 829–841.

CASE STUDY

A 65-year-old retired accountant is scheduled to undergo elective radical pros-
tatectomy for cancer of the prostate, under general anesthesia. During the preoperative evaluation, he complains of difficulty breathing (dyspnea), especially
during exertion. He is 6 ft tall and weighs 130 lb. He says he has smoked at least
one pack of cigarettes a day since he was in his late teens. He reports that he does
have a moderate cough but does not usually produce much sputum and he sometimes gets what he calls chest colds, during which breathing is difficult for him.
His skin does not show any evidence of a bluish color (cyanosis) often associated
with some pulmonary diseases.

The following data were obtained during the patient's pulmonary function
tests:

Spirometry (BTPS)	Predicted	Actual	% predicted
FVC, liters	4.54	4.50	99
FEV$_1$, liters	3.57	2.59	72
FEV$_1$/FVC, %	78	57	
FEV$_3$/FVC, %	97	82	
FEF$_{25-75}$, liters/s	3.64	1.35	37
PEF, liters/s	8.52	7.21	84
FIVC, liters	4.54	3.76	82
PIF, liters/s	4.03	4.39	108

Repeating these tests after administration of a bronchodilator had no effect.

Lung Volume (BTPS)	Predicted	Actual	% predicted
VC, liters	4.54	4.50	99
TLC, liters	6.61	8.27	125
RV, liters	2.09	3.77	180
RV/TLC, %	31	45	—
FRC, liters	3.90	5.32	136
ERV, liters	1.81	1.55	85
IC, liters	2.70	2.95	109

Diffusion (STPD)	Predicted	Actual	% predicted
DLCO, ml CO/min/mmHg	31	22	71

The spirometry data indicate *airway obstruction*. Although the forced vital capacity (FVC) is nearly that predicted, the forced expiratory volume in the first second (FEV$_1$) is low, as are the ratios of the forced expiratory volumes in the first second and first 3 s to the FVC (FEV$_1$/FVC; FEV$_3$/FVC). The forced expiratory flow during the second and third quarters of the forced vital capacity maneuver (FEF$_{25-75}$) is also much lower than the predicted value. The peak expiratory flow (PEF) is only slightly decreased below that predicted. The forced inspiratory vital capacity (FIVC) and the peak inspiratory flow (PIF) were not abnormal. The administration of a bronchodilator had no effect.

The total lung capacity (TLC) and functional residual capacity (FRC) were above those predicted, and the residual volume (RV) was nearly double that predicted. The vital capacity (VC), expiratory reserve volume (ERV), and inspiratory capacity (IC) were not abnormal. The carbon monoxide diffusing capacity (DLCO) was much lower than predicted.

The cause of the pattern of obstruction appears to be predominately *emphysema*. The lack of airflow obstruction on inspiration rules out a *fixed obstruction* such as those caused by some kinds of tumors or by aspiration of a foreign body (which is ruled out by the patient's history). An airway hyperactivity component (e.g., *asthma*) is also unlikely because of a lack of response to the bronchodilator and a lack of episodic history, although this could be tested with a bronchoprovocator. The two most common forms of chronic obstructive pulmonary disease (COPD) are *chronic bronchitis* and *emphysema*. They often appear in the same patient, but one or the other often predominates. In this case the symptoms and signs of chronic bronchitis—copious sputum production, cough, cyanosis, and a bloated appearance—are not obvious.

Emphysema destroys alveolar walls, including their pulmonary capillaries. This decreases the surface area for gas exchange, thus decreasing the DLCO. The destruction of alveolar walls also decreases the elastic recoil of the lungs, resulting in an increased FRC and TLC and less traction holding small airways open during forced expiration. This causes more compression and collapse of airways, which decreases the FEV$_1$/FVC, FEV$_3$/FVC, FEF$_{25-75}$, and increases the RV.

Preoperative room air arterial blood gases later revealed a pH of 7.37, a PCO$_2$ of 53 torr, PO$_2$ of 78 torr, a bicarbonate of 31 meq/liter, and a Hb saturation of 92 percent. The patient had received preoperative training with an incentive spirometer. The remainder of the preoperative evaluation was essentially negative, except for a hematocrit of 55 percent. An elevated hematocrit (polycythemia) is common for patients with COPD.

This patient tolerated anesthesia and the surgical procedure fairly uneventfully, but at the end of the operation, the pulse oximeter showed desaturation of the hemoglobin when the patient was allowed to breathe spontaneously. For this reason, the patient was left intubated and started on mechanical ventilation in the intensive care unit.

The initial ventilator settings were for a tidal volume of 800 ml, a rate of 10/min, an F$_1$O$_2$ of 40 percent, and a continuous positive airway pressure (CPAP, which is a combination of intermittent positive-pressure ventilation and positive end-expiratory pressure) of 3 cmH_2O with the ventilator mode on intermittent mandatory ventilation (IMV). IMV is a mode of ventilation in which the ventilator provides a certain number of breaths per minute and the patient can breathe spontaneously between machine breaths. CPAP is usually set at minimal levels for patients with COPD to reduce the risk of overinflation of the lungs. On these ventilator settings, the patient had the following blood gases: a pH of 7.55, a PCO_2 of 34 torr, PO_2 of 92 torr, a bicarbonate of 31 meq/liter, and a Hb saturation of 97 percent.

As the patient's condition stabilized, weaning from the ventilator was attempted, but as long as the arterial PCO_2 was maintained in the range of 35 to 45 torr, the patient did not exert any spontaneous ventilatory efforts. After 10 h on the ventilator without spontaneous ventilatory efforts, the ventilator rate was reduced to 6/min. When the PCO_2 was allowed to rise to 55 torr, the patient began to breathe spontaneously and was able to be weaned and extubated.

Problem   Why wouldn't the patient breathe spontaneously with the initial ventilator settings?

Answer   The reduction in arterial CO_2 and the accompanying metabolic alkylosis removed the patient's ventilatory drive. Metabolism of lactate from the intravenous solution produces bicarbonate, causing further metabolic alkylosis. Hypocapnia, alkalosis, and narcotics (administered perioperatively) all reduce the drive for breathing. If an elevated arterial CO_2 is rapidly and extremely reduced, the resultant alkalosis can cause tetany.

STUDY QUESTIONS

1 Which of the following statements concerning the compliance of the respiratory system is correct?
   a The sum of the compliances of both lungs is less than that of either lung alone.
   b The total compliance of the lungs and the chest wall is equal to the sum of the compliance of the lungs and the compliance of the chest wall.
   c Alveoli are more compliant at large volumes than they are at small volumes.
   d Lungs with low compliance have high elastic recoil.
   e The lungs of a person with emphysema are less compliant than those of a normal person when they are at the same lung volume.

2 At the functional residual capacity, if intrapleural pressure is -5 cmH$_2$O, what is alveolar elastic recoil pressure?
   a -5 cmH$_2$O
   b 5 cmH$_2$O
   c 0 cmH$_2$O
   d 10 cmH$_2$O
   e -10 cmH$_2$O

3 Which of the following would be expected to *decrease* static pulmonary compliance (that is, shift the static pressure-volume curve of the lungs downward and to the right)?
   a Diffuse alveolar atelectasis
   b Decreased functional pulmonary surfactant
   c Pulmonary vascular congestion
   d Diffuse alveolar interstitial fibrosis
   e One lung collapsed secondary to pneumothorax

4 Which of the following would be expected to *increase* the resistance to airflow offered by the airways?
   a Forced expiration to the residual volume
   b Stimulation of the sympathetic innervation of the airways
   c Breathing through the mouth instead of the nose
   d Breathing a gas mixture that is less viscous than air
   e Increased alveolar septal traction on small airways

5 Which of the following are associated with restrictive pulmonary diseases?
   a Low total lung capacity (TLC)

     b Low functional residual capacity (FRC)

     c Low residual volume (RV)

     d Low forced vital capacity (FVC)

     e Low ratio of the forced expiratory volume in the first second to the total forced vital capacity (FEV_1/FVC)

6 Which of the following statements concerning a healthy person breathing normally in the upright posture is correct?

     a There is more ventilation in upper lung regions than in lower lung regions during normal breathing.

     b Alveoli in lower lung regions are larger than those in upper lung regions.

     c Airway closure occurs in lower lung regions before it occurs in upper lung regions.

     d Most of the residual volume is in lower lung regions.

     e Most of the inspiratory reserve volume is in upper lung regions.

7 A woman's tidal volume is 600 ml. Her anatomic dead space is 100 ml. Her arterial P_{CO_2} is 42 torr, her end-tidal P_{CO_2} is 40 torr, and her mixed expired P_{CO_2} is 28 torr. Her breathing frequency is 20 breaths per minute.

    A What is her physiologic dead space?

       a   0 ml

       b   100 ml

       c   200 ml

       d   300 ml

       e   400 ml

    B What is her alveolar dead space?

       a   0 ml

       b   100 ml

       c   200 ml

       d   300 ml

       e   400 ml

    C What is her minute ventilation ($\dot{V}_E$)?

       a   1000 ml/min

       b   2000 ml/min

       c   8000 ml/min

       d 10,000 ml/min

       e 12,000 ml/min

    D What is her alveolar ventilation ($\dot{V}_A$)?

       a   1000 ml/min

       b   2000 ml/min

       c   8000 ml/min

       d 10,000 ml/min

       e 12,000 ml/min

    E How much of her alveolar ventilation is reaching perfused alveoli?

       a   1000 ml/min

       b   2000 ml/min

       c   8000 ml/min

       d 10,000 ml/min

       e 12,000 ml/min

8 In zone 2 of the lung:

     a $P_A > Pa$.

     b $Pv < P_A$.

     c Alveoli are ventilated but not perfused.

     d Alveoli constitute alveolar dead space.

     e The effective during pressure for blood flow is $Pa - Pv$.

9 Which of the following will *decrease* pulmonary vascular resistance?

     a Inhaling from the FRC to the TLC

     b Exhaling from the FRC to the RV

     c Increasing the output of the right ventricle from 5 to 7 liters/min

     d Decreasing the inspired oxygen concentration from 100 to 10 percent

     e Positive-pressure ventilation

10 Which of the following statements concerning the blood supply of the lungs is correct?

     a The lungs normally receive about 15 percent of the left ventricular output via the bronchial circulation.

     b Upper (less gravity-dependent) regions of the lung are relatively better perfused than are lower regions.

     c Much less of the total resistance to blood flow offered by the pulmonary vessels is in the capillaries and veins than is the case in the systemic circulation.

     d During exercise, as cardiac output increases, more pulmonary capillaries are recruited, thus increasing the surface area available for gas exchange.

     e All of the above statements are correct.

11 If a man at sea level breathes ambient air, any of his alveoli that are ventilated but not perfused:

     a Have P_{CO_2}'s of about 0 torr.

     b Have infinite $\dot{V}/\dot{Q}$'s

     c Have P_{O_2}'s of about 149 torr.

     d Will cause an arterial-alveolar P_{CO_2} gradient.

     e All of the above statements are correct.

12 A woman's arterial oxygen content is 18 ml O_2/100 ml blood and the oxygen content of blood sampled from her pulmonary artery is 14 ml O_2/100 ml blood. If her pulmonary end-capillary oxygen content is calculated to be 22 ml O_2/100 ml blood and her cardiac output is 6 liters/min, what is her pulmonary venous admixture in milliliters per minute?

     a 1333 ml/min

     b 2200 ml/min

     c 2500 ml/min

     d 3000 ml/min

     e 3800 ml/min

13 A person with a large absolute (true) intrapulmonary shunt (>35 percent) would be expected to:

     a Have a low arterial P_{O_2} while breathing room air at sea level.

     b Respond to an $F_{I_{O_2}}$ of 0.4 with a dramatic increase in arterial P_{O_2}.

     c Have an alveolar-arterial P_{O_2} gradient of less than 5 torr.

     d Have an elevated mixed venous P_{O_2}.

     e All of the above are correct.

14 Which of the following would be expected to *increase* the diffusing capacity?

     a $\dot{V}/\dot{Q}$ mismatch

     b Increased pulmonary capillary blood volume

    c Emphysema
    d Interstitial pulmonary edema
    e Decreased cardiac output

15 A man has 18 g of hemoglobin per 100 ml of blood. At an arterial P_{O_2} of 50 torr ($P_{CO_2} = 40$ torr, pH 7.40) his hemoglobin is 85 percent saturated with oxygen.

  A What is his oxygen carrying capacity?
    a 12.06 ml O_2/100 ml blood
    b 17.09 ml O_2/100 ml blood
    c 20.10 ml O_2/100 ml blood
    d 20.50 ml O_2/100 ml blood
    e 24.12 ml O_2/100 ml blood

  B What is his arterial oxygen content (*not* including physically dissolved oxygen)?
    a 12.06 ml O_2/100 ml blood
    b 17.09 ml O_2/100 ml blood
    c 20.10 ml O_2/100 ml blood
    d 20.50 ml O_2/100 ml blood
    e 24.12 ml O_2/100 ml blood

16 Which of the following would be expected to shift the oxyhemoglobin dissociation curve to the left (that is, for any given P_{O_2} the percent oxyhemoglobin will be greater)?
    a Decreased blood 2, 3 DPG concentration
    b Decreased blood temperature
    c Increased blood pH
    d Decreased blood P_{CO_2}
    e All of the above are correct.

17 Which of the following would be expected to shift the CO_2 response curve to the left (that is, produce greater alveolar ventilation at the same Pa_{CO_2})?
    a Narcotic overdose
    b Slow-wave sleep
    c Hypoxia
    d Deep anesthesia
    e Chronic airway obstruction

18 The central chemoreceptors:
    a Do not normally respond to hypoxia.
    b Are on the blood side of the blood-brain barrier.
    c Are responsible for less than half of the steady-state response to elevated CO_2.
    d Show increased activity in response to elevated CSF bicarbonate concentration.
    e All of the above statements are correct.

19 The ventilatory response to hypoxia:
    a Is initiated by the arterial chemoreceptors.
    b Is usually enhanced by hypercapnia.
    c Is not pronounced at Pa_{O_2}'s > 60 torr.
    d Can cause respiratory alkalosis.
    e All of the above statements are correct.

20 The ventilatory response to hydrogen ions produced outside the brain:
    a Arises in the central chemoreceptors.
    b Does not begin until [H^+]'s exceed 60 neq/liter.
    c Is initiated by the arterial chemoreceptors.
    d Is not important in compensating for metabolic acidosis.
    e All of the above statements are correct.

ANSWERS

1   Answer *d* is correct. Compliance is inversely related to elastic recoil, so the less the compliance, the greater the elastic recoil. Answer *a* is incorrect because the two lungs are arranged in parallel and compliances in parallel add directly. Therefore, the sum of the compliances of the two lungs is greater than that of either lung alone. Answer *b* is incorrect because the lungs and the chest wall are arranged in series and their compliances are added as reciprocals. Therefore, 1/total compliance is equal to 1/compliance of the lungs plus 1/compliance of the chest wall. Answer *c* is incorrect. Alveoli are more compliant at smaller volumes than they are at larger volumes. Answer *e* is incorrect. Emphysematous lungs are more compliant than those of a normal person at the same volume because emphysema destroys the alveolar septa responsible for much of the elastic recoil of the lungs.

2   Answer *b* is correct because the alveolar pressure is equal to the sum of the intrapleural pressure and the alveolar elastic recoil pressure. Thus, at the functional residual capacity when alveolar pressure is equal to 0 cmH$_2$O, alveolar elastic recoil pressure should be equal and opposite to the intrapleural pressure.

3   Answers *a*, *b*, *c*, *d*, and *e* are all correct. Atelectasis of alveoli throughout the lungs (answer *a*) or localized to one lung (answer *e*) removes units arranged in parallel and inflates noncollapsed units to larger volumes at which they are less compliant. Decreased functional pulmonary surfactant (answer *b*) both increases the effects of surface tension in the lungs and tends to cause diffuse alveolar atelectasis. Pulmonary vascular congestion (answer *c*), that is, engorgement of the pulmonary blood vessels with blood, "stiffens" the lungs and therefore makes them less compliant. Fibrosis of the pulmonary interstitium (answer *d*) decreases pulmonary compliance primarily by a proliferation of collagen, which is quite elastic.

4   Answer *a* is correct because a forced expiration to the residual volume increases the resistance to airflow by causing *dynamic compression* of the airways and also by decreasing alveolar septal *traction* on small airways. As the alveolar volume decreases, the alveoli have less elastic recoil and exert less traction. Answer *e* is therefore incorrect because increased alveolar septal traction on small airways should decrease airways resistance. Answer *b* is incorrect because stimulation of the sympathetic innervation of the airways activates B$_2$ receptors and therefore generally dilates the bronchioles, especially if their muscular tone is already elevated. It is stimulation of the *parasympathetic* innervation of the airways that causes bronchoconstriction. An-

swer c is incorrect because the resistance to airflow is normally much greater if one is breathing through the nose rather than through the mouth. Answer d is incorrect because resistance is directly proportional to viscosity and length; it is *inversely* proportional to the fourth power of the radius.

5   All but answer e are correct. Restrictive pulmonary diseases are characterized by an inability to expand the lungs. This can result from fibrosis or other problems making the alveoli themselves difficult to expand (e.g., sarcoidosis, occupational lung diseases, insufficient pulmonary surfactant); air or fluid outside the lungs but inside the chest wall, impeding lung expansion and/or interfering with the ability to generate negative intrapleural pressure (e.g., pneumothorax); or musculoskeletal or neuromuscular disorders (e.g., kyphoscoliosis, obesity, myasthenia gravis, Guillain-Barré syndrome). The FRC is usually decreased (answer b) because of increased inward elastic recoil of the lungs, decreased outward elastic recoil of the chest wall, or both. Decreased surfactant and some of the neuromuscular diseases may also decrease the FRC by causing atelectasis. The TLC is decreased (answer a) because of increased inward recoil of the lungs and/or increased inward recoil of the chest wall at higher thoracic volumes, or because of decreased effectiveness of the inspiratory muscles. The RV is usually decreased (answer c) because of increased inward lung recoil, decreased outward chest wall recoil, or accumulation of air or liquid in the intrapleural space. An exception might be seen in neuromuscular diseases that lead to decreased expiratory muscle function. The FVC is usually decreased (answer d) because the TLC is decreased so there is less volume to blow out. This may be exacerbated by muscle dysfunction. However, the FEV_1/FVC is usually normal or even slightly elevated (answer e). A decreased FEV_1/FVC indicates *obstructive* pulmonary diseases, that is, pulmonary diseases caused by increased resistance to airflow.

6   Answer c is correct. In a healthy person breathing normally in the upright posture intrapleural pressure is more negative in upper thoracic regions than it is in more gravity-dependent regions. This results in larger alveoli in upper lung regions than those in lower lung regions (answer b), so more of the FRC will be found in upper lung regions. Because the smaller alveoli in the lower regions are more compliant (that is, they are on a steeper portion of the pressure-volume curve), they are better ventilated than those in upper lung regions (answer a). Inspiring to the TLC from end inspiration will therefore fill alveoli in lower lung regions more than those in upper lung regions, so most of the IRV is in lower lung regions (answer e). During a forced expiration from the FRC to the RV, alveoli in lower lung regions, which begin at smaller volumes and are also more compliant, empty more rapidly than those in upper lung regions. Most of the RV therefore remains in upper lung regions (answer d) even though airway closure first occurs in lower regions (answer c), because of the greater intrapleural pressures in lower thoracic regions and because the smaller alveoli exert less traction on the small airways.

7A   Answer c is correct. Use the Bohr equation to calculate the physiologic dead space (V_DCO_2):

$$\frac{V_DCO_2}{V_T} = \frac{PaCO_2 - P_{\bar{E}}CO_2}{PaCO_2}$$

$$\frac{V_DCO_2}{V_T} = \frac{42 \text{ torr} - 28 \text{ torr}}{42 \text{ torr}}$$

$$\frac{V_DCO_2}{V_T} = 0.333$$

$$V_DCO_2 = 0.33 \times 600 \text{ ml}$$

$$V_DCO_2 = 200 \text{ ml}$$

B   Answer *b* is correct. The physiologic dead space V_DCO_2 equals the anatomic dead plus the alveolar dead space, so the alveolar dead space is equal to 200 ml − 100 ml, or 100 ml.

C   Answer *e* is correct. The minute ventilation $\dot{V}_E$ is equal to the product of the breathing frequency *n* and the tidal volume V_T:

$$\dot{V}_E = n(V_T)$$

$$\dot{V}_E = 20 \text{ breaths/min} \times 600 \text{ ml/breath}$$

$$\dot{V}_E = 12,000 \text{ ml/min}$$

D   Answer *d* is correct. Alveolar ventilation $\dot{V}_A$ is equal to the product of the breathing frequency *n* and the alveolar volume V_A. The alveolar volume is equal to the tidal volume minus the anatomic dead space V_D:

$$\dot{V}_A = n(V_T - V_D)$$

$$\dot{V}_A = 20 \text{ breaths/min} (600 \text{ ml/breath} - 100 \text{ ml/breath})$$

$$\dot{V}_A = 20 \text{ breaths/min} (500 \text{ ml/breath})$$

$$\dot{V}_A = 10,000 \text{ ml/min}$$

E   Answer *c* is correct. The alveolar ventilation reaching perfused alveoli equals the minute volume minus the ventilation wasted on the physiologic dead space, that is, both the anatomic and alveolar dead space:

12,000 ml/min − 20 breaths/min (200 ml/breath) =
12,000 ml/min − 4000 ml/min   = 8000 ml/min

8   Only answer *b* is correct. In zone 2 of the lung, pulmonary artery pressure Pa exceeds alveolar pressure P_A, so answer *a* is incorrect. Alveolar pressure does exceed pulmonary venous pressure Pv, so answer *b* is correct. Because P_A > Pv in zone 2, P_A is the effective downstream pressure for pulmonary perfusion. Therefore, answer *e* is incorrect. It is in *zone 1* where alveoli are ventilated but not perfused because P_A > Pa. Such alveoli would constitute alveolar dead space. Therefore, answers *c* and *d* are incorrect for zone 2.

9   Only answer *c* is correct. Increasing the right ventricular output should decrease pulmonary vascular resistance by recruiting and distending pulmonary blood vessels. Pulmonary vascular resistance is normally lowest at the FRC and increases at both higher and lower lung volumes. Therefore, answers *a* and *b* are both incorrect. Decreasing the F_IO_2 from 1.00 to 0.10 causes hypoxic pulmonary vasoconstriction, so answer *d* is incorrect. Positive-pressure ventilation increases both alveolar and intrapleural pressure, compressing both the alveolar and extraalveolar vessels, respectively. The increase in intrapleural pressure also compresses the great veins, which restricts venous return and decreases right ventricular output, thus derecruiting pulmonary vessels and causing less distention. Thus positive-pressure ventilation increases pulmonary vascular resistance, and answer *e* is incorrect.

10   Answer *d* is correct. The lungs normally receive about 2 percent of the left ventricular output via the bronchial circulation, so answer *a* is incorrect. Lower regions of the lung are relatively better perfused than are the upper regions because greater hydrostatic pressures in lower lung regions result in more distention and recruitment of blood vessels and thus decrease the resistance to blood flow. Answer *b* is therefore incorrect. The total resistance to blood flow offered by the pulmonary circulation is much more evenly distributed among the arteries, capillaries, and veins than it is in the systemic circulation. Answer *c* is therefore incorrect.

11   All of the statements are correct (answer *e*). Alveoli that are ventilated but not perfused constitute alveolar dead space and have infinite $\dot{V}/\dot{Q}$'s. Such alveoli have P_{O_2}'s and P_{CO_2}'s identical to those of inspired air (149 and 0 torr, respectively, at sea level). Because such alveoli contribute no CO_2 to the mixed expired alveolar (that is, end-tidal) air, there will be an arterial-alveolar P_{CO_2} gradient.

12   Answer *d* is correct. Use the shunt equation to calculate pulmonary venous admixture

$$\frac{\dot{Q}s}{\dot{Q}T} = \frac{Cc'_{O_2} - C'a_{O_2}}{Cc'_{O_2} - C\bar{v}_{O_2}}$$

$$\frac{\dot{Q}s}{\dot{Q}T} = \frac{(22 - 18) \text{ ml } O_2/100 \text{ ml blood}}{(22 - 14) \text{ ml } O_2/100 \text{ ml blood}}$$

$$\frac{\dot{Q}s}{\dot{Q}T} = 0.5$$

$$\dot{Q}s = 0.5 \ (6000 \text{ ml/min})$$

$$\dot{Q}s = 3000 \text{ ml/min}$$

13   Answer *a* is correct. A large intrapulmonary shunt effectively results in large volumes of mixed venous blood entering the pulmonary veins and therefore decreasing the Pa_{O_2}. True intrapulmonary shunts are refractory to increased $F_{I_{O_2}}$'s because the hemoglobin in the blood perfusing well-ventilated areas of the lung is almost completely saturated with O_2 at a normal $F_{I_{O_2}}$ of 0.21. Any additional small volume of O_2 physically dissolved in this blood will be taken up by the hemoglobin of the shunted blood, so there will be nearly no increase in Pa_{O_2}. Therefore, answer *b* is incorrect. The (A-a)D$_{O_2}$ (answer *c*) will increase above 5 torr, which is at the low end of the normal range, because the P_{O_2} of the ventilated alveoli should be normal (or even elevated if the hypoxemia is sufficient to stimulate the arterial chemoreceptors), but the arterial P_{O_2} will be low. Mixed venous P_{O_2} should also be low as the tissues extract oxygen from the arterial blood, which already has a low P_{O_2}. Thus answer *d* is incorrect.

14   Only answer *b* is correct. Recall Fick's law for diffusion as you answer this question. $\dot{V}/\dot{Q}$ mismatch (answer *a*) decreases the diffusing capacity because it decreases the effective surface area for diffusion. Decreased cardiac output (answer *e*) also decreases the surface area for diffusion by derecruiting pulmonary vessels—this is opposite to what happens with an increased pulmonary capillary blood volume. Emphysema (answer *c*) also decreases the surface area for diffusion by destroying alveoli and blood vessels. Interstitial pulmonary edema (answer *d*) decreases the diffusing capacity by increasing the thickness of the barrier.

15A O_2 carrying capacity $= 1.34$ ml O_2/g Hb times 18 g Hb/100 ml blood or 24.12 ml O_2/100 ml blood. Answer e is therefore correct.

   B The arterial O_2 content is 85 percent of the O_2 carrying capacity or 20.50 ml O_2/100 ml blood. Answer d is therefore correct.

16 Answer e is correct.

17 Only answer c is correct. Narcotic overdose (a), slow-wave sleep (b), deep anesthesia (d), and chronic airway obstruction (e) all *decrease* the ventilatory response to CO_2.

18 Only answer a is correct. The central chemoreceptors are on the brain side of the blood-brain barrier, so answer b is incorrect. They are said to be responsible for approximately 80 percent of the steady-state response to CO_2, so answer c is also incorrect. Increased CSF bicarbonate ion concentration would be expected to depress the activity of the central chemoreceptors, so answer d is incorrect.

19 Answer e is correct. Hypoxemia sufficient to stimulate the arterial chemoreceptors increases alveolar ventilation, causing a decrease in Pa_{CO_2} and respiratory alkalosis (answer d). The central chemoreceptors are not sensitive to hypoxia, so the response is initiated in the arterial chemoreceptors (answer a). The response is not pronounced until the Pa_{O_2} is less than 50 to 60 torr (answer c) and it is usually enhanced by elevated Pa_{CO_2}'s (answer b).

20 Only answer c is correct. Answer a is incorrect because hydrogen ions do not cross the blood-brain barrier easily and so they would not be available to stimulate the central chemoreceptors. The ventilatory response to hydrogen ions can certainly be demonstrated at $[H^+]$'s lower than 60 neq/liter, so answer b is incorrect. The response is an important compensatory mechanism for metabolic acidosis, so answer d is incorrect.

ADDITIONAL STUDY QUESTIONS

1 A patient is admitted for an intestinal bypass procedure for treatment of morbid obesity. His height is 65 in., and his weight is 134 kg. He is diagnosed as having the Pickwickian syndrome. You would expect his pulmonary functions test to show:

   a Alveolar hyperventilation, anemia, and hypoxemia

   b Alveolar hyperventilation, erythrocytosis, and hypoxemia

   c Decreased expiratory reserve volume and higher intraabdominal pressure when supine

   d Lower work of breathing

   e Unimproved respiratory condition after weight reduction

2 If a patient is allowed to spontaneously breathe 100% oxygen under anesthesia:

   a Intrapulmonary shunting will increase.

   b The arterial oxygen tension will always increase.

   c The P_{O_2} will rise because of increased dead space.

   d Lung units with high ventilation/perfusion (V/Q) ratios will become shunt units.

   e The oxygen tension will rise owing to an increase in functional residual capacity.

3 The carbon dioxide response curve describes the pattern of ventilation following challenge by various concentrations of carbon dioxide. Which of the following is true?

   a The patient under general inhalational anesthesia will show the same effects regardless of the agent.

    b The slope of the response may change, but the position of the curve remains the same.

    c The position and slope are the same in adults and infants.

    d Increased work of breathing leads to a steeper slope.

    e With increasing halothane concentration, the curve is depressed and shifts to the right.

4 Which of the following statements concerning the effects of general anesthesia on functional residual capacity in the supine position is false?

    a Soon after induction of general anesthesia, FRC is reduced.

    b The change in FRC is about 18 percent.

    c The change is progressive with time.

    d The reduction in FRC can lead to hypoxemia.

    e The change in FRC is not affected by muscle paralysis.

5 In the adult, the tracheobronchial tree:

    a Divides at an uneven angle, making foreign bodies more apt to go to the left side.

    b Divides into right and left bronchi, the left bronchus being narrower and longer.

    c Is relatively fixed and immovable with respiration.

    d Is lined with squamous epithelium.

    e Is protected by circular cartilaginous rings throughout.

6 The adult human larynx:

    a Lies at the level of the second through fifth cervical vertebrae.

    b Is narrowest at the level of the cricoid cartilage.

    c Is innervated solely by the recurrent laryngeal nerve.

    d Is protected anteriorly by the wide expanse of the cricoid cartilage.

    e Is lined with stratified squamous epithelium.

ANSWERS

1 The correct answer is *c*. Obesity is associated with decreased FRC and increased intraabdominal pressure. Pickwickian syndrome causes hypoxia, erythrocytosis, and hypoventilation.

2 The correct answer is *a*. Although in theory breathing 100% O_2 should eliminate the contribution of shuntlike units to low arterial P_{O_2}, the development of absorption atelectasis will actually convert these units to true shunt.

3 The correct answer is *e*. All of the commonly used inhalant anesthetics depress the response to CO_2 in a dose-dependent manner, with halothane having somewhat less effect than enflurane and isoflurane.

4 The correct answer is *c*. The change in FRC is not progressive with time. It happens almost immediately, probably because of loss in muscle tone.

5 The correct answer is *b*. Aspirated foreign bodies tend to go to the right. The trachea moves with ventilation and is lined with ciliated columnar epithelium. The trachea has C-shaped cartilage while the only true cartilagenous ring in the airway is the cricoid.

6 The correct answer is *e*. The large thyroid cartilage protects the larynx anteriorly. The larynx is lined with stratified squamous epithelium and in the adult is narrowest at the glottis. The adult larynx is anterior to C 3–6.

APPENDIXES

I. SYMBOLS USED IN RESPIRATORY PHYSIOLOGY

P	Partial pressure of a gas (torr)
V	Volume of a gas (ml)
$\dot{V}$	Flow of gas (ml/min, liter/s)
Q	Volume of blood (ml)
$\dot{Q}$	Blood flow (ml/min)
F	Fractional concentration of a gas
C	Content or concentration of a substance in the blood (milliliters per 100 ml of blood)
S	Saturation in the blood (%)
I	Inspired
E	Expired
$\bar{E}$	Mixed expired
A	Alveolar
T	Tidal
D	Dead space
a	Arterial
v	Venous
$\bar{v}$	Mixed venous
c	Capillary
c$'$	End capillary

II. THE LAWS GOVERNING THE BEHAVIOR OF GASES

1. **Avogadro's hypothesis** Equal volumes of different gases at equal temperatures contain the same number of molecules. Similarly, equal numbers of molecules in identical volumes and at the same temperature will exert the same pressure. (One mole of any gas will contain 6.02×10^{23} molecules and will occupy a volume of 22.4 liters at a temperature of 0°C and a pressure of 760 mmHg.)

2. **Dalton's law** In a gas mixture the pressure exerted by each individual gas in a space is independent of the pressures of other gases in the mixture, e.g.,

    $$P_A = P_{H_2O} + P_{O_2} + P_{CO_2} + P_{N_2}$$

    $P_{gas,1} = \%$ of total gases $\times P_{tot}$

3. **Boyle's law**

    $P_1 V_1 = P_2 V_2$ (at constant temperature)

4. **Charles' law or Gay Lussac's law**

$$\frac{V_1}{V_2} = \frac{T_1}{T_2} \quad \text{(at constant pressure, with T the absolute temperature in } °K)$$

5. **Ideal gas law**
   $$PV = nRT$$

6. **Henry's law** The weight of a gas absorbed by a liquid with which it does not combine chemically is directly proportional to the pressure of the gas to which the liquid is exposed (and its solubility in the liquid).

7. **Graham's law** The rate of diffusion of a gas (in the gas phase) is inversely proportional to its molecular weight.

8. **Fick's law of diffusion**
   $$\dot{V}_{gas} = \frac{A \times D \times (P_1 - P_2)}{T}$$

   $$D \propto \frac{\text{solubility}}{\sqrt{\text{molecular weight}}}$$

III. FREQUENTLY USED EQUATIONS

1. The alveolar air equation
   $$PA_{O_2} = PI_{O_2} - \frac{PA_{CO_2}}{R}$$

2. The Bohr equation
   $$\frac{VD_{CO_2}}{V_T} = \frac{Pa_{CO_2} - P\bar{E}_{CO_2}}{Pa_{CO_2}}$$

3. Components of alveolar pressure
   $$P_A = P_{ip} + P_{elas}$$

4. The diffusing capacity equation
   $$D_{Lx} = \frac{V_x}{P_{x1} - P_{x2}}$$

5. The Fick equation
   $$\dot{V}_x = \frac{A \times D \times P_{x1} - P_{x2}}{T}$$

6. The Henderson-Hasselbalch equation
   $$pH = pK' + \log \frac{[HCO_3^-]}{.03 \times P_{CO_2}}$$

7. Oxygen carrying capacity of hemoglobin
   1.34 ml O_2/g Hb

8. The shunt equation
   $$\frac{\dot{Q}_s}{\dot{Q}_T} = \frac{Cc'_{O_2} - Ca_{O_2}}{Cc'_{O_2} - C\bar{v}_{O_2}}$$

9. Solubility of oxygen in plasma
   0.003 ml O_2/100 ml blood/mmHg P_{O_2}

IV. TABLE OF NORMAL RESPIRATORY AND CIRCULATORY VALUES

	Term newborn	1 Year	8 Year	Adult
Breaths/min	40	25	18	12
Tidal volume (ml/kg)	7	8	7	7
Dead space (ml/kg)	2	2	2.8	2
Alveolar ventilation (ml/kg)	130	120	80	60
Vital capacity (ml/kg)	40	45	60	60
Functional residual capacity (ml/kg)	28	25	40	35
Heart rate/min	133 ± 18	120 ± 2	85 ± 10	75 ± 5
Cardiac index (L/min/m^2)	2.5 ± 0.6	2.5 ± 0.6	4.0 ± 1.0	3.7 ± 0.3
Systolic blood pressure (mmHg)*	73 ± 8	96 ± 30	100 ± 15	122 ± 30
Diastolic blood pressure (mmHg)	50 ± 8	66 ± 25	56 ± 9	75 ± 20
Oxygen consumption (ml/kg/min)	6.0 ± 10	5.2 ± 0.1	4.9 ± 0.9	3.4 ± 0.6

* The lower limit for normal systolic blood pressure can be approximated by the formula 70 + (2 × age in years) for pediatric patients; the lower limit for normal systolic blood pressure for term newborns is 60 mmHg.

INDEX

Page numbers followed by an *f* indicate figures; numbers followed by a *t* indicate tables.